FABRICATION PROCESS MANUAL

for Orthotic Intervention for the Hand and Upper Extremity

SPLINTING PRINCIPLES AND PROCESS

THIRD EDITION

FABRICATION PROCESS MANUAL

for Orthotic Intervention for the Hand and Upper Extremity

SPLINTING PRINCIPLES AND PROCESS

THIRD EDITION

MaryLynn A. Jacobs, MBA, MS, OTR/L, CHT
Senior Director, National Hand Therapy Services
ATI Physical Therapy
Bolingbrook, Illinois

Noelle M. Austin, MS, PT, CHT
Owner/Educator
CJ Education & Consulting, LLC
Nashville, Tennessee

Hand Therapist
STAR Physical Therapy
Nashville, Tennessee

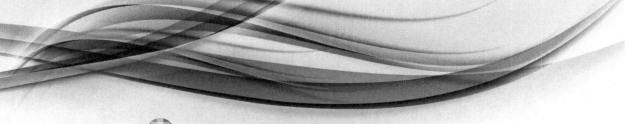

Wolters Kluwer

Philadelphia • Baltimore • New York • London
Buenos Aires • Hong Kong • Sydney • Tokyo

Acquisitions Editor: Matt Hauber
Senior Development Editor: Amy Millholen
Editorial Coordinator: Vinoth Ezhumalai
Production Project Manager: Barton Dudlick
Design Coordinator: Steve Druding
Manufacturing Coordinator: Margie Orzech
Prepress Vendor: TNQ Technologies

Third edition

Library of Congress Cataloging-in-Publication Data

ISBN-13: 978-1-9751-7235-0

Cataloging in Publication data available on request from publisher.

shop.lww.com

Dedication

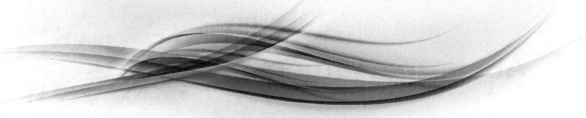

To our families and all the patients we have treated throughout the years
and to

Judy C. Colditz, OT/L, CHT, FAOTA

A master clinician, a skilled teacher, a committed leader, a mentor to many, and an expert orthotic fabricator.

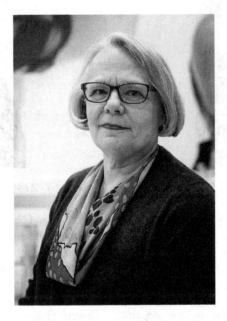

"When You Learn It, Teach It"

This is Judy's motto and if you have had the unique opportunity to attend one of her in-person courses, hear her present at professional meetings, read any of her articles/chapters from an extensive list of her publications, viewed her educational videos, or had the occasion to learn from her at hand conferences, you are able to fully appreciate this motto. She teaches with passion, intrigue, depth of knowledge, and relentless energy.

Judy has had an enormous and lasting impact on the field of Hand Therapy through her various professional contributions. To name a few, she has taught us the value of the intrinsics, the intricacies of the dorsal apparatus, a casting technique to mobilize stiffness (CMMS), and further enhanced our knowledge of the thumb CMC joint.

Judy's commitment to hand therapy has extended beyond her clinical work and into leadership roles. She has been president of both the International Federation of Societies of Hand Therapists (IFSHT) and the American Society of Hand Therapists (ASHT), helping to advance and shape Hand Therapy policy.

We are enormously grateful for Judy's ongoing support and guidance throughout our careers and encouraging our passion for teaching and writing—she kindly wrote the foreword to our second edition. In this latest edition, we are especially thankful for her generous sharing of her various Clinical Pearls that are scattered throughout this textbook and the fabrication manual derived from her world-known Clinical Pearl series from her company HandLab.

Through her 40+ years of hand therapy work, she has pushed us all to be better, think deeper, think "what else," be innovative, and always stay intellectually challenged. We are hopeful that future generations will continue to be inspired by her work and live by her motto of "when you learn it, then teach it".

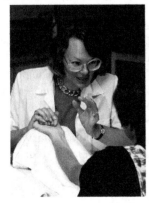
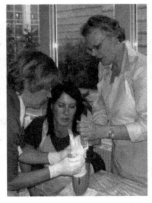
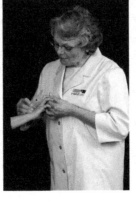
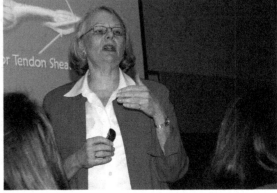

About the Authors

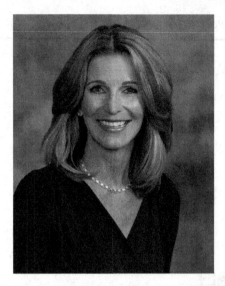

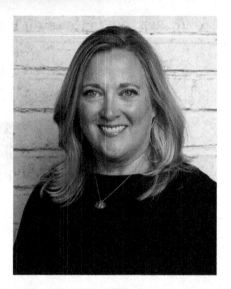

MaryLynn Jacobs earned a Bachelor of Science in Rehabilitation Medicine from Springfield College, Springfield, MA; a Master of Science in Occupational Therapy from Boston University, Boston, MA; and a Master in Business Administration in Entrepreneurial Thinking and Innovative Practices from Bay Path University, Longmeadow, MA. She has been a certified hand therapist (CHT) for most of her professional career.

Her academic, clinical, and business expertise spans well over three decades. She has developed several hand therapy departments, consulted to physician practices, industry, hospitals, home health care agencies, and software development companies. She has been teaching hand therapy and upper extremity orthosis/splinting courses across the country for over 35 years.

MaryLynn coedited and coauthored *Orthotic Intervention of the Hand and Upper Extremity, Splinting Principles and Process* published by Lippincott Williams and Wilkins, 2003/2013/2021. MaryLynn has contributed to the hand therapy literature with several journals, newspaper articles and coauthored *Orthotics in the Management of Hand Dysfunction in Orthotics and Prosthetics in Rehabilitation*, second edition, Saunders/Elsevier, 2005.

MaryLynn cofounded Attain Therapy + Fitness, a private practice, Physical and Occupational Therapy Company with a large footprint in Western MA. In 2015, Attain Therapy + Fitness merged with ATI Physical Therapy. Presently she is the Senior Director of National Hand Therapy services, overseeing the growth and development of hand therapy throughout ATI Physical Therapy nationwide. She is a member of the American Society of Hand Therapists (ASHT), past ASHT chair of the Legislation and Reimbursement Committee, and past chair of ASHT's Practice Management Committee. She is on several advisory boards as a board member of the Springfield College Board of Trustees, Springfield, Massachusetts.

Noelle M. Austin, MS, PT, CHT, is a graduate of Quinnipiac University, Hamden, CT with a Bachelor of Science in Physical Therapy and later obtained her Master of Science from the University of Connecticut, Storrs, CT with a special focus on Allied Health Education. She owns CJ Education and Consulting, LLC, offering private clinical education events on orthotic fabrication, as well as consulting services related to orthotic product development. Noelle was initially certified by the Hand Therapy Certification Commission as a Certified Hand Therapist (CHT) in 1996, and most recently recertified in 2021. She is an active member of the American Society of Hand Therapists. Noelle has been teaching the art and science of orthotic fabrication for over 25 years. In addition to conducting conferences both nationally and internationally, she has presented multiple sessions at Annual ASHT meetings, various State Chapter meetings, and for Hand Therapy Special Interest Groups on the topic of orthotic fabrication.

Noelle has been practicing in Hand Therapy for 30 years and most recently accepted a position with STAR Physical Therapy in the Nashville TN area. She was previously employed at OrthoVirginia in Lynchburg and ProPT in Hamden, CT. She has also been adjunct faculty/guest lecturer in the Physical Therapy Programs at Lynchburg College in Virginia and Sacred Heart University in Connecticut, presenting lectures/labs on the topics of hand anatomy/kinesiology, examination/intervention, and orthotic fabrication. Noelle also consults with Kinetec USA as a Senior Clinical Specialist, assisting in product development and education with their Manosplint thermoplastics.

Noelle is coauthor and coeditor of the book: *Orthotic Intervention for the Hand and Upper Extremity: Splinting Principles and Process* published by Lippincott Williams and Wilkins, 2003/2013/2021. In addition, she authored the chapter "Wrist and Hand Complex" in the fourth/fifth/sixth edition of *Joint Structure and Function: A Comprehensive Analysis* (Levangie and Norkin) published by FA Davis in 2005/2011/2019. Noelle also authored "Orthotics in the Management of Hand Dysfunction" in the second and third edition of *Orthotics and Prosthetics in Rehabilitation* (Lusardi and Nielsen) published by Elsevier 2007/2012.

Foreword

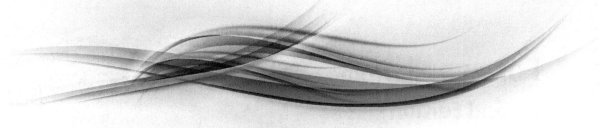

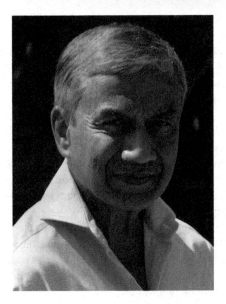

It is with the utmost respect and best wishes that I am honored to write this Foreword for the Third Edition of *Orthotic Intervention for the Hand and Upper Extremity: Splinting Principles and Process.*

In 2021, I will be entering into the fifth decade of my clinical practice and synchronously, this latest edition will be available to healthcare practitioners such as physical therapists, occupational therapists, hand therapists, physicians, surgeons, and clinical nurse specialists. This is the second time I have had the opportunity to write a chapter in this textbook on orthotics for arthritic conditions. Over the years, I have admired MaryLynn Jacobs and Noelle Austin for working tirelessly in compiling the previous two editions, and again with this third edition. Having compared the previous two editions, I found the third editions (main text and the *Fabrication Process Manual*) both to have new improved, simplified, and innovative orthotic prescription, fabrication, and application techniques.

As a clinician, educator, administrator, and researcher, and having practiced for five decades, I have witnessed the understanding of orthotic applications and how they have evolved significantly over time. Historically, after World War I, orthoses were primarily used for fracture fixation, providing rest to the healing tissues and/or correction of deformities. Over the years, with greater understanding of anatomy, healing processes, tissue engineering, and biomechanics, the orthotic fabrication and its clinical application has made a world of difference in restoring motion of human joints.

This third edition offers substantial clinical reasoning considering all avenues that are necessary to regain and restore extremity function. I find this textbook extremely valuable to clinicians and healthcare practitioners who are either prescribing or fabricating orthotics for their patients or clients. The extensive descriptions presented in the main textbook and the *Fabrication Process Manual* enable the clinician to have an edge on problem identification and evidence-based clinical reasoning for achieving specific orthotic goals. The step-by-step illustrations and instructions for the various mobilization orthoses empowers the practitioner to custom tailor the orthotic fabrication, and make necessary alterations for the best clinical outcome. Moreover, the chapters included in these books assist the healthcare provider in making the correct judgment of orthotics prescription and applications.

The Third Edition of *Orthotic Intervention for the Hand and Upper Extremity: Splinting Principles and Process* presents descriptions of a wide variety of diagnoses. This textbook and its companion manual undoubtedly are a valuable resource for healthcare practitioners. In addition, these books offer highlights of anatomical and mechanical principles, and biomechanics of normal and altered pathomechanics; discusses associated indications and precautions; and promotes clinical reasoning skills by presenting a wide variety of expert pearls and patient case studies. This wide-ranged approach allows practitioners to confidently present their clinical reasoning to referring physicians and surgeons and utilize techniques in their clinical practice to promote and advance the hand therapy profession for greater recognition.

This publication has many new and well-thought-out added features, including new chapters on Relative Motion Orthoses and Prosthetics, a separate *Fabrication Process Manual* for every orthotic design, full-color images with a larger format, Expert Pearls shared by the international experts, surgeons' comments, addressing Frequently Asked Questions by the practitioners for specific clinical diagnoses, instructional videos, and the printable patterns for orthotic fabrication. These additions to the textbook make the third edition a most desirable resource material for the practitioner of all levels. Reading this book, as well as exploring the extensive references, will undoubtedly bring the professionals a long way in improving their knowledge and skills that are necessary in an evidence-based clinical practice environment.

I know that the compilation of material presented in this third edition by MaryLynn Jacobs and Noelle Austin will help improve clinical practice for this generation and many generations to come.

With due respect and best wishes.

Shrikant J. Chinchalkar, MThO, BScOT, OTR, CHT, OTReg(ON)
Roth-McFarlane Hand & Upper Limb Centre
St. Joseph's Health Care London
London, Ontario,
Canada

Foreword (from Second Edition)

As a therapist who has written about and taught hand splinting (now accurately called orthotic fabrication) for many years, I commend MaryLynn A. Jacobs and Noelle Austin on giving you, the reader, this second edition of *Splinting the Hand and Upper Extremity: Principles and Process*, which now has the updated title of *Orthotic Intervention for the Hand and Upper Extremity: Splinting Principles and Process*.

This book is your doorway into the complex, skill-based, real world of orthotic intervention for the upper extremity. Therapists who want to specialize in treating upper extremity patients must have a wide range of knowledge and ability in orthotic intervention by developing an understanding of the underlying anatomical principles, how tissue heals and matures, how to apply mechanical principles to orthotic design, how to skillfully handle orthotic tools and materials, and how to evaluate and determine the need for and the appropriate design of an orthosis. Then they must be able to design, fabricate, fit, adjust, and describe for billing, as well as reevaluate the effectiveness of the orthotic intervention. This book delivers all of this information and more to the reader.

WHY SHOULD YOU READ THIS BOOK?

I have observed therapists in the clinic wanting a book, which will give them a pattern for an orthosis and how to construct it but nothing more. But an orthosis is only part of the treatment approach and cannot be separated from a comprehensive understanding of the pathology and how a therapist can influence the outcome. This book combines the "how to" with the "why" and directs you to resources, which can further your understanding. To appreciate the entire therapy process and not just the construction, an orthosis should be every therapist's goal.

A number of features of this book set it apart from others on this subject. Not all orthoses need to be made of low-temperature thermoplastics, and the authors' discussion of casting, taping, use of neoprene, and prefabricated orthoses completes your armamentarium to address the wide range of specific patient needs. The real-life "Clinical Pearls" included throughout the book give you insight from experienced clinicians who have learned on-the-job tips and tricks to increase efficiency and patient comfort.

For therapists who are looking for a starting point, the section on "Orthotic Fabrication" gives you a step-by-step design and construction process, while concurrently the section on "Orthotic Intervention for Specific Diagnoses and Populations" provides deeper insight to the appropriate orthotic intervention for specific diagnostic problems. The case study accompanying each chapter in this latter section illustrates direct application to a specific situation.

Reading this book as well as some of the recommended references will take you a long way toward gaining orthotic skills. In our current busy clinic climate, time to practice and learn orthotic skills is scarce, and we must find innovative methods and resources to build and maintain this skill set.

WHY WAS I WILLING TO WRITE THIS FOREWORD?

I wrote this because it matters that we, as therapists, develop and maintain a high level of orthotic intervention skills for our patients as part of our treatment spectrum. No one else can integrate the use of an orthosis into the treatment but us. My recommendation is to keep this book at your bedside as well as next to your treatment area. Read a few pearls each day and incorporate them into your clinical practice or make an unfamiliar orthosis on a coworker as self-training. You will build your skill and knowledge arsenal each day.

Who knows… perhaps you will contribute to the text on orthotic intervention for the next generation.

Judy C. Colditz, OTR/L, CHT, FAOTA
HandLab
Raleigh, North Carolina
June 1, 2013

Preface

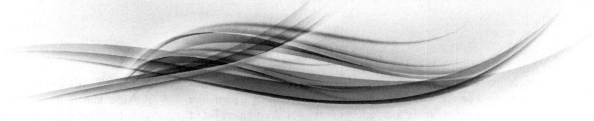

Orthotic Intervention for the Hand and Upper Extremity: Splinting Principles and Process, Third Edition, along with the complementary *Fabrication Process Manual*, was inspired by clinicians and students who, in our teaching experience, were requesting one resource that would clarify all appropriate traditional orthosis fabrication/splinting, casting, and taping managements for upper extremity diagnoses. Although an upper extremity therapist tends to fabricate thermoplastic orthoses most of the time, there are many situations when casting, taping, neoprene, or even a prefabricated orthosis is a more appropriate choice. These books are unique in that they provide orthosis patterns for most upper extremity diagnoses as well as in-depth discussions and instructions for choosing and fabricating with these other options. This feature truly distinguishes these books from all others currently on the market. We do not delve into the specifics of rehabilitation techniques and surgical interventions; instead, we provide contemporary overviews of the various diagnoses described to clarify a particular rationale specific to an orthosis design or evidence-based protocol. New authors have contributed to the following chapters: **Concepts of Orthotic Fundamentals, Tissue Healing, Prefabricated Orthoses, Taping Techniques, Stiffness, Arthritis, Flexor Tendon Injuries, Peripheral Nerve Injuries, Burns, The Musician,** and **Hand and Upper Extremity Transplantation.** New chapters include: **Relative Motion Orthoses, Upper Extremity Prosthetics, Orficast® and Orficast® More, Delta-Cast®,** and **Tendon and Nerve Transfers.**

ORGANIZATION HIGHLIGHTS AND FEATURES

The main text is divided into three sections. **Section I** focuses on the **Fundamentals of Orthotic Fabrication.** Much of the mystery surrounding orthotic fabrication can be eliminated if the therapist has a good working knowledge of appropriate nomenclature (to interpret referrals), upper extremity anatomy, tissue healing guidelines, and a concrete understanding of mechanical principles. This section provides the foundation necessary to plan and create an orthosis. **Chapter 1** presents a modified version of the American Society of Hand Therapists (ASHT) orthosis nomenclature, various types of orthoses, and objectives for orthosis intervention which are used consistently throughout the book. **Chapter 2** systematically reviews the bony and neuromuscular anatomy, specifically as it relates to the application of orthoses. **Chapter 3** describes the stages of healing, factors that influence healing, and the relationship of specific stages of healing to orthosis selection and application. **Chapter 4** defines the fundamental mechanical terms and concepts pertinent to orthosis design and fabrication and discusses the clinical relevance and application of these basic principles using specific examples. **Chapter 5** surveys the proper equipment crucial to effective orthosis fabrication. **Chapter 6** outlines the entire process of creating an accurate orthosis design, from obtaining an appropriate referral to properly dispensing the device. It also introduces the PROCESS concept used in the *Fabrication Process Manual*.

Section II entitled **Optional Methods** describes alternative interventions for immobilization, mobilization, or restriction of a body part. Because of time constraints, monetary issues, or perhaps lack of product availability, it is not always practical or appropriate to make an orthosis from thermoplastic materials. The chapters included in this section provide information on alternative means of orthotic fabrication. **Chapter 7** presents how to integrate relative

motion orthoses into everyday practice. **Chapter 8** provides an overview of upper extremity prosthetics. **Chapter 9** outlines the considerations and options related to the use of prefabricated orthoses, including information on how to become an educated consumer on the availability, application, and modification of these devices. **Chapters 10 to 12** describe casting as a treatment technique that has the ability to provide outcomes that no other orthotic intervention approach can offer—including traditional casting, Orficast® and Delta-Cast® techniques. This new content familiarizes the clinician with the characteristics of casting products and outlines the ideal material to be chosen that best meets the patient's needs. **Chapter 13** provides information on the most common taping methods: traditional athletic taping, McConnell taping, and elastic therapeutic taping. Each technique is described with specific instructions and multiple clinical examples. **Chapter 14** is a noteworthy chapter because neoprene is becoming increasingly popular. This unique content reviews the basic information regarding the benefits of neoprene, qualities of neoprene materials, and a variety of thought-provoking options and alternatives for orthotic management.

Each chapter in **Section III** on **Orthotic Intervention for Specific Diagnoses and Populations** goes into depth regarding the following: stiffness, fractures, arthritis, extensor and flexor tendon injuries, peripheral nerve injuries, tendon and nerve transfers, the athlete, adult neurologic dysfunction, the pediatric patient, burns, the musician, and upper extremity transplantation.

After an overview of the specific topic, these chapters include common orthotic interventions and specific considerations. Many chapters include tables that clarify information and decrease redundancy within the text. **Case Studies** and **Chapter Review Questions** accompany each chapter and are meant to stimulate clinical reasoning and synthesize information reviewed in the text. **Expert Pearls** are a new feature in these chapters which provide unique ideas regarding intervention for that population. The addition of **MD notes** and **Field Notes** in Section III allows for alternative perspectives from the world of hand surgery/therapy.

The *Fabrication Process Manual* is a hands-on working manual and organized into four chapters that cover immobilization (**Chapter 1**), mobilization (**Chapter 2**), restriction (**Chapter 3**), and nonarticular (**Chapter 4**) orthoses.

Each chapter includes pattern illustrations and accompanying photography of the orthosis described. Most of the pattern descriptions include **Clinical Pearls**, **Pattern Pearls,** and newly added **Expert Pearls** that apply to that particular orthosis. The Clinical and Pattern Pearls relate to our personal experience and the Expert Pearls were contributed by our colleagues working in the field of Hand Therapy. They include fabrication and orthosis modification tips as well as insight for improving cost containment and maximizing time efficiency. Most orthosis patterns have alternative design options in the event that the therapist cannot fabricate a custom orthosis. Common diagnoses and general positioning are recommended. However, one must appreciate that the diagnoses appropriate for an orthosis and the recommended positioning can be varied and depend on many factors. The pattern designs illustrated are suggestions of the ones we have found simple to visualize and use. The Pattern Pearls give alternative pattern designs that we have used in our clinical practice. The therapist is encouraged to modify the pattern according to specific patient needs. The manual is meant as a guideline for orthosis construction—use your creativity to individualize each device. The pearls are not always unique to a particular orthosis, and many apply to a variety of orthoses. A complete list of Clinical/Pattern/Expert Pearls is provided at the front of the book to help the student locate specific points of interest.

Appendix A is a list of orthotic vendors/resources that offer equipment, materials, and prefabricated orthoses. **Appendices B** and **C** provide examples of forms used in a clinical setting. The **Index** allows the reader to access information about orthoses by their common names as well as by the ASHT terminology.

FEATURES OF THE MANUAL

*   **Expert Pearls:** New feature added in both main text and manual, generously shared by dozens of hand therapy experts from around the world including unique orthotic ideas, tips, and material usage. This unique feature includes select pearls authored by Judy Colditz, OT/L, CHT, FAOTA.
*   **Clinical Pearls:** Appearing in main text and manual, these illustrate tips on ways to modify the design or alter the fabrication process to improve efficiency or maximize patient specificity.
*   **Pattern Pearls:** Presented in manual, these provide alternative pattern designs or other orthotic options.
*   **Discussion Points:** At the end of *Fabrication Process Manual* chapters, these questions challenge students to use critical thinking to recall concepts and theories learned in these chapters.
*   **Printable Patterns:** Available online to allow for easy accessibility and ability to resize for lab/clinic use. Orthotic fabrication for a spectrum of diagnoses and special populations (available with *Fabrication Process Manual* only).

*   **Full Color/Large Format:** This updated presentation of images provides a more intimate view of the orthoses presented.

This book reviews numerous pattern designs and other options for orthotic management for the upper extremity. Although this endeavor documents a spectrum of orthotic management, the possibilities for different options extend far beyond a single text. New challenges face the clinician daily; and it is with each patient that we learn something new, building on our previous knowledge. This book is meant to stimulate clinical skills and clinician creativity, encouraging the integration of principles and process from which a clinician can create new orthoses.

ADDITIONAL RESOURCES

Fabrication Process Manual for Orthotic Intervention for the Hand and Upper Extremity includes additional resources for both instructors and students that are available on the book's companion website at http://thePoint.lww.com.

Instructor Resources

Approved adopting instructors will be given access to the following additional resources:
*   Image Bank
*   Answers to Discussion Points

Student Resources

*   Videos detailing the fabrication process and common orthoses
*   Checklist
*   Printable Orthotic Patterns
*   Appendix A: Care and Use of Your Custom Orthosis

Expert Pearl Contributors

Natalie Alfaro, OT, CHT
Macquarie Hand Therapy
Australia

Baptiste Arrate, OT
Institut Sud Aquitain de la Main et du Membre Supérieur
France

Michele Auch, OTR/L, CHT,
ATI Physical Therapy
Illinois

Larissa Póvoa Alves Barradas, OT
Hamato Rehabilitation
Brazil

Nancy Beaman, MBA, OTR/L, CHT
ATI Physical Therapy
Massachusetts

Jeanine Beasley, EdD, OTR, CHT, FAOTA
Grand Valley State University
Michigan

Theresa Bell-Nagle, OTR/L, CHT
2 Thumbs Up Hand Therapy
Massachusetts

Carolyn Brown, OTR/L, CLT, OTD candidate
Hospital for Special Care
Quinnipiac University
Connecticut

Laura Carter, OT, Hand Therapist
Advanced Health and Hand Therapy
Australia

Sabrina Cassella, MEd, OTR/L, CHT
ATI Physical Therapy
Massachusetts

Melissa Cepeda, OTR/L
Peak Physical Therapy & Wellness
Colorado

Ana Candice Coelho, PT, Hand Therapist
Quiros Reabilitação Integrada
Brazil

Michelle Coil, MOT, OTR, CHT, PYT, CEAS
Virtual Hand Care
Texas

Diane Coker, PT, DPT, CHT
South County Orthopedic Specialists
California

Judy Colditz, OT/L, CHT, FAOTA
HandLab/BraceLab
North Carolina

Laura Conway, OTR, CHT, COMT UE
Select Medical
Florida

Bruce Curtis, OT
Performance Health
Illinois

Mary Anne Dykstra, OTR/L, CHT
ATI Physical Therapy
Illinois

Chantal Etcheverry, OT
Institut Sud Aquitain de la Main et du Membre Supérieur
France

Sheri B. Feldscher, OTR/L, CHT
Philadelphia Hand to Shoulder Center
Pennsylvania

Debbie Fisher, MS, OTR, CHT
Baylor Scott and White Institute of Rehab
Texas

Angela Frigerio, OT, CHT
Pacific Hand Therapy
Australia

Ginny Gibson, OTD, OTR/L, CHT
Samuel Merritt University
California

Trish Griffiths, OT, Hand Therapist
Christian Barnard Memorial Hospital
South Africa

Amanda Hall, PT, MPT, PCS, ATP
The HSC Pediatric Center
The Center
Washington Dc

Emma Hirst, OT, Hand Therapist
The Hand Therapy Group
New Zealand

Clyde Johnson, PT, CHT
Bellevue Bone and Joint Orthopedics
Washington

Joanna Jourdan, OT
HLO Handtherapie and Ergotherapeutin
Germany

Saba Kamal, OTR, CHT
Hands-On-Care,
California

Magdalena Kolasińska, PT
Józef Piłsudski University of Physical Education
Poland

Hannah Leaman, OTR/L, OTD
University of Virginia Medical Center
Virginia

Julianne Lessard, OTR/L, CHT
ATI Physical Therapy
Massachusetts

Niamh Masterson, OT, Hand Therapist
UrbanRehab
Australia

Grégory Mesplié, PT
Institut Sud Aquitain de la Main et du Membre Supérieur
France

Andrea Moser, OT, Hand Therapist
Trauma Hospital Klagenfurt
Private practice – St. Veit/Glan
Austria

Alfred Ninja, OTR/L, CHT
Fortis Hand Therapy Clinic
Kenya

Anna Ovsyannikova, MD, Hand Therapy
University Clinic
Russia

Jill Peck-Murray, MOTR/L, CHT
Rehab Education
California

Kirsten C. Pedersen, OT
K.C. Pedersen / Ergoklinikken
Denmark

Beth Perko, OTR/L, CHT
OrthoVirginia
Virginia

Bob Phillips, OTR/L, CHT
Optim Orthopedics
Georgia

Ceri Pulham, OT, CHT
Norwest Hand Therapy
Australia

Lisa Ray, OTR/L, CHT
OrthoVirginia
Virginia

Kerry Raymond, MS, OTR, CHT, CFCE
Key Therapy Services
New Hampshire

Kathy Riley, PT, CHT
University of Virginia/Healthsouth
Virginia

Kim Rosinski, OTR/L, CSCS, CHT
NovaCare Rehabilitation
Pennsylvania

Veruschka Moreira Coêlho Savoldeli, OT
Hamato Rehabilitation
Brazil

Debby Schwartz, OTD, OTR/L, CHT
Orfit Industries America
New Jersey

Erfan Shafiee, OT, Hand Therapist
University of Western Ontario
Canada

Mary Sommer, OTR/L, CHT
ATI Physical Therapy
Washington

Kimberly Goldie Staines, OTR, CHT
Michael E. DeBakey Veterans Affairs Medical Center
Texas

Alison Taylor, OTR/L, CHT, CKTP, CKTI
Baylor Scott & White Health
Texas

Janine Thomas, OTR/L, CHT, COMT
OrthoVirginia
Virginia

Hoang Tran, OT/L, CHT
Hands on Therapy Services
CHT Secrets
Florida

Ngaire Turnbull, OT, Hand Therapist
Hand Spark
Australia

Kathy Villacres, OTR/L, CHT
Hand and Arm Therapy Specialists
Ohio

Anne Wajon, PT, CHT
Macquarie Hand Therapy
Australia

Karol Young, OTD, OTR/L, CHT
HandLab/BraceLab
North Carolina

Acknowledgments

The undertaking of this third edition would not be possible if it were not for the patience and guidance provided by our experienced team at Wolters Kluwer including: Matt Hauber, Acquisitions Editor; Amy Millholen, Development Editor; Cody Adams and Vinoth Ezhumalai, Editorial Coordinators; Barton Dudlick, Production Project Manager; Steve Druding, Design Coordinator; Margie Orzech, Manufacturing Coordinator. We truly value their time and experience with assisting us in updating the design of this new edition including dividing the original text into two separate books. We want to thank them for allowing us the space to expand our content including the overwhelming task of organizing the hundreds of additional color photographs and contributions from dozens of therapists. We truly appreciate the hard work provided by Oviya Balamurugan, Project Manager at TNQ Technologies during this revision; she successfully conquered the daunting task of creating a user-friendly format to present the images and information.

No book is solely the work of its authors. We would like to thank all the patients who were so generous in allowing us to photograph them and provide such a plethora of clinical examples for our book. We would like to express our gratitude to the many therapists and physicians we have worked with over the years who contributed to our knowledge base, professional growth, and clinical skills. So many of you have urged and supported us to always dig deeper and be as creative as possible! Your trust in our expertise and appreciation for what we do has fueled the underlying passion for the writing of this book. We also want to acknowledge the generosity of therapists from around the world who were eager to contribute their unique ideas that will provide the reader with so many options when it comes to orthosis selection.

We would like to specially thank Performance Health, especially Paul England, former Director of Marketing, Orthopedics for the generous support in supplying the majority of thermoplastic materials and components used in the Fabrication Manual for the professional photographs. We have thoroughly enjoyed working with TailorSplint which has stood the test of time since our first edition. Thanks so much!

Finally, we would like to express our sincere thanks to our families who have been so patient and understanding during the writing process—from our first edition nearly 20 years ago to this third edition. Without their love, support, and ongoing patience, we would not have been able to tackle such a huge, detail-oriented task successfully.

Contents

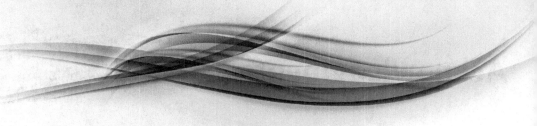

CLINICAL PEARLS

EXPERT PEARLS

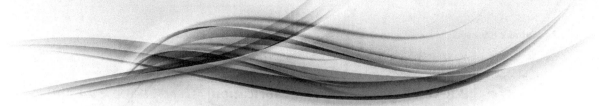

Orthotic Fabrication Process Manual

MaryLynn A. Jacobs, MBA, MS, OTR/L, CHT
Noelle M. Austin, MS, PT, CHT

This manual contains the instructions for orthotic fabrication. The orthoses have been organized into four chapters according to the type of orthosis: **IMMOBILIZATION** (Chapter 1), **MOBILIZATION** (Chapter 2), **RESTRICTION** (Chapter 3), and **NONARTICULAR** (Chapter 4). Before delving into orthotic fabrication, it is important to note that the patterns given here should not be approached as if they were a recipe from a cookbook, blindly used for every patient. The patterns are a collection of frequently used designs intended to be modified to meet each specific patient's needs and diagnosis requirements. Therapists must tailor their approaches to orthotic fabrication according to the unique needs of each patient. Again, these patterns are to be used as *basic guidelines only*. More detailed information about orthotic fabrication for specific patient populations and diagnoses can be found in Section III of the main textbook.

To be consistent when naming orthoses, this text will continue to support and integrate historical nomenclature; however, the language set forth by the Centers for Medicare & Medicaid Services (CMS) takes precedence and will be fully described and incorporated into naming all orthoses. The authors of Chapter 1 have taken the modified ASHT Splint Classification System (1992) and the current CMS L-Code orthotic descriptions and created a modified, streamlined classification system that will be used for the primary name of each orthosis described in this book.

The fabrication instructions for each orthosis will also include the **Common Names** of each orthosis design, which will allow the reader to cross-reference and use the terms preferred in a specific clinical setting. Under the heading "**Alternative Orthosis Options**," other orthoses are noted that may be used as a substitute or alternative if, for some reason, the described orthosis is not appropriate because of the specific circumstances of the patient or diagnosis.

The patterns for the orthoses also include the most common reason for application, **Primary Function**, and other uses listed under the heading "**Additional Functions**." The reader may use the cross-reference index (**found in the back of this book**) to locate a specific pattern. "**Common Diagnoses and General Optimal Positions**" are outlined for each orthosis. As noted, these lists are intended to be general guidelines. For example, only the most common diagnoses

for each orthosis are noted. The fabrication method of each orthosis follows the **PROCESS** acronym, which is described in detail in Chapter 6 (main textbook) as well as on the foldout bookmark.

The PROCESS acronym is defined as follows (Table 1):

P—Pattern creation
R—Refine pattern
O—Options for material
C—Cut and heat
E—Evaluate fit while molding
S—Strapping and components
S—Survey completed orthosis

This manual includes **Pattern Pearls** that are alterations/modifications made to the pattern. These alterations in the pattern may include ways to accommodate for use with different materials or modify the existing pattern to meet the specific needs of the patient.

Clinical and **Expert Pearls** are found throughout the manual (and main textbook). These Pearls can be "tricks of the trade" and/or "clinical tips" that stimulate *clinician creativity*, *critical thinking*, and *problem-solving* when attempting to fabricate the best option for the patient and the circumstances surrounding the diagnosis. Clinical Pearls are from the authors of the textbook, and Expert Pearls are from outside contributors. Many of the Pearls shown throughout the manual can be applied to various orthoses/conditions and not just to the orthosis they are located adjacent to in the text. See the list of Clinical and Expert Pearls at the beginning of the book to locate a specific "pearl" of interest.

In this revised text, the clinical, expert, and pattern pearls are numerous and well detailed via accompanying color photographs. These photographs and additional instructions further highlight how the fabricator should consider modifying the specific orthosis to meet the patient's unique orthotic requirements. The Clinical and Expert Pearl photographs are of actual patients gathered from the authors and their colleague's years of clinical practice. Many of these pearls are not "perfect" in construction/design; however, the authors felt they are wonderful teaching tools as is. These imperfections reflect what happens in daily practice given the shortage of time, materials, and perhaps lack of experience. On the appropriate orthoses, the authors have noted the problematic areas with suggestions for improvements.

Most of the orthoses shown in this manual (except for many of the Pearls) were fabricated using TailorSplint™ thermoplastic material (Performance Health, Warrenville, IL). A nonperforated material was used for the professionally photographed orthoses to minimize distractions and improve visualization of details. The therapist is encouraged to use the most appropriate material for the diagnosis and patient; more information may be found under the heading "Options for Materials" and in Chapter 5 (main textbook).

TABLE 1	P-R-O-C-E-S-S of Orthotic Fabrication	
P	Pattern creation	• Obtain referral with specific custom orthosis information from physician. • Perform upper extremity examination. • Determine specific needs and decide on type of orthosis to fabricate. • Trace pattern on paper towel per orthosis diagram and cut it out. Use anatomic landmarks highlighted on pattern to aid in accurate pattern creation.
R	Refine pattern	• Check fit of paper pattern by trying it on patient's extremity (or on unaffected extremity if warranted). • Mark areas that need adjustment (i.e., add or delete material).
O	Options for materials	• Decide on type of thermoplastic and strapping material. • Transfer pattern to thermoplastic material using wax pencil or pen.
C	Cut and heat	• Partially heat thermoplastic material until soft enough to cut pattern accordingly. • Place patient's extremity in desired position and heat thermoplastic material to appropriate temperature. • Apply any padding to high-risk bony areas prior to molding. • Fully heat thermoplastic material, dry water off, and check temperature on your own skin before applying to patient.

E	Evaluate fit while molding	• Mold orthosis to patient, and remember to:
		  • Use gravity to assist whenever possible.
		  • Incorporate arches.
		  • Provide adequate length and width.
		  • Evenly distribute pressure while molding.
		  • Handle thermoplastic material gently.
		• Mark areas to be trimmed with fingernail edge or pen, and carefully remove orthosis from patient.
		• Trim designated areas.

S	Strapping and components	• Determine optimal means of securing orthosis to extremity. • Provide adequate width in strapping and consider foam for key straps to obtain optimal positioning. • Place orthosis on patient's limb and apply appropriate strapping. • Affix specific components—such as hinges or outriggers—per pattern instructions.
S	Survey completed orthosis	• Flare edges and round sharp corners of orthosis. This is best completed by selectively dipping 1–2 mm of material's edge into warm water. • Round corners of strapping. • Provide patient with written handouts describing the orthosis' purpose, precautions, proper care, and wearing schedule. • Instruct in functional use and diagnosis-specific exercises within the orthosis if appropriate. • Check that patient is able to don and doff the orthosis independently. Patients may benefit from digital photographs of proper orthosis application. • Provide information on replacements for stockinette, straps, or other items. • Consider taking digital photographs of completed custom-fabricated orthosis for patient records and to verify accurate accounting and billing to payers. • Schedule follow-up visit to reevaluate and modify orthosis as appropriate.

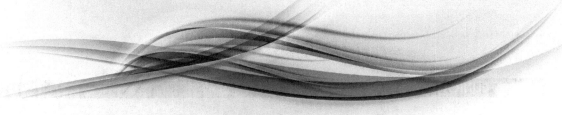

1

Immobilization Orthoses

MaryLynn A. Jacobs, MBA, MS, OTR/L, CHT
Noelle M. Austin, MS, PT, CHT

GENERAL CLINICAL PEARLS RELATED TO IMMOBILIZATION ORTHOSES

PATTERN CREATION/REFINE PATTERN

CLINICAL PEARL 1–X1

Transferring Pattern to Material

There are many ways to transfer the paper towel pattern to the thermoplastic material. The main goal is to avoid an unsightly orthosis with pen markings along the edges. **A,** Here are some techniques: **B,** Allow the paper towel to adhere to the wet material during the cutting process, use a wax pencil to outline the design, or scratch the thermoplastic material with an awl to draw the pattern. **C,** If using a marker, draw the outline a little larger and cut on the inside to prevent makings from showing on final orthosis.

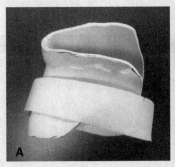
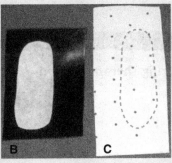

CLINICAL PEARL 1–X2

Pattern Considerations for Border Digits

To provide for better stability of the orthosis on the hand and to achieve increased purchase of distal joints, include a portion of the metacarpal (and overlying thenar and hypothenar eminences) within the orthosis. This is especially helpful when applying orthoses on small hands **(A-C).**

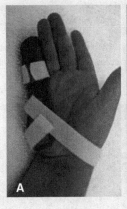
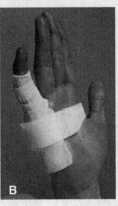
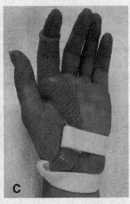

CLINICAL PEARL 1-X3

Pin Care

For patients with complicated injuries that require pin care during the immobilization period, consider fabricating a removable window for easy access to the pins **(A and B)**. This technique eliminates the need to remove the entire orthosis when inspecting pin sites. While molding the material over the pin(s), use a piece of gauze or cotton batting to prevent the thermoplastic material from adhering to the pins; this also provides a protective bubble to ensure the material will not place undue pressure directly over the area. **C and D,** Material can also be pushed out enough to create a space for the pins to not abut the material, yet the hardened thermoplastic can provide adequate protection. **E and F,** This patient needed full protection over the pins that were stabilizing the SF volar plate reconstruction. The therapist applied sterile gauze over the pins allowing the safe fabrication of a thermoplastic cap to be worn during healing.

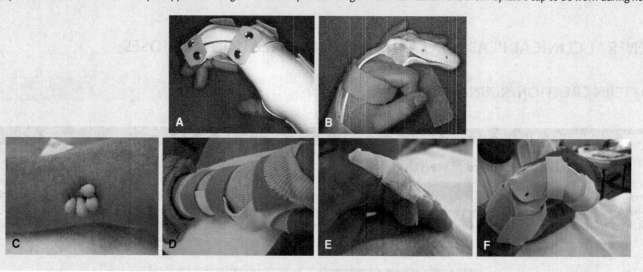

CLINICAL PEARL 1-X4

Orthoses for Use During Therapy Session

A thermoplastic volar hand piece with an integrated hook can hold a weight to apply a passive stretch during a therapeutic intervention technique such as shown with ultrasound.

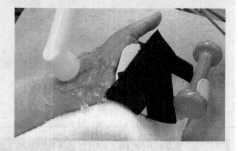

OPTIONS FOR MATERIALS

CLINICAL PEARL 1-X5

Elastic-Based Materials Allow for Remolding

Consider an elastic-based material when fabricating an orthosis on an edematous extremity or when it is known that an orthosis will need to be modified during the rehabilitation because of diagnosis-specific issues. When reheated, the memory characteristic in these materials allows the material to closely return to its original shape **(A and B)**.

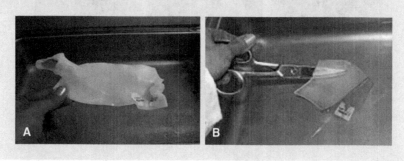

CLINICAL PEARL 1–X6

Material Thickness

Choose thickness of material based on rigidity needed **(A)** 1/16", **(B)** 1/8"—always trying to make orthosis as low profile/light weight as possible. Circumferential design allows for thinner materials.

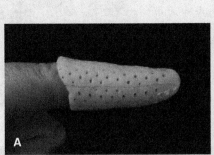
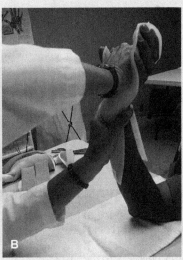

CLINICAL PEARL 1–X7

Using Scrap Thermoplastic Material

Scrap pieces of thermoplastic material come in handy for many different situations. **A and B,** Material can be molded around a pen/pencil, eating utensil, or tools to build up the handle; **(C)** fabrication of small platforms to enhance AROM exercises; **(D)** to create homemade rivets or washers; **(E and F)** or for securing or guiding mobilization components onto bases; **(G–I)** create exercise tools to enhance motion and strength facilitate digit and wrist strength. **J,** Roll scrap material into a think tube and cut into small segments—use for in-hand manipulation activities to promote functional grasp and pinch. Vary the size from large to small increasing the level of difficulty.

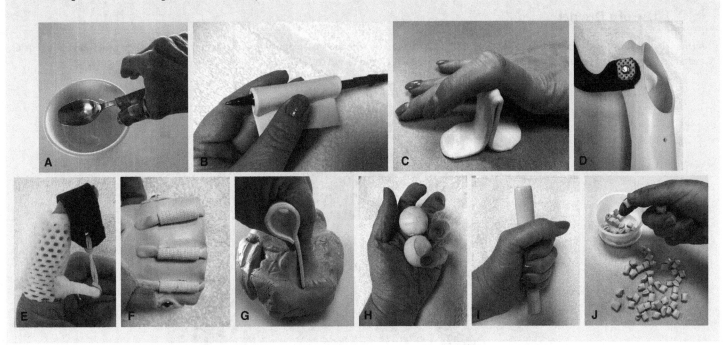

CLINICAL PEARL 1–X8

Reusing Old Orthoses

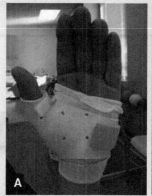 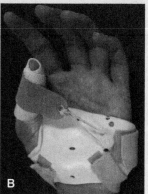

To save money and materials, reuse old orthoses to fabricate new ones when appropriate. For example, during the initial phases of healing after a UCL injury, the patient may require a thumb immobilization orthosis for protection **(A)**. Once the fracture has healed, the patient may experience joint stiffness at the thumb MP and/or IP joints that requires mobilization. The original immobilization orthosis can be remolded into a mobilization orthosis by simply trimming the thumb region and attaching components **(B)**.

CLINICAL PEARL 1–X9

Cutting Thermoplastic Material

A, If scissors are not used properly (incorrectly using the tips of scissors and "snipping"), jagged edges will occur making it challenging to smooth out the orthosis borders after completion. **B,** Use long strokes, getting the warm thermoplastic material into the depth of the blades. **C,** To make a slit in the thermoplastic material: A spot heater can be used when it is too cumbersome to partially heat a thermoplastic material to make either a hole or a slit as shown here. This is particularly true when working with a large piece of material. Shown is the use of a spot heater to warm the middle section of the pattern in order to create the "slit" used in this dorsal volar forearm immobilization orthosis. Once warmed, sharp scissors are able to cut through the material without creating jagged edges.

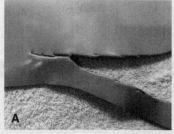 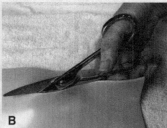 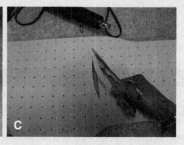

CLINICAL PEARL 1–X10

Use of a Dremel

A Dremel is a helpful tool to have in the clinic. **A and B,** This can be used to perforate solid material in a specific area to prevent skin issues and assist with air exchange; **(C and D)** cut holes in areas unreachable with a hole punch; **(E and F)** and cut slits in material for creative strapping techniques.

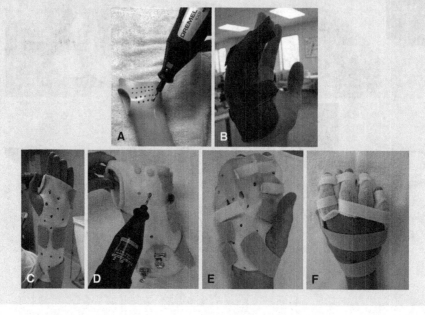

EXPERT PEARL 1–1

Homemade Rivet
KIMBERLY GOLDIE STAINES, OTR, CHT
Texas

Therapists are often intimidated by securing rivets, or they may not have them in the clinic. Homemade rivets are easy to make—simply take a small scrap of thermoplastic, heat it and roll it, push it through the hole in the orthosis **(A and B)**, adhere to the inside, and press down to prevent any potential pressure areas **(C)** (make sure to remove any protective coating on the material to ensure a secure connection). On the outside, slip the thermoplastic piece through a hole in the strapping and press down to form the smooth "rivet" head **(D-F)**.

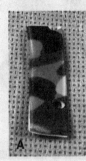
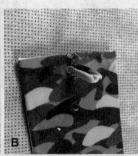
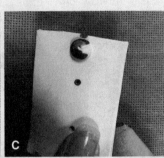
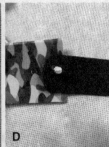
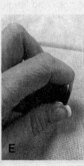
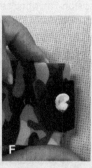

CUT AND HEAT

CLINICAL PEARL 1–X11

Quality Scissors

Not all scissors are appropriate for every task. Having various types of scissors on hand can make the fabrication process a lot easier. **A,** Gingher Super Shears are best used for cutting out orthosis patterns on warm thermoplastic material and may not be effective for small detailed cutting. **B,** Unlimited Scissors are an excellent alternative for detailed cutting in small areas. **C,** When serial static finger orthoses are fabricated using a circumferential method of application, small Serial Cast Cutter Scissors are extremely useful for easy removal; the blunt nose prevents any risk of injury for the patient. **D,** Fiskars® Non-Stick Scissors are ideal for cutting adhesive products because of the protective coating. **E,** Pinking Shears can be an excellent addition to a utility drawer. Using these scissors to cut stockinette off a roll can prevent and/or prolong the fraying of this material. (All available through Performance Health.)

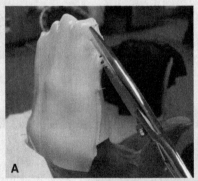
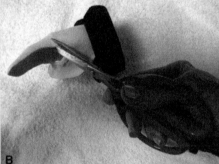
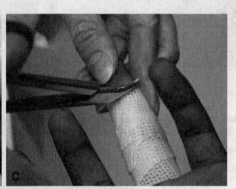
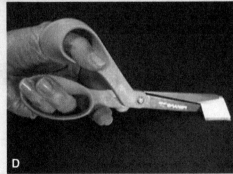
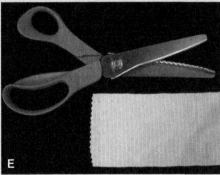

CLINICAL PEARL 1–X12

Caring for Scissors

First, investing in quality scissors is a must for the frequent orthotic maker. Proper care of the scissors is crucial to ensure their effective use. Being sure the scissors are regularly sharpened will make the task easier and also save your thumbs from undue stress. Designating scissors "thermoplastic only" and "strapping only" prevents the strapping material's adhesive from sticking to the thermoplastic when cutting and trimming warm material. Use solvent, adhesive remover, alcohol wipes, or nail polish remover to clean the adhesive from scissors. Furthermore, sharpen the scissors often to achieve smooth edges when cutting materials (Rolyan® Self-Bonding Solvent; Performance Health) **(A and B)**.

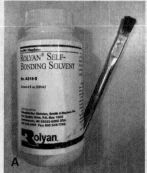
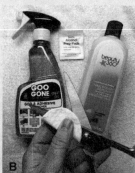

CLINICAL PEARL 1–X13

Tips for Heating Thermoplastic Materials

Use a designated heating device such as a commercially available heat pan or skillet. The addition of pan netting **(A)** as well as a spatula can prevent thermoplastics from sticking to the bottom of the unit. Empty and clean the unit regularly. Adding a small amount of liquid soap to the water can help "soften" any potentially hard water, making thermoplastics less sticky and easier to handle. Avoid using a hot pack unit to heat the materials; they are not hygienic or heat controlled. Also, be sure to partially heat the material for approximately 30 seconds prior to cutting out the pattern to save your own thumbs from the potential wear and tear of the repetitive forceful cutting of hard thermoplastics. **B,** Another heating trick is to heat the material in sections so that you always have control over the material. You can consider partially heating a section, trimming it, and then moving on to the next section. **C,** To smooth out borders of an orthosis, just dip the edges in the heating pan approximately ¼", for a few seconds just to partly heat. The material can then tolerate pressure to flare and eliminate rough borders.

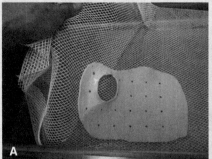
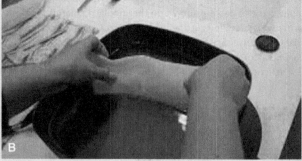
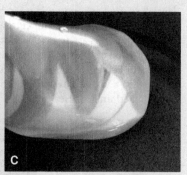

CLINICAL PEARL 1–X14

Heating Large Piece of Material Evenly

Warm a section of material that will fit into the heating pan **(A)**, making sure that there is netting on the bottom of the heating pan. Once it begins to soften, cover the section that is in the water completely with a paper towel **(B)**. Then gently allow the remaining section to fold over the paper towel into the water **(C)**. Pull the entire folded piece out of the water using the netting. Gently unfold and apply to patient.

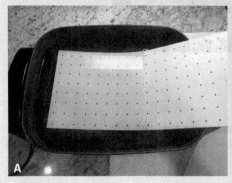
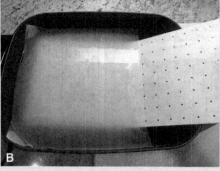
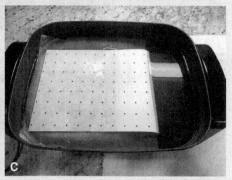

CLINICAL PEARL 1–X15

Handling Warm Thermoplastic Material

A, The surface used to dry off warmed thermoplastic material after removal from the heat pan can cause unsightly ridges or markings, especially with materials that are very contouring. Consider using a smooth pillowcase versus a textured terry cloth towel. Consider partially heating material to cut the pattern out which will result in a self-sealed edge that minimized need for contouring later. Lift the heated material out of the heating pan with a spatula or lift with netting to prevent overstretching. To prevent towel markings, place the warm material on a pillowcase before molding it onto the patient's extremity. **B,** If marker is used, cut along the inside of the line to avoid permanent orthosis markings. Note the long strokes made with the Gingher scissors; **(C)** good quality scissors are being used to cut "pinched" warm material which in turn will create a bonded seam. **D,** On occasion, a warm, larger piece of material will need to be cut. Use quality scissors with long stokes and handle the material with as much of your hands surface area as possible. This will help prevent undue stretching.

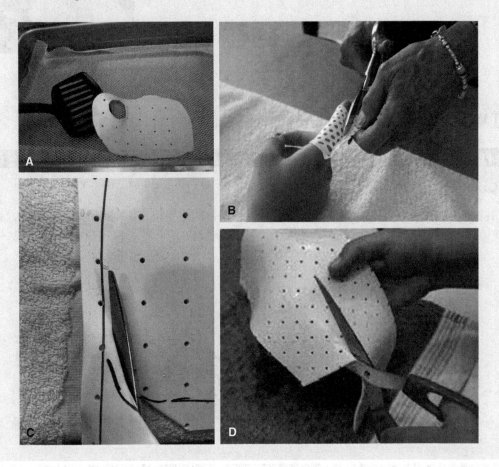

CLINICAL PEARL 1–X16

Temperature of Material

Be sure to dry the material fully and check the temperature prior to applying to the patient's extremity. If the material is too hot, lay it on a cold countertop to facilitate the cooling process prior to molding. If they are sensitive to heat, utilize a stockinette to protect their skin.

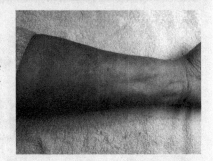

Adjusting Orthosis
DIANE COKER PT, DPT, CHT
California

When adjustment is needed in a tight region of an orthosis, heating the area by immersion in water may potentially oversoften adjacent areas or cause loss of orthotic shape. Consider this alternative—heat the scissors with a heat gun—this also reduces the amount of force needed to cut through the thermoplastic.

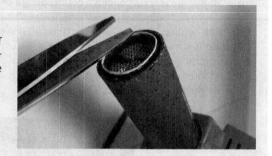

EVALUATE FIT WHILE MOLDING

CLINICAL PEARL 1–X17

Avoid "Grabbing"

Ideally, if the patient is positioned in a gravity-assisted fashion, the therapists should not have to be overly hands-on during the molding process. Utilize soft strokes when molding (**A**) the material versus forceful grabbing which can cause ridges in the end orthosis potentially irritating the extremity (**B**).

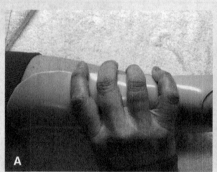
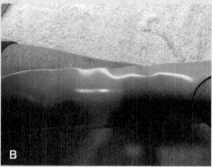

CLINICAL PEARL 1–X18

Using a Wrap or Stockinette Sleeve to Aid Fabrication

A–C, A light elasticized wrap (Ace™), prewrap, and elasticized or cotton stockinette can aid in the fabrication and setting of a forearm-based orthosis, especially when positioning the joints is a challenge or when there is no assistant available to help with positioning. Use the wrap proximally to allow for hands-on positioning distally. Be sure to watch for compression forces at the forearm borders of the orthosis; leave a small amount of thermoplastic exposed (**D**); just before the orthosis sets up, remove the wrap/sleeve and gently flare the borders away from the skin.

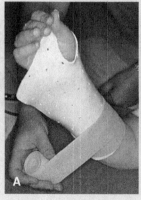
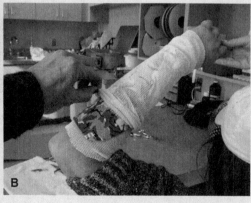
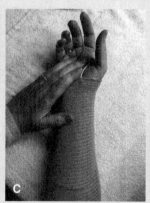
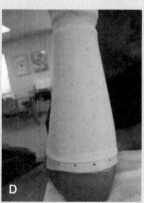

CLINICAL PEARL 1–X19

Fabricating an Orthosis Over Edema Management Products and Wound Dressings

During orthosis fabrication, the thermoplastic material can inadvertently adhere to the edema products (Coban™) and/or wound dressing **(A and B)**. The dressing could potentially be pulled off the healing tissue causing disruption to the healing wound. To avoid that risk, place a piece of stockinette over the wrap or dressing before molding the orthosis to the area **(C-E)**. Once the orthosis is completely set, simply cut off the stockinette and remove the orthosis.

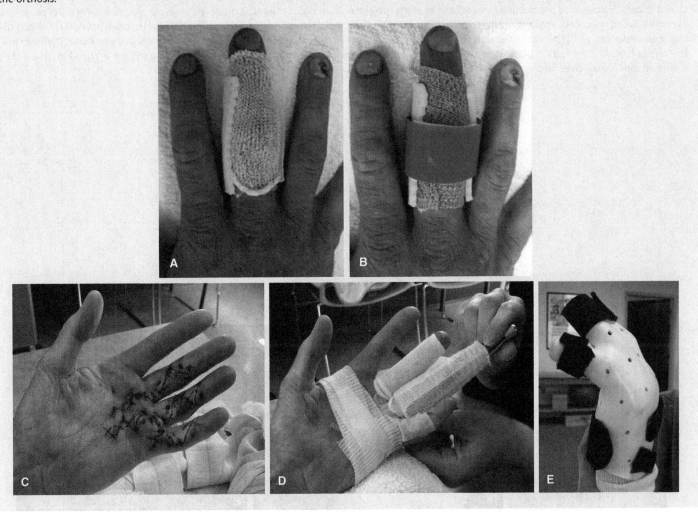

CLINICAL PEARL 1–X20

Techniques for Adding Clamshell Piece

Many orthoses can be modified by molding an additional piece of thermoplastic material dorsally to create a "clamshell" orthosis commonly used with wrist and wrist/thumb immobilization orthoses **(A and B)**. This modification can provide additional protection and more rigid immobilization of the region. First, fabricate the volar orthosis per the instructions, but do not apply the strapping. Next, create the pattern for the dorsal piece, allowing approximately ½" of overlap of the dorsal piece over the molded volar segment. Prepad any bony prominences such as the ulnar styloid process to help prevent irritation. Use a coated material if possible to prevent unwanted adherence of the two pieces. If uncoated material is the only choice, use a stockinette or a wet paper towel over the volar segment while molding the dorsal piece. Other examples of dorsal protection provided for **(C)** distal phalanx crush injury, **(D)** thumb proximal phalanx pinning, and **(E)** multiple metacarpal fractures with pinning. **F–H,** Note the prepadded ulna styloid using a high-dense foam. The light cotton stockinette is holding the foam in place while a second piece of warm thermoplastic is molded over the hardened base to form a "clamshell." The orthosis is finished with 2" elasticized loop closures.

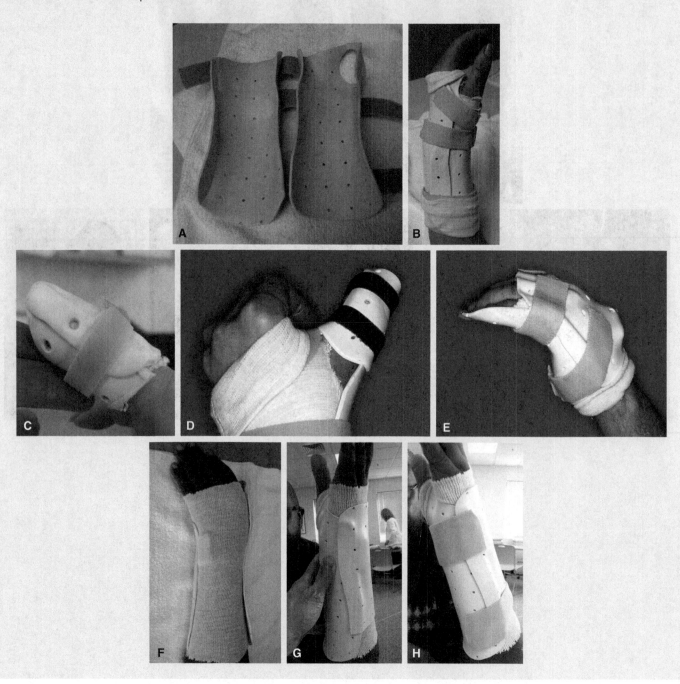

CLINICAL PEARL 1-X21

Flaring Versus Rolling of Edges

A and B, A flaring force should be gently applied to the warmed edge (approximately ¼") by the therapist's thenar and hypothenar regions. When deciding how to finish the edges, consider the advantages of flaring and the disadvantages of rolling. Rolling does not allow for simple modifications, such as widening the opening for the thumb or shortening the distal border to allow unimpeded MCP joint motion. Rolling back of a previously rolled region may lead to a bulky, unsightly orthosis. **C,** Flaring provides for easy adjustments and a neater looking orthosis.

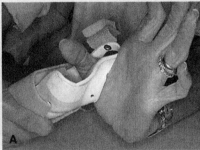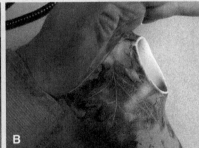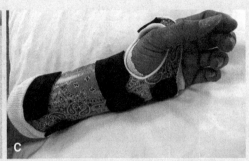

CLINICAL PEARL 1-X22

Overstretching of Material

Caution should be taken when intending to overlap material for a closure technique. If not enough material is estimated, then overstretching and material breakdown will occur.

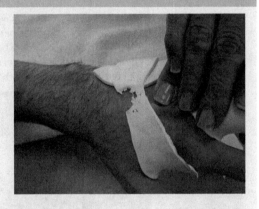

CLINICAL PEARL 1-X23

Facilitating Cooling

Consider using cold water to speed the cooling process if required. Cold sprays are also available for this purpose. If you remove the orthosis prior to it fully setting, there is a risk of losing proper fit so be cautious.

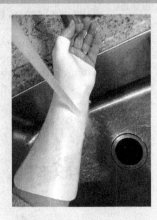

Removeable Foam
KATHY RILEY, PT, CHT
Virginia

Foam padding can often increase the comfort or function of an orthosis; however, some foams bottom out and need to be frequently replaced. Adhering the foam to Moleskin helps to easily remove the foam at a later date replacement **(A-C)**.

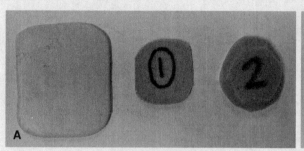
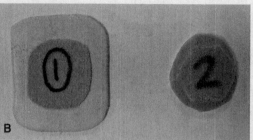
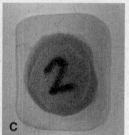

STRAPPING AND COMPONENTS

CLINICAL PEARL 1–X24

Strapping Material Choices

Strapping comes in different colors, widths, and properties. The majority of orthoses can be secured using standard hook-and-loop closure, which is the most economical choice. Instead of buying various widths, purchase multiple colors of 2″ loop and cut these down to fit the needs of the orthosis, keeping the scraps for later use. Using 1″ adhesive hook allows for securing of both 1″ and 2″ loop without any extra trimming of the adhesive necessary. In certain circumstances, providing specialty straps may be indicated, such as the use of soft strapping for the arthritic patient **(A)**, thin strapping for between digits **(B)**, elasticized loop for functional orthoses, allowing for muscle movement beneath the straps **(C)**, and soft conforming neoprene which is further described in detail in Chapter 14 **(D and E)**.

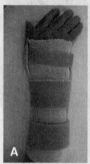
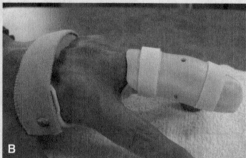
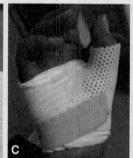
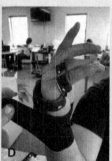
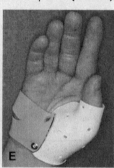

CLINICAL PEARL 1–X25

Cutting Straps to Avoid Pressure on "At-Risk" Sites

Careful trimming of soft straps to avoid pressure on sensitive areas can greatly assist in orthosis compliance. **A,** This neoprene strap avoids pressure on the pin site. **B and C,** These 2″ foam straps have been cut strategically to pass from volar to dorsal, allowing gentle radial deviation pressure on the proximal phalanges without irritating the digital web spaces. Both these materials tend to not fray. **D,** This strap is placed under the orthosis to "lift" pressure the thermoplastic border of this orthosis creates on this very fragile skin.

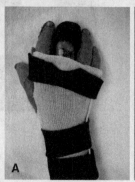
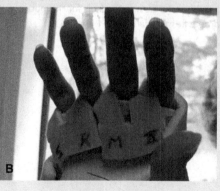
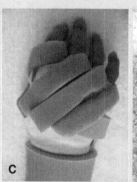
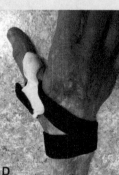

CLINICAL PEARL 1–X26

Foam Beneath Strapping

Application of strategically placed foam can be extremely helpful in obtaining the desired joint positions. **A,** Note the foam on the distal strap encouraging PIP joint extension as the pressure is applied volarly in this dorsal orthosis for a patient after Dupuytren release. **B,** In this volar design, gentle dorsal application of a strap and foam protect the thumb IP joint post pinning and reconstruction. **C,** Note the addition of foam under the distal phalanx volarly as well as the PIP joint dorsally to obtain full PIP extension. **D,** With volar forearm-based orthoses, the strap just proximal to the wrist crease is the most important, and the addition of foam will further encourage the wrist in the desired position, preventing wrist flexion within the orthosis. **E,** Slits cut into rectangle of 2″ foam strapping and slid onto 1″ strapping material can help improve pressure distribution as well as provide softer material against the skin.

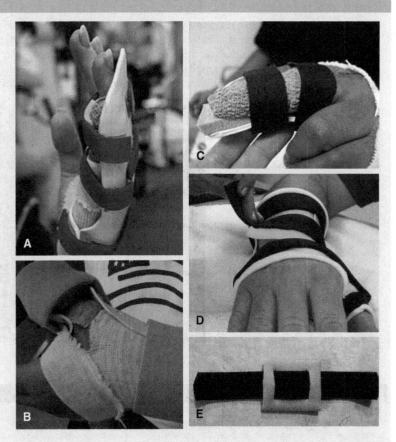

CLINICAL PEARL 1–X27

Rotating Rivet for Flexibility in Strap Orientation

A and B, A thin piece of adhesive-backed Moleskin, adhesive loop, or similar material can be applied to both sides of a strap where the rivet is to be placed. A hole punch is then used to create a hole through the layers of strap, Moleskin, and thermoplastic material. The rivet stem and cap is then closed with the blunt-nosed pliers; however, caution is taken to set the rivet with a gentle force. The rivet should be able to allow the strap to swivel in various directions as shown.

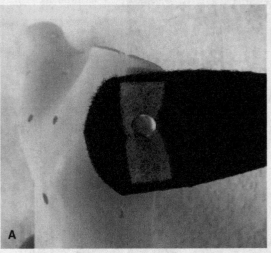

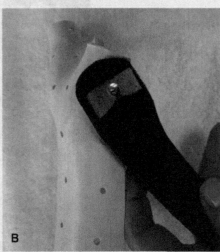

CLINICAL PEARL 1–X28

Various Stockinette/Liner Choices

A, Several choices are available that add a layer of protection between the skin and the material. These liners help absorb perspiration and prevent any skin irritation that can occur at the skin-material interface. They can be removed multiple times a day and washed. The choices include materials such as cotton, elastic (for edema-reducing compression properties), polyester, and/or a combination of these. Removable liners offer a more hygienic option compared to semipermanent adhesive liners that need to be removed frequently if soiled. For long-term use, consider using a men's silk sock by cutting the end off and adding a hole for the thumb. **B,** If available, sewing a longitudinal segment as shown will create a thumb design to be worn with thumb orthoses.

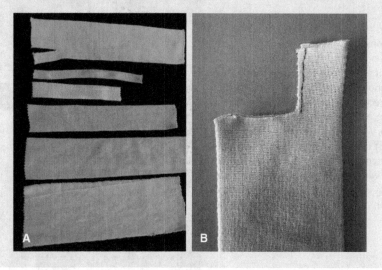

CLINICAL PEARL 1–X29

Edging Thermoplastic and Casting Material

A, One method is to use 1/16″ material to line the orthosis border. This works particularly well with perforated material because the edges of the cut holes can irritate the skin. Cut 1/16″ material in 1½″- to 2″-wide strips by the length required to go around the periphery of the orthosis. Apply solvent to the orthosis base to remove the protective coating and allow adherence of the strip. Once the strip is thoroughly heated, gently stretch (to disrupt the coating) and quickly place it along the orthosis border. The strip must be gently stretched and pinched over the edges to flatten out. This application must be done quickly and accurately because thin materials set readily. **B,** Other methods include (from left to right) Rolyan® Polycushion® Padding, Microfoam™ tape, and elastic therapeutic tape (Kinesio® Tex Tape, Performance Health) to line the borders. These methods work well for "quick fixes." **C,** Microfoam™ tape also can be used for smaller areas to provide relief from irritating edges as commonly seen in the first web space or to cushion the proximal or distal borders as show with this humeral fracture brace. **D,** Terry-Net™ Adhesive Fleece Edger (Essity) can be used with both Delta-Cast products as well as thermoplastics—especially helpful when perforated edges become problematic.

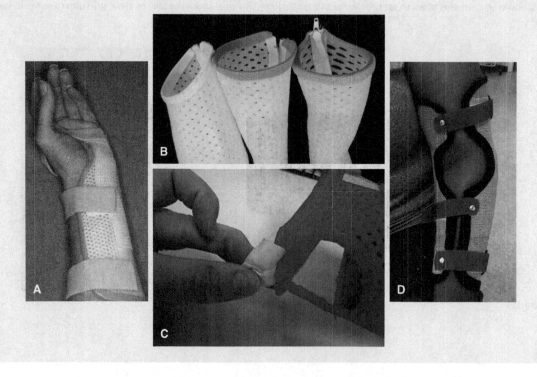

CLINICAL PEARL 1–X30

Thermoplastic Tapes or Scrap Materials as Reinforcement Strips

Heated thermoplastic tape materials such as QuickCast2 **(A)** and Orficast® **(B)** or thin strips of leftover thermoplastic material **(C)** can be used to add additional reinforcement to a weak area, secure a seam, or a region that has been "thinned out" by overzealous stretching/molding.

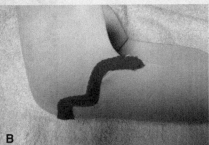
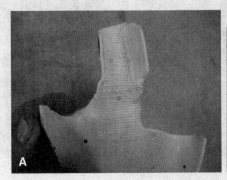
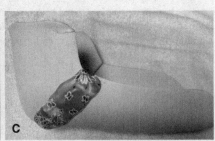

 CLINICAL PEARL 1–X31

Elastomer Scar Molds Integrated into Orthosis

Scar management products such as Rolyan® 50/50 Mix™ Elastomer Putty (Performance Health) can be integrated into orthotic designs. Perforated thermoplastics **(A-C)** allow for the material to set within the holes, securing the elastomer in place during the setting process. When using nonperforated materials, mold around one or more borders to assist in holding the product in the correct position. **D,** shows scar mold within QuickCast2 circumferential orthosis.

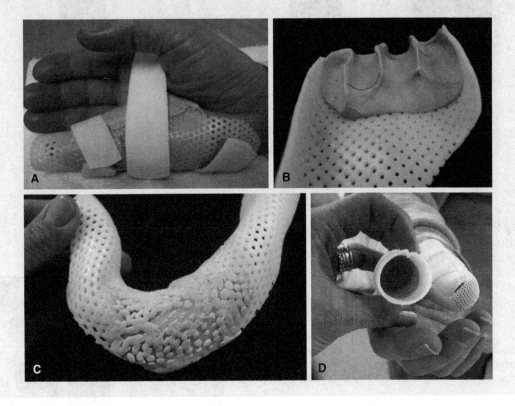

EXPERT PEARL 1–4

Strap Application

HANNAH LEAMAN, OTR/L, OTD
Virginia

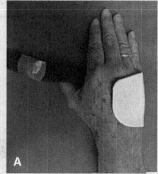
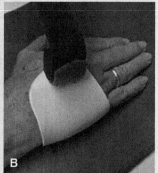

To be sure, all hook strapping is covered by corresponding loop material—place the adhesive hook on the loop strap **(A)**, remove the adhesive paper cover, and then wrap the strap at the angle needed for the strap to lie flat **(B)**.

EXPERT PEARL 1–5

Custom Trimming Stockinette

HANNAH LEAMAN, OTR/L, OTD
Virginia

When dispensing a hand-based orthosis with fingers included, it can be more comfortable to wear a stockinette. To improve fit and provide custom finger coverage, create an extra hole to allow full AROM of the fingers not immobilized in the orthosis. Refer to templates for cutting stockinette.

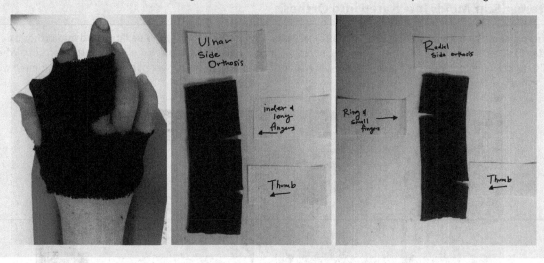

EXPERT PEARL 1–6

Padding Sleeve Opening

JANINE THOMAS, OTR/L, CHT, COMT
Virginia

Use a thin strip of a soft padding folded over the hole in wrist sleeve to improve patient comfort **(A and B)**. This also prevents the sleeve from fraying as well as reduces any pressure area sometimes caused by elasticized products.

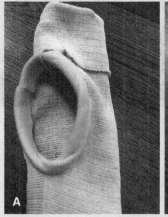
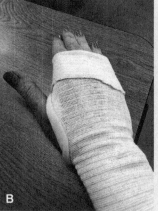

SURVEY COMPLETED ORTHOSIS

CLINICAL PEARL 1–X32

Forearm Trough Height

The forearm trough borders should be high enough to completely support and stabilize forearm. The deeper this trough, the more rigid the orthosis design and the more comfortable for the patient. Use the 45° angle technique (Clinical Pearl 1–49) to estimate two-thirds the circumference of the forearm. Once applied, be sure the borders are not too high; the straps should not "float" on top of the forearm but should sit flush against this area to secure the orthosis on the extremity **(A and B)**. The addition of foam beneath the straps can help secure the position. Inspect the borders with the orthosis off the patient as well by looking down the shaft of the orthosis, proximal to distal, checking for symmetry, and matching heights.

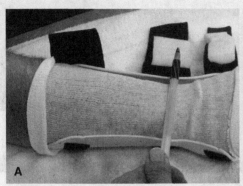
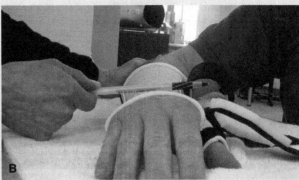

CLINICAL PEARL 1–X33

Color Stain Test

When a patient complains of irritation from an orthosis, have him or her mark the area on the skin using a washable marker or lipstick and then put the orthosis back. When it is removed again, the color can be seen on the thermoplastic and the therapist can visualize the specific part that needs to be adjusted.

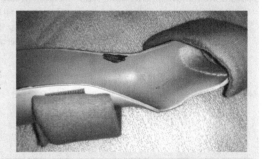

CLINICAL PEARL 1–X34

Final Strap Check

With the orthosis on the patient, check that all hook material on the orthosis is fully covered by the loop. This will prevent the hook from sticking to clothing, bedding, and the like. Make sure all hook-and-loop material is rounded on the edges to prevent areas from lifting off the orthosis. Finally, assess the mechanics of the orthosis; if a joint is to be mobile, use strapping to firmly secure the proximal or distal joints as shown in **(A)**. Also consider that the straps should be placed strategically throughout, taking full advantage of the length of the orthosis as shown in **(B)**.

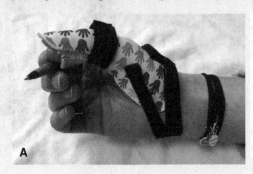
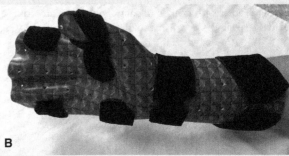

CLINICAL PEARL 1–X35

Keeping Orthosis Dry

With some specific diagnoses, an orthosis may have to be worn 24 hours a day, including during bathing. It can be challenging for the patient to keep the area completely dry. For finger-based designs, options include using a glove **(A)** or finger cot (available at local drugstores); for longer orthoses, try long bags, including newspaper or umbrella sleeves or protective wraps such as Saran™ or Glad® ClingWrap **(B)**. An elastic or adhesive tape proximally will help prevent area from getting wet. Patient should be told to remove wrap after bathing and alert the therapy office if the area/orthosis gets wet; this will need to be addressed in a timely manner to prevent any issues of maceration and potential skin breakdown.

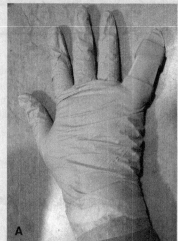
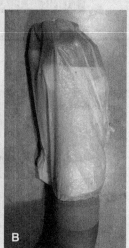

CLINICAL PEARL 1–X36

Cleaning of an Orthosis

Adhesive removers (Goo Gone), rubbing alcohol, soft nonabrasive cleansers (Soft Scrub), and specialized scrubbers called Mr. Clean Magic Eraser can all be used to clean marks and remove adhesives off an orthosis. Antibacterial wipes such as Lysol® Disinfecting Wipes can also be used as a quick way to cleanse the inside of an orthosis to remove any sweat or remove odors.

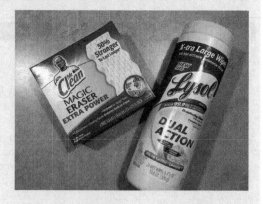

CLINICAL PEARL 1–X37

Removing Odors From an Orthosis

Various products such as Febreze can be used to control odor from an orthosis. Other techniques have been described such as soaking the device in a solution of 50% water and vanilla extract or water and baking soda.

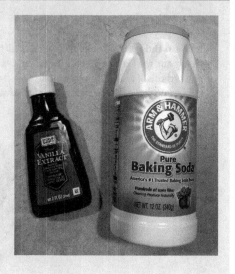

1 Digit- and Thumb-Based Orthoses

DISTAL INTERPHALANGEAL IMMOBILIZATION ORTHOSIS (FO) (Fig. 1–1)

COMMON NAMES

- Distal interphalangeal (DIP) extension splint
- DIP resting splint
- Static DIP extension splint
- Mallet finger splint

ALTERNATIVE OPTIONS

- Aluminum-padded splint
- Stax finger splint
- Finger cast
- Ring design splints

PRIMARY FUNCTIONS

- Immobilize DIP joint to allow healing of involved structure(s).
- Rest a painful and/or inflamed DIP joint.

ADDITIONAL FUNCTIONS

- Promote gliding of flexor digitorum superficialis (FDS) tendon by restricting movement of DIP joint during active flexion exercises.
- Statically position DIP joint flexion contracture at maximum extension to facilitate lengthening of tissue (mobilization).
- Restrict proximal interphalangeal (PIP) hyperextension.

Common Diagnoses	General Optimal Positions
Zone I extensor tendon injury and/or repair (mallet finger)	0° to +10° hyperextension
Distal phalanx fracture	Tolerable extension
Partial fingertip amputation	Tolerable extension
Crush injury to distal phalanx	Tolerable extension
Nail bed injury and repair	Tolerable extension
DIP joint osteoarthritis	Position of comfort

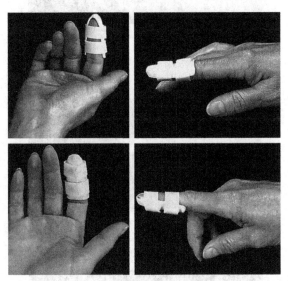

FIGURE 1–1

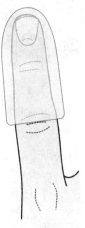

FIGURE 1–2

FABRICATION PROCESS

Pattern Creation (Fig. 1–2)

- Mark for proximal border just distal to middle digital crease.
- Allow extra ¼″ to ½″ of material around borders, depending on digit circumference.

Refine Pattern

- Proximal border should allow nearly full PIP joint motion.
- Lateral borders should encompass two-thirds circumference of digit to prevent undue compressive stress from straps and maximize rigidity. If borders are too generous, there may be too much digit mobility allowed within orthosis.

Options for Material

- Consider nonremovable circumferential design or cast for young children or questionably compliant patients.
- Perforated thermoplastics may prevent skin maceration; consider using them for patients who require full-time use.

- Use thinnest material possible that provides necessary strength to decrease bulk (1/16″).
- Materials that can be reheated and remolded several times are a good option if ongoing modifications become necessary to accommodate for fluctuations in edema or changes in desired joint position.

Cut and Heat

- Position patient's forearm supinated (volar design) and pronated (dorsal design) for gravity-assisted molding.
- If using elasticized edema wraps or dressings under orthosis, apply to digit before heating material. (Use layer of tubular gauze over any dressing to prevent adherence.)

Evaluate Fit While Molding

Dorsal Design

- Place material on dorsal aspect of digit just distal to PIP joint. Maximizing length of orthosis will improve stability and leverage.
- Avoid applying direct pressure over dorsum of DIP joint while molding, which may cause pressure areas. Incorporate thin padding if necessary.

Volar Design

- Place material on volar aspect of digit just distal to PIP joint crease.
- Apply slight DIP extension force (patient may aid in extending tip by using his or her other hand to gently position tip via fingernail).
- Pinch together excess material distally then trim to shape of fingertip, aiding to further protect a sensitive or painful tip.

Strapping and Components

- Use two ½″ straps or one 1″ strap to secure over DIP joint.
- Extra-thin ½″ strapping material can help decrease bulk between digits.
- May consider various tapes (such as paper tape or Microfoam™ tape, Performance Health) to secure the orthosis because these work very well.

Dorsal Design

- Place straps at proximal border and over distal phalanx.

Volar Design

- Place straps at proximal border and directly over DIP joint.
- Thin padding under distal strap may reduce migration and improve comfort.

Survey Completed Orthosis

- Smooth material borders; avoid rolling and flaring, which may irritate adjacent soft tissues or interfere with PIP joint movement.
- Check for mobility of uninvolved joints.

 ## PATTERN PEARLS 1–1 TO 1–10

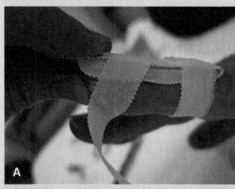

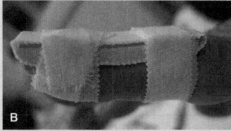

FIGURE PP1–1 A and B, Dorsal AlumaFoam® with tape; note angle of distal tape to contour at tip.

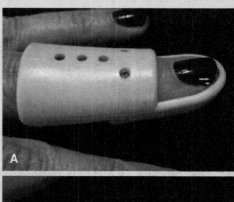

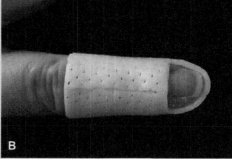

FIGURE PP1–2 A and B, Stax-type splint: prefabricated and custom.

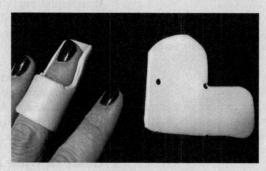

FIGURE PP1–3 L-pattern.

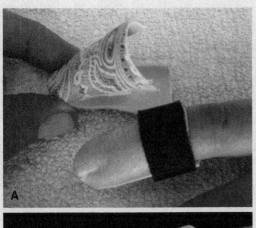

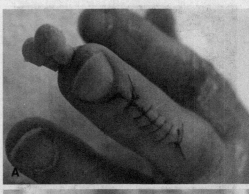

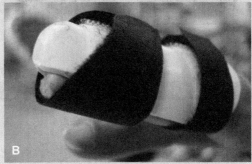

FIGURE PP1–5 A and B, Incorporating postsurgical pin.

FIGURE PP1–4 A and B, Bivalve or Tong design.

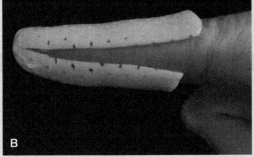

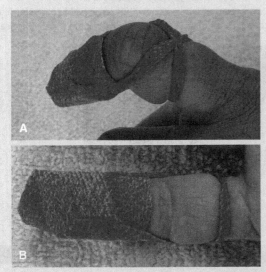

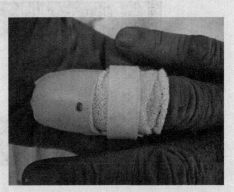

FIGURE PP1–7 Nail bed protector.

FIGURE PP1–6 A and B, Circumferential with proximal anchor strip.

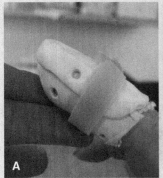

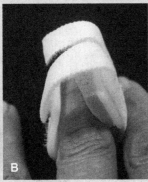

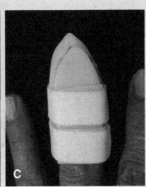

FIGURE PP1–8 Clamshell designs.

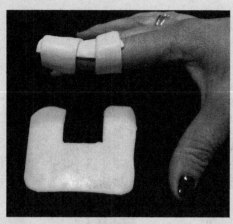

FIGURE PP1–9 U-pattern.

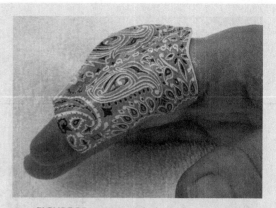

FIGURE PP1–10 Dorsal edge to ease removal.

CLINICAL PEARL 1–1

Management of Mallet Finger

When treating a mallet finger, the DIP joint should be positioned in neutral to slight hyperextension uninterrupted for approximately 6 to 8 weeks during the healing process. Preventing skin breakdown on the dorsum of the DIP joint is imperative. If using a removable design, reliable patients may be instructed to carefully remove for hygiene and skin inspection while maintaining DIP extension; all other patients should be seen regularly by the therapist for skin inspection. Consider a circumferential design using thermoplastic material, plaster, or an alternative casting product. Circumferential designs may help eliminate bulk at the fingertip, control edema, and deter removal when compliance is questionable **(A)**. Some products may be used without a liner and can be worn while bathing without risk of material breakdown, making it a good choice for children and athletes. Elasticized wraps/tapes can also be used over finger orthoses to keep them clean and/or to better secure the proximal portion of the orthosis if the therapist is concerned that it will become loose if edema subsides. Leaving a window/opening at the distal end will allow the clinician and patient to monitor for adequate blood flow should this be a concern **(B)**.

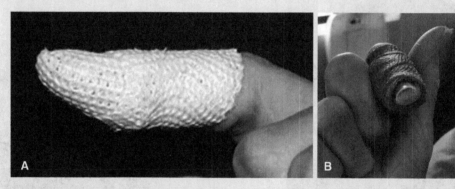

CLINICAL PEARL 1–2

Protective Fingertip Caps

Create a contour at tip of digit by pinching the excess distal material together while warm, then cut to the shape of the tip, forming a protective cap **(A and B)**. Carefully smooth the seam while the material is warm to prevent separation. May need to use solvent and heat gun to be sure area stays adhered **(C)**. This closed design protects the area after crush, nail bed injury, or amputations **(D–F)**.

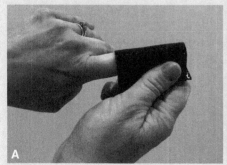

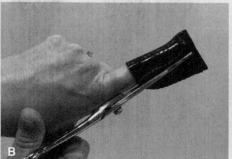

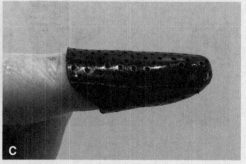

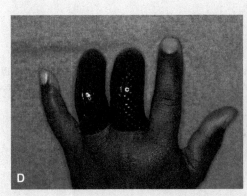

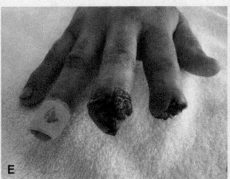

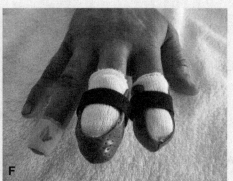

CLINICAL PEARL 1–3

Securing Circumferential DIP Orthoses

Elasticized tapes, adhesive or nonadhesive (such as Coban™ **(A)** or Microfoam™ **(B)** tape, Performance Health), can be used to secure a circumferential DIP orthosis.

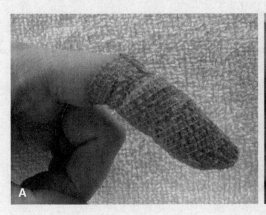

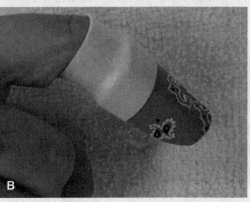

EXPERT PEARL 1–7

Digit Strap
SABRINA CASSELLA, MED, OTR/L, CHT
Massachusetts

"One" strap design for digit immobilization allows ability to tighten both ends to customize fit.

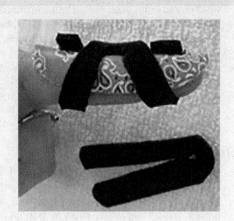

PIP IMMOBILIZATION ORTHOSIS (FO) (Fig. 1–3)

COMMON NAMES

- Finger splint
- PIP resting splint
- Static PIP extension splint
- Finger gutter splint

ALTERNATIVE OPTIONS

- Aluminum-padded splint
- Finger cast
- Ring design splints

PRIMARY FUNCTIONS

- Immobilize PIP joint to allow healing of involved structure(s).
- Rest a painful and/or inflamed PIP joint.

ADDITIONAL FUNCTIONS

- Promote gliding of flexor digitorum profundus (FDP) tendon by restricting movement of PIP joint during active flexion exercises.
- Statically position PIP joint flexion contracture at maximum extension to facilitate lengthening of tissue (mobilization).

- Restrict specific amount of extension (e.g., dorsal dislocation of PIP joint) or flexion (e.g., zones II and III extensor tendon injury) to protect healing structures (restriction).

Common Diagnoses	General Optimal Positions
Zones III and IV extensor tendon injury	0°
Boutonniere deformity	0°
PIP joint sprain	0°
PIP joint intra-articular fracture	0°
PIP joint arthritis	Position of comfort
PIP joint arthroplasty	0°

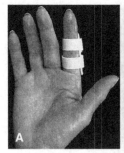 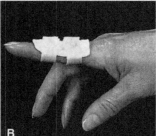 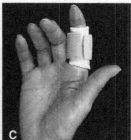 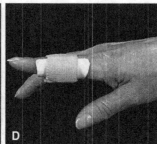

FIGURE 1–3

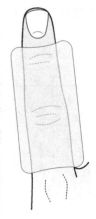

FIGURE 1–4

FABRICATION PROCESS

Pattern Creation (Fig. 1–4)

- Mark for proximal border at proximal digital crease and distal border at distal digital crease.
- Appreciate the proximal oblique angle of the border digits (index and small) because this angle should be incorporated into the pattern to allow increased stability via a longer lever arm and better strap placement.
- Proximal border should be oblique, providing for long lever to maximize mechanical advantage.
- Allow extra ¼″ to ½″ of material around borders, depending on digit circumference.
- Consider including DIP joint if digit is small (children, small adults) to improve ability of orthosis to secure desired PIP joint position or mobilize PIP joint to improve leverage.

Refine Pattern

- Proximal border should allow unrestricted MCP joint motion.
- Distal border should allow unrestricted DIP joint motion.
- Lateral borders should encompass two-thirds circumference of digit to prevent undue compressive stress from straps and maximize rigidity. If borders are too generous, there may be too much digit mobility allowed within orthosis.
- Web space areas should have adequate rooms to allow unrestricted motion of adjacent digits.
- May extend pattern distally to include DIP joint.

Options for Materials

- Consider using 3/32″ thermoplastic material (perforated or non-perforated); it is light and thin but still provides stability to PIP joint.
- Perforated thermoplastics may prevent skin maceration; consider using them for patients who require full-time use.
- Materials that can be reheated and remolded several times are a good option if ongoing modifications become necessary to accommodate for fluctuations in edema or changes in desired joint position.
- A circumferential design fabricated with plaster, digit casting products, or thermoplastic material can help when addressing the small finger PIP joint. Small surface area can make it difficult for the traditional design to obtain adequate purchase.

Cut and Heat

- Position patient's forearm supinated (volar design) and pronated (dorsal design) for gravity-assisted molding.
- If using elasticized edema wrap or dressings under orthosis, apply to digit before heating material. (Use layer of tubular gauze to prevent adherence.)
- Thin padding over PIP joint may be incorporated into dorsal design if necessary; apply before heating material.

Evaluate Fit While Molding

Dorsal Design

- Place material on dorsal aspect of digit just proximal to dorsal DIP joint skin folds and distal to MCP joint. Maximizing length of orthosis will improve stability and leverage.
- Allow gravity to form lateral borders. Avoid grabbing or wrapping material around digit.
- Avoid applying direct pressure over dorsum of PIP joint while molding, which may cause pressure areas.

Volar Design

- Place material on volar aspect of digit, just clearing DIP joint crease and slightly distal to MCP joint crease.
- Allow gravity to form lateral borders; avoid grabbing or wrapping material around digit.
- If used to address flexion contracture, carefully mold with even, gentle pressure throughout length of orthosis in direction of extension.
- Important to note: With PIP flexion contractures, the clinician will need to incorporate the longest lever arm possible; therefore, including the DIP (especially true with short digits) and proximal edge of the proximal phalanx is critical. When including the DIP, positioning in gentle flexion is preferable in order to prevent hyperextension forces at the PIP joint.

Strapping and Components

- Use two ½″ straps or one 1″ strap to secure orthosis directly over PIP joint.
- Proximal strap should have slight oblique orientation.
- Extra-thin ½″ strapping material can help decrease bulk between digits.

Dorsal Design

- Place straps at proximal border and over middle phalanx.

Volar Design

- Place straps over proximal and middle phalanx.
- Place one strap with piece of foam directly over PIP joint if maintaining PIP extension is a priority.
- Thin padding under distal strap may reduce migration and improve comfort.
- Proximal straps for border digits will have a slight oblique orientation.

Survey Completed Orthosis

- Smooth material borders; avoid rolling or flaring, which may irritate adjacent soft tissues and web spaces or interfere with MCP and/or DIP joint movement.
- Check for mobility of uninvolved joints.

 PATTERN PEARLS 1–11 TO 1–18

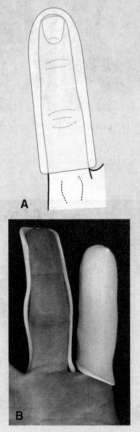

FIGURE PP1–11 **A and B,** Combined PIP/DIP orthosis.

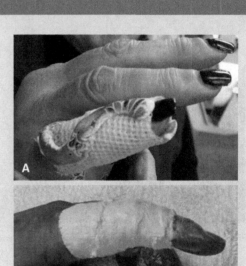

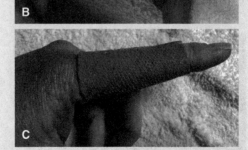

FIGURE PP1–12 **PIP** Casting Options. **A,** QuickCast 2 (Performance Health) with thermoplastic strip for reinforcement. **B,** Plaster of paris PIP cast. **C,** Orficast®.

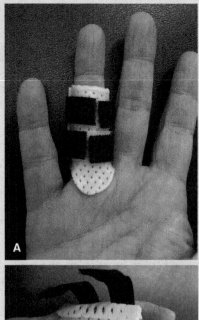

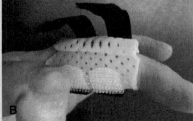

FIGURE PP1–13 A and B, For shorter digits, extend pattern proximally and notice overlapped on one side allowing for adjusting tension.

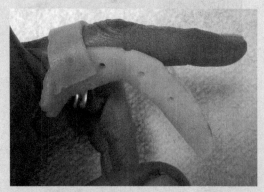

FIGURE PP1–15 Volar flexion restriction orthosis for extensor tendon injury.

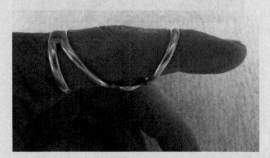

FIGURE PP1–17 Silver Ring™ Splint to restrict extension for swan-neck deformity.

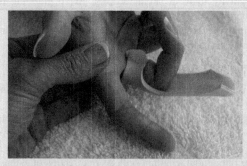

FIGURE PP1–14 Dorsal extension restriction orthosis for volar plate injury.

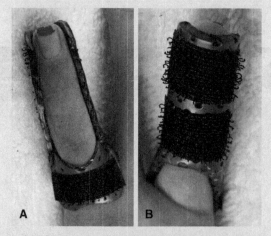

FIGURE PP1–16 A and B, Dorsal/volar digit orthosis PIP.

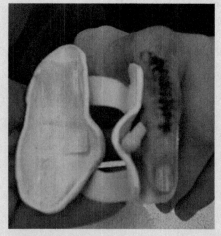

FIGURE PP1–18 Bivalve design to protect pins.

CLINICAL PEARL 1–4

Digit Exercise Orthoses

An orthosis that immobilizes all the PIP and DIP joints in extension can aid in directing the forces of flexion to the MCP joints during active flexion exercises **(A)**. This can be used as an exercise tool to increase active MCP flexion, which is often lacking after MCP joint arthroplasty. An orthosis that immobilizes the PIP joint in extension can aid in directing the force of flexion to the DIP joint during active flexion exercises **(B)**. This can be used as an exercise tool to increase active DIP flexion, to maximize FDP tendon glide, and/or to stretch tight oblique retinacular ligaments. An orthosis that immobilizes the DIP joint in extension can aid in directing the force of flexion to the PIP joint during active exercises. This can be used as an exercise tool to increase active PIP flexion and/or maximize FDS tendon glide **(C)**. An orthosis that immobilizes the MCP joints in extension can encourage differential flexor tendon gliding as well as actively stretch the intrinsic muscles in the hand. Note the clamshell design and the slight hyperextension of the MCP joints. This design further isolates FDS and FDP tendon gliding **(D and E)**. Exercise orthoses can be used to isolate and strengthen a specific muscle as shown here with focus on the opponens and flexor pollicis brevis muscles **(F)** or the extensor pollicis longus **(G)**.

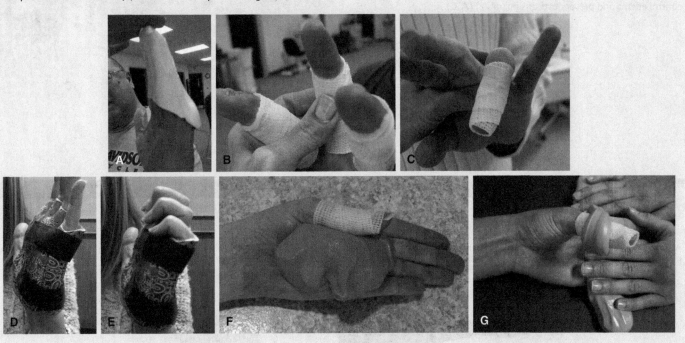

CLINICAL PEARL 1–5

Small Finger PIP Orthoses

With short fifth digits, the clinician may find it helpful to incorporate a portion of the fifth metacarpal. This provides a longer lever arm and increases the stability and position of the orthosis onto the hand. Shown is **(A)** QuickCast 2 (Performance Health) material; **(B)** a night orthosis for a child with camptodactyly; **(C)** notice foam on the dorsum of the PIP strap to encourage PIP extension.

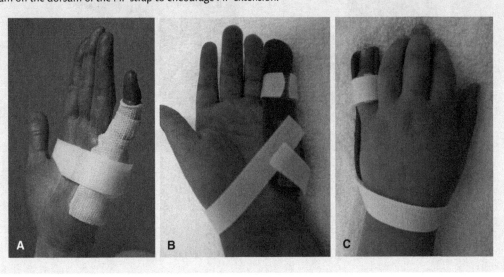

CLINICAL PEARL 1–6

Spiral Design With "Cling Wrap" for Edema

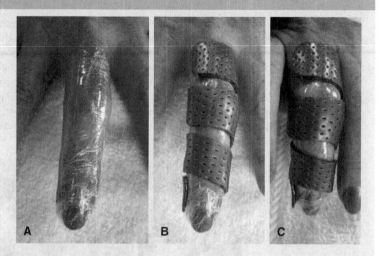

A spiral design orthosis fabricated with 1/16″ Orfit® (North Coast Medical, Morgan Hill, CA) material was used to allow limited IP motion 8 weeks after PIP joint arthroplasty. The plastic wrap was used under the orthosis to control edema and prevent orthosis migration (**A-C**).

CLINICAL PEARL 1–7

Edema Wrapping

Addressing edema in the digit can be a key intervention and often includes the use of wrapping with Coban™ or similar. There are a few techniques that can be used to apply this product: (**A**) circumferentially and (**B–D**) pinch and trim technique.

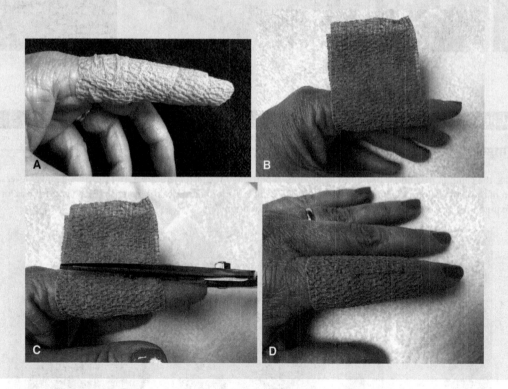

CLINICAL PEARL 1–8

Strapping Alternatives for PIP Orthoses

A–D, Shown are variations of split strap designs with either traditional loop (**A**) or with neoprene materials (**B–D**). The wider straps can be used to increase the surface area for attachment of the loop material onto the hook, thus providing more stability and less mobility of the orthosis of the digit. To prevent migration of digit-based orthoses, elasticized wraps can be used to secure the orthosis to the hand (**E**), or if using a thermoplastic tape, the tape can be lightly wrapped around the hand web space for securing onto the hand (**F**). Circumferential products can also be used such as Silipos® Digital Caps (**G**) and edema Finger Sleeves (**H**).

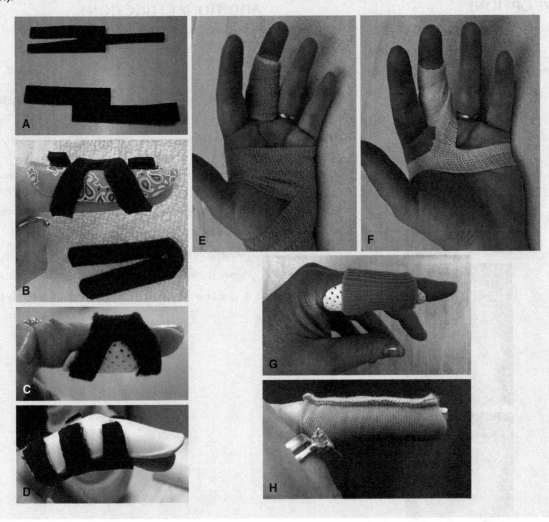

EXPERT PEARL 1–8

Hook Adherence Around Contours
THERESA BELL-NAGLE, OTR/L, CHT
Massachusetts

Cut a dart out of the hook so that the adhesive will stick better when laying over a curved region of orthosis (**A**). This technique will make it much less likely to peel off (**B**).

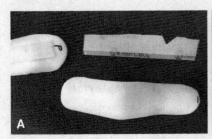
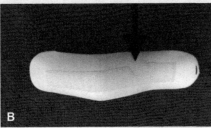

THUMB INTERPHALANGEAL IMMOBILIZATION ORTHOSIS (FO) (Fig. 1–5)

COMMON NAMES

- Thumb IP extension splint
- Static thumb splint

ALTERNATIVE OPTIONS

- Aluminum-padded splint
- Stax splint
- Thumb cast
- Ring design orthosis

PRIMARY FUNCTIONS

- Immobilize thumb IP joint to allow healing of involved structure(s).
- Rest a painful and/or inflamed thumb IP joint.

ADDITIONAL FUNCTIONS

- Statically position IP joint flexion contracture at maximum extension to facilitate lengthening of tissue (mobilization).
- Restrict IP hyperextension.

Common Diagnoses	General Optimal Positions
Zone TI extensor tendon injury (mallet)	+5 to +15° hyperextension
Distal phalanx fracture	0° to +15° hyperextension (depends on flexor pollicis longus [FPL] status)
Crush injury to distal phalanx	0° to slight hyperextension
Nail bed injury and repair	0°
Partial tip amputation	Tolerable ext
IP joint sprain	0° to slight hyperextension
IP joint arthritis	Position of comfort

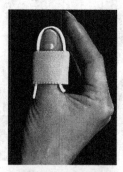
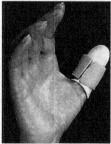
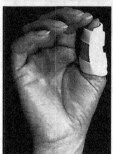

FIGURE 1–5

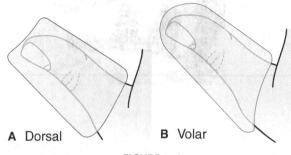

A Dorsal **B** Volar

FIGURE 1–6

FABRICATION PROCESS

Pattern Creation (Fig. 1–6)

- Mark for proximal border at proximal thumb crease.
- Proximal border has an oblique angle and should be incorporated into orthosis, providing for long lever to maximize mechanical advantage.
- Allow extra ¼″ to ½″ of material around borders, depending on thumb circumference.
- Dorsal design may improve function of thumb by providing partial sensory input.

Refine Pattern

Dorsal Design

- Extend proximal border to middle of dorsal MP joint skinfolds.
- Lateral borders should encompass two-thirds circumference of digit to prevent undue compressive stress from straps and maximize rigidity. If

borders are too generous, there may be too much digit mobility allowed within orthosis.
- Taper lateral borders slightly volar and distal to avoid irritation at first web space.
- Proximal border has an oblique angle and should be incorporated into orthosis.

Volar Design

- Extend proximal border just distal to volar MP joint crease.
- Taper lateral borders slightly dorsal and proximal to form oblique border.

Options for Materials

- Consider nonremovable circumferential orthosis or cast for young children or questionably compliant patients.
- Perforated thermoplastics may prevent skin maceration; consider using them for patients who require full-time use.

- Use thinnest material possible that provides necessary strength to decrease bulk (1/16″ or 3/32″).
- Materials that can be reheated and remolded several times are a good option if ongoing modifications become necessary to accommodate for fluctuations in edema or changes in desired joint position.

Cut and Heat

- Position patient's forearm supinated (volar design) and pronated (dorsal design) for gravity-assisted molding.
- IP joint position depends on diagnosis.
- If using elasticized edema wrap or dressings under orthosis, apply to thumb before heating material. (Use layer of tubular gauze to prevent adherence.)

Evaluate Fit While Molding

Dorsal Design

- Place material on dorsal aspect of thumb to middle of dorsal MP joint skinfolds. Maximizing length of orthosis will improve stability and leverage.
- Avoid applying direct pressure over dorsum of IP joint while molding, which may create pressure spots. Thin padding may be incorporated if necessary.
- Allow gravity to form lateral borders; avoid grabbing or wrapping material around digit.
- Slightly flare material about the MP joint.

Volar Design

- Place material on volar aspect of thumb, just clearing volar MP joint crease.
- Apply slight IP extension pressure (patient may aid in extending tip by using his or her other hand to gently lift tip via fingernail).

Strapping and Components

- Use two ½″ straps or one 1″ strap to secure over DIP joint.
- Proximal strap should have slight oblique orientation.
- Extra-thin ½″ strapping material can help decrease bulk between digits.
- May consider paper tape to secure as well.

Dorsal Design

- Place straps at proximal border (as close to MP flexion crease as possible without interfering with MP joint flexion) and over distal phalanx.

Volar Design

- Place straps at proximal border and directly over IP joint.
- Thin padding under distal strap may reduce migration and improve comfort.

Survey Completed Orthosis

- Smooth material borders; avoid rolling and flaring, which may irritate adjacent soft tissues or interfere with MP joint movement.
- Check for mobility of uninvolved joints.

 PATTERN PEARLS 1–19 TO 1–25

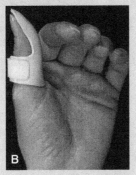

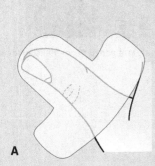

FIGURE PP1–19 A and B, Thumb IP orthosis with tab.

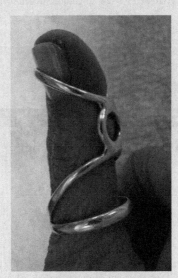

FIGURE PP1–20 Silver Ring™ Splint (Silver RIng Splint Company, Charlottesville, VA) to prevent IP joint deviation with pinch.

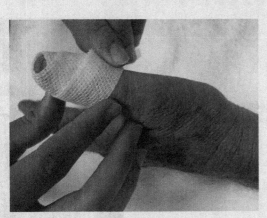

FIGURE PP1–21 Thumb IP Orthosis using QuickCast 2.

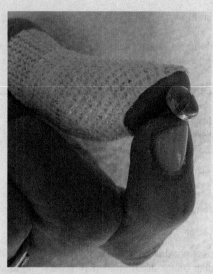

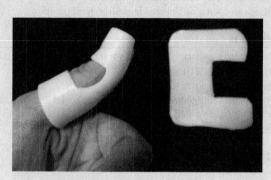

FIGURE PP1–23 U-pattern.

FIGURE PP1–22 Circumferential orthosis with volar free for sensation.

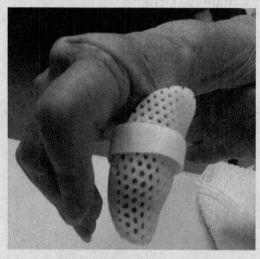

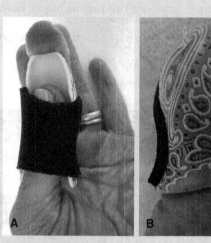

FIGURE PP1–25 A and B, Permanently embedded neoprene strap for easy don/doff.

FIGURE PP1–24 Circumferential design.

 CLINICAL PEARL 1–9

TheraBand®-Assisted Molding

TheraBand® (Performance Health) can be applied volarly to the distal phalanx while molding a volar DIP or thumb IP orthosis. This technique aids in positioning the DIP in hyperextension and precludes the need to apply direct pressure dorsally at the DIP joint.

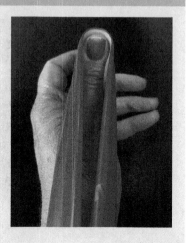

2 Hand-Based Orthoses

DORSAL MCP/PIP/DIP IMMOBILIZATION ORTHOSIS (HFO) (Fig. 1–7)

COMMON NAMES

- Hand-based digit extension splint
- Hand-based digit resting splint
- Static finger splint
- Dorsal hand splint

PRIMARY FUNCTIONS

- Immobilize the MCP, PIP, and/or DIP joint(s) to allow healing or rest of the involved structure(s).

ADDITIONAL FUNCTIONS

- Restrict specific amount of extension (e.g., after digital nerve repair) to protect healing structures.

Common Diagnoses	General Optimal Positions
Intra-articular fracture of PIP/DIP joint	MCP: 60° flexion; PIP/DIP: 0°
Dupuytren surgical and nonsurgical	All joints maximal extension; 3 to 6+ months: maximum extension at night only
Trigger finger	MCP: 0°; PIP/DIP: free
Tenosynovitis	Position of comfort, intrinsic plus
Infection	Position of comfort, intrinsic plus
MCP/PIP joint volar plate injury	MCP/PIP: 20°–30° flexion

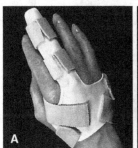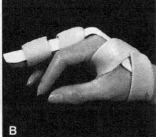

FIGURE 1–7

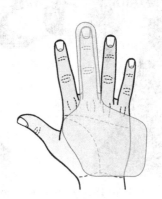

FIGURE 1–8

FABRICATION PROCESS

Pattern Creation (Fig. 1–8)

- Consider dorsal design if patient presents with volar wound/incision to allow for air circulation.
- Mark for proximal border at dorsal wrist crease.
- Allow extra ¼″ to ½″ of material around borders, depending on digit circumference.
- Be sure the proximal portion of the orthosis has adequate surface area for strap application.
- For small finger (SF), consider including ring finger (RF) to provide greater protection, better stabilization, and improved comfort.
- If MCP is to be flexed, allow extra material distally to accommodate for flexion angle. If material must be stretched over MCP joint, a weakened and unstable orthosis may result.
- Draw pattern with fingers slightly abducted. Be sure to provide enough surface area to accommodate all immobilized digits. Remember, material can always be trimmed away after initial molding is completed.

Refine Pattern

- Proximal border should allow full wrist motion and clearance of ulnar styloid.
- Lateral borders should encompass two-thirds circumference of digit to prevent undue compressive stress from straps and maximize rigidity. If borders are too generous, there may be too much digit mobility allowed within orthosis.
- Allow adequate room in digit web space areas to allow unrestricted motion of unaffected digits.

Options for Materials

- Use drapable material to achieve intimate fit over MCP joints to prevent migration and improve comfort.
- Coated material will allow for overlapped ulnar border to pop apart after setting fully.
- Perforated thermoplastics may help prevent skin maceration; consider using them for patients who require full-time use of orthosis.
- Materials that can be reheated and remolded several times are a good option if ongoing modifications become necessary to accommodate for fluctuations in edema, changes in motion, or bulk of dressings.

Cut and Heat

- Position patient's forearm pronated for gravity-assisted molding.
- If using elasticized wrap or dressings under orthosis, apply to digit before heating material.
- To prevent adherence to dressings, consider the following:
  - A layer of tubular gauze or stockinette over dressings that can be removed with the orthosis when set
  - Lightly and evenly spread a thin layer of lotion over dressings
- Thin padding may be incorporated dorsally across MCP joint(s) if necessary; apply before heating material.

Evaluate Fit While Molding

- Place material over dorsum of hand and gently pull tab through first web space and temporarily adhere to ulnar border, being sure to place material just proximal to distal palmar crease (DPC).
- Lateral borders of the digit should form a deep trough (instead of a flat pan), which will act to strengthen and support the molded orthosis.
- Contour dorsal MCP area well.

- Avoid applying direct pressure over dorsum of MCP and PIP joints while molding.
- Consider light rolling of the material edges about the dorsum of the MCP joints when using thin material. This is especially applicable when the orthosis is fabricated to include only one digit.

- If applying a stiff loop material through the web space, consider "fringing" the edges to increase contour of the strap as it traverses through the web space.
- Consider using rivets to secure one end of proximal strap to minimize space needed for hook material.

Strapping and Components

- Apply straps at DIP joint, around proximal phalanx, at overlapped ulnar border, and about wrist to prevent migration.
- Watch for radial sensory nerve irritation that may occur with a tight wrist strap

Survey Completed Orthosis

- Smooth material borders; avoid rolling or flaring, which may irritate adjacent soft tissues and web spaces or interfere with unaffected/adjacent joint movement.
- Check mobility of uninvolved joints.

 PATTERN PEARLS 1–26 TO 1–32

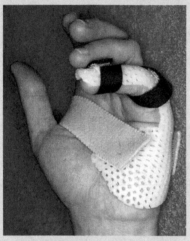

FIGURE PP1–26 Digit extension restriction orthosis.

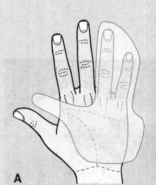

FIGURE PP1–27 A and B, RF/SF orthosis used post-Dupuytren release.

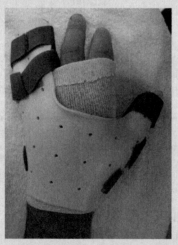

FIGURE PP1–28 RF/SF and thumb orthosis used post-Dupuytren release.

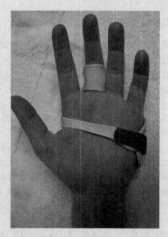

FIGURE PP1–29 Volar/dorsal MCP joint orthosis for trigger finger.

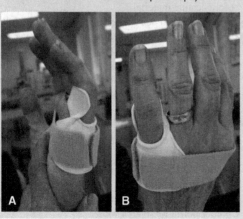

FIGURE PP1–30 A and B, Volar/dorsal MCP joint orthosis for trigger finger.

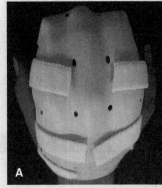
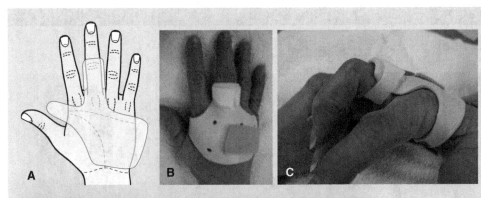
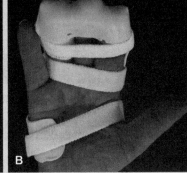

FIGURE PP1–31 **A–C,** Dorsal MCP joint orthosis.

FIGURE PP1–32 **A and B,** Dorsal-based tip protector.

 CLINICAL PEARL 1–10

Strapping Through Web Spaces

Trim strapping material to contour through the web spaces to prevent the borders from irritating these sensitive areas (**A**) may be helpful to cover the edge with a thin lining material to decrease likelihood of soft tissue irritation (**B**). Note that many elasticized strapping materials may fray if trimmed. Another specialty strap is a thin material to decrease bulk between the digits (**C**). Neoprene is an alternative strapping material that contours nicely and can be trimmed without risk of fraying (**D**). Trim soft foam straps by "feathering" the edges to prevent skin irritation (**E**).

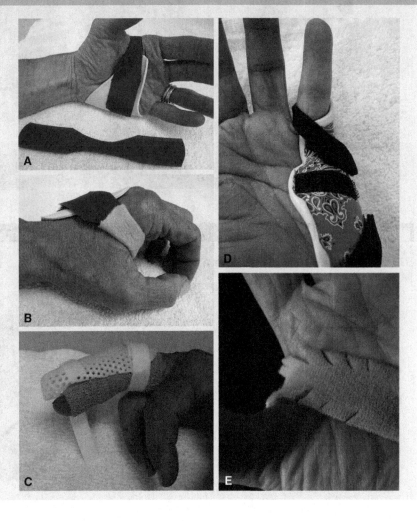

CLINICAL PEARL 1–11

Flaring or Clearing for the MCP Joint

A, When applying material *dorsally* across MCP joints, be sure to flare material away from bony prominences. Note: In this orthosis, the material over the DIP protects a distal tip injury. **B** and **C,** in both these orthoses, the *volar* web spaces between MCP joints is cleared. This will allow free movement of adjacent digits without tissue irritation.

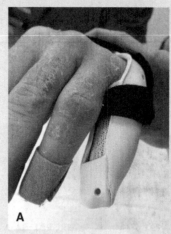
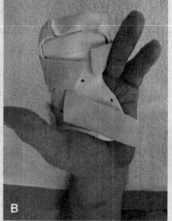
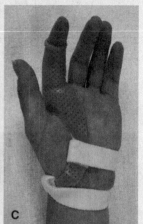

CLINICAL PEARL 1–12

Split Strap Alternative

A, This "split" strap is cut from neoprene material and conforms well as it traverses through the first web and base of the thumb of this dorsal design.
B and C, "Split" strap for volar wrist can help maximize pressure distribution dorsally and increase comfort.

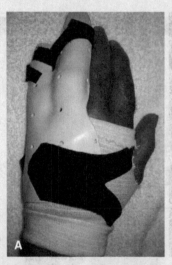
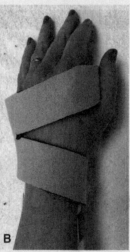
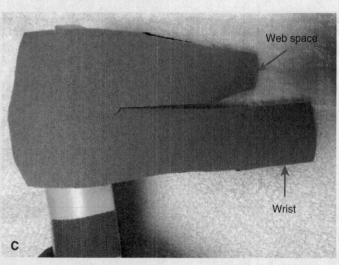

CLINICAL PEARL 1–13

Dorsal Weave for Strap Application

Slits can be made in a dorsal hand orthosis to direct straps into extension. This is especially helpful when digits vary in degrees of contracture. Note the clearance of the dorsal web space.

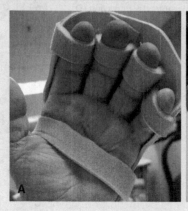
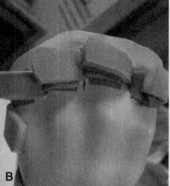

VOLAR MCP/PIP/DIP IMMOBILIZATION ORTHOSIS (HFO) (Fig. 1–9)

COMMON NAMES

- Hand-based digit extension splint
- Hand-based digit resting splint
- Static finger splint
- Volar resting splint
- Volar hand splint
- Finger gutter splint

PRIMARY FUNCTIONS

- Immobilize the MCP, PIP, and/or DIP joint(s) to allow healing or rest of the involved structure(s).

ADDITIONAL FUNCTIONS

- Statically position MCP joint contracture at maximum flexion or extension to facilitate lengthening of tissue (mobilization).
- Restrict specific amount of flexion (e.g., after zone IV extensor tendon repair) to protect healing structures (restriction).

Common Diagnoses	General Optimal Positions
Intra-articular fracture of PIP or DIP joint	MCP: 60° flexion; PIP/DIP: 0°
Fracture of proximal and/ or middle phalanx	MCP: slight flexion; PIP/DIP: 0°
Dupuytren surgical and nonsurgical	All joints maximal extension; 3 to 6+ months: maximum extension at night only
MCP joint sprain	MCP: 60°–80° flexion; PIP/DIP: 0°
Trigger finger release	MCP: 0°; PIP/DIP: free
Tenosynovitis	Position of comfort, intrinsic plus
Infection	Position of comfort, intrinsic plus
Crush injury	MCP: 60°–80° flexion; PIP/DIP: 0°
Zone IV extensor tendon injury	MCP/PIP/DIP: 0°
Sagittal band injury and repair	MCP: 0° with slight deviation to side of injury or repair; PIP/DIP: free
Ulnar nerve injury	PM use: MCP: 60°–80° flexion; PIP/DIP: 0°

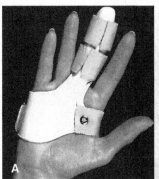 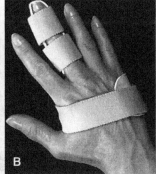

FIGURE 1–9

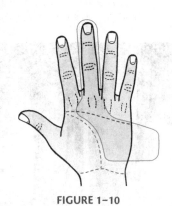

FIGURE 1–10

FABRICATION PROCESS

Pattern Creation (Fig. 1–10)

- Consider volar design if patient has dorsal wound/incision or extruding pins to allow for air circulation.
- Mark for proximal border at volar wrist crease.
- Allow extra ¼″ to ½″ of material around borders, depending on digit circumference.
- Be sure proximal portion of the orthosis has adequate surface area for strap application.
- For SF, consider including RF to provide greater protection, better stabilization, and improved comfort.
- Draw pattern with fingers slightly abducted. Be sure to provide enough surface area to accommodate all immobilized digits. Remember, material can always be trimmed away after initial molding is completed.

Refine Pattern

- Proximal border should allow full wrist motion.
- Radial border should allow nearly full thumb motion.
- Lateral borders of the involved digit(s) should encompass two-thirds circumference of digit to prevent undue compressive stress from straps and maximize rigidity. If borders are too generous, there may be too much digit mobility allowed within orthosis.
- Allow adequate room in digit web space areas to allow unrestricted motion of unaffected digits.
- May modify pattern to exclude PIP and/or DIP joints if necessary.

Options for Materials

- Coated material will allow for overlapped ulnar border to pop apart after setting fully.
- Perforated thermoplastics may prevent skin maceration; consider using them for patients who require full-time orthosis use.
- Materials that can be reheated and remolded several times are a good option if ongoing modifications become necessary to accommodate for fluctuations in edema, changes in motion, or bulk of dressings.

Cut and Heat

- Position patient's forearm supinated for gravity-assisted molding.
- If using elasticized wrap or dressings under orthosis, apply to digit before heating material. (Use layer of tubular gauze or stockinette to prevent adherence.)

Evaluate Fit While Molding

- Lateral borders of the digit should form a deep trough (instead of a flat pan), which will act to strengthen and support the molded orthosis.
- Remember that when addressing index finger (IF), thumb mobility is somewhat hindered because of necessary contouring about thumb web to obtain proper stabilization.

Strapping and Components

- Apply straps at DIP joint, over PIP joint proximal phalanx, at overlapped ulnar border, and about wrist to prevent migration.

- Consider using rivets to secure one end of proximal strap to minimize space needed for hook material.
- Padding under proximal phalanx strap may reduce migration and rotation, maintain MCP joint position, and improve comfort.

Survey Completed Orthosis

- Smooth material borders; avoid rolling or flaring, which may irritate adjacent soft tissues and web spaces or interfere with unaffected/adjacent joint movement.
- Check mobility of uninvolved joints.

 PATTERN PEARLS 1–33 TO 1–39

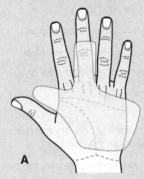 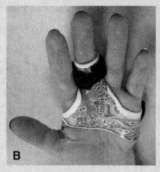 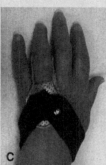 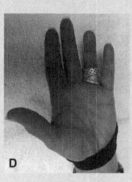 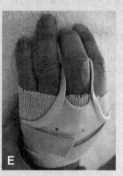

FIGURE PP1–33 A and B, Volar design. **C–E,** Volar/dorsal designs made by cutting slit at MCP joint level—both can be used for trigger finger.

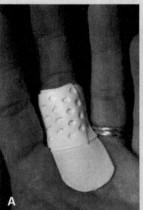 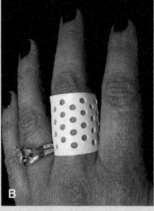

FIGURE PP1–34 A and B, "Ring" design for trigger finger.

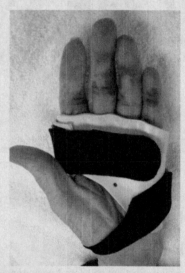

FIGURE PP1–35 All MCP joints included for active intrinsic stretching.

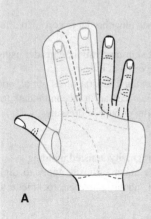 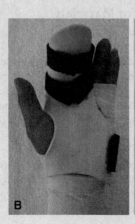 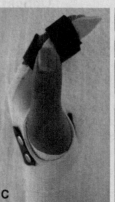 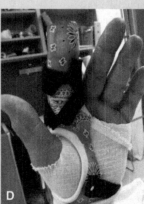

FIGURE PP1–36 A–C, IF/MF thumbhole design; **D,** IF only.

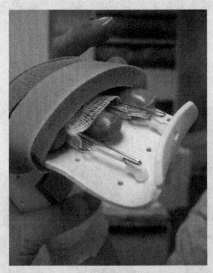

FIGURE PP1–37 Protecting pins with distal edge.

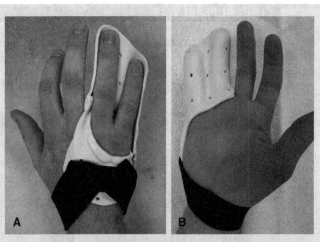

FIGURE PP1–38 **A and B,** Volar/dorsal design.

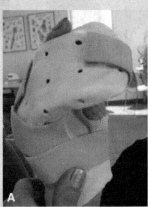 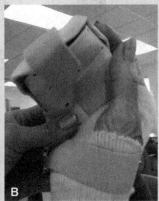

FIGURE PP1–39 **A and B,** Clamshell design for additional protection.

CLINICAL PEARL 1–14

Thermoplastic Strap Through Web Space

Orthotic material can be used as an alternative method for securing both volar and dorsal hand-based orthoses. This is especially useful in the thenar web space because it eliminates the need for loop traversing through this potentially sensitive region as well as decreasing the amount of hook needed on the orthosis itself **(A)**. The material can be lightly stretched to "thin" it out. Be sure to keep a narrow width in order to not impede IF MCP flexion **(B)**.

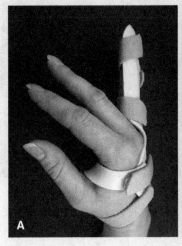 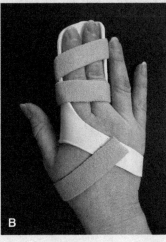

CLINICAL PEARL 1–15

Strapping Around Wrist to Prevent Migration

An elasticized wrist strap such as neoprene or elasticized loop can be used to secure a hand-based orthosis onto the hand **(A–C)**. Rivets can be helpful to anchor the strap onto the base because surface area may be limited. Rivets also aid in maintaining orientation of the strap **(A and C)**.

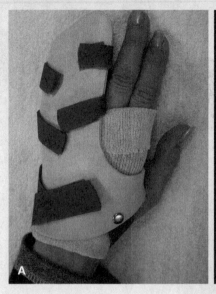 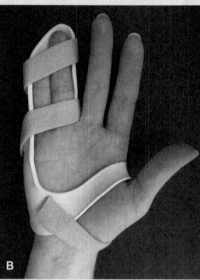 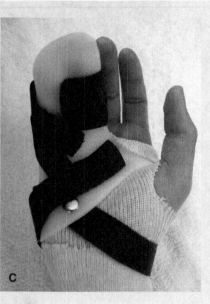

CLINICAL PEARL 1–16

Rolling Material Through Web Spaces

Avoid cutting material to accommodate for web space areas. This may significantly alter the rigidity. Instead, carefully roll and flatten a small border of the warm material back onto itself, just enough to clear for mobility of the adjacent digits **(A and B)**.

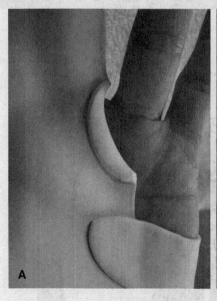 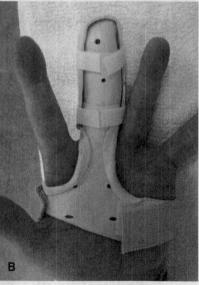

CLINICAL PEARL 1–17

Contouring Around Thumb to Increase IF Stability

Allowing unimpeded thumb mobility when immobilizing the IF is challenging, because to adequately stabilize this digit, a portion of the thenar eminence must be included in the orthosis. The contouring technique shown provides good stability along the radial volar aspect yet allows functional thumb mobility **(A and B)**.

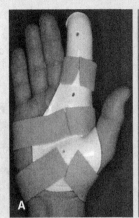

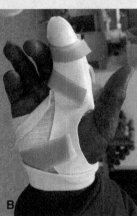

CLINICAL PEARL 1–18

Using Foam on Straps

Utilize foam beneath key straps to improve joint positioning. This acts as a gentle "dynamic" force to keep the joints at the desired angles. This can be used with dorsal designs **(A and B)** or volar designs **(C and D)**.

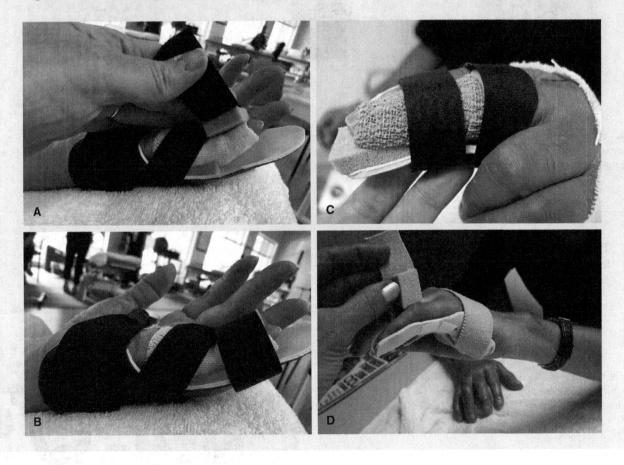

RA Prefabricated Orthosis

MARY SOMMER, OTR/L CHT
Washington

This prefabricated orthosis was dispensed by the patient's rheumatologist during a routine office visit. The patient brought the orthosis to a therapy session where it was adapted to better control the deforming forces of the hand.

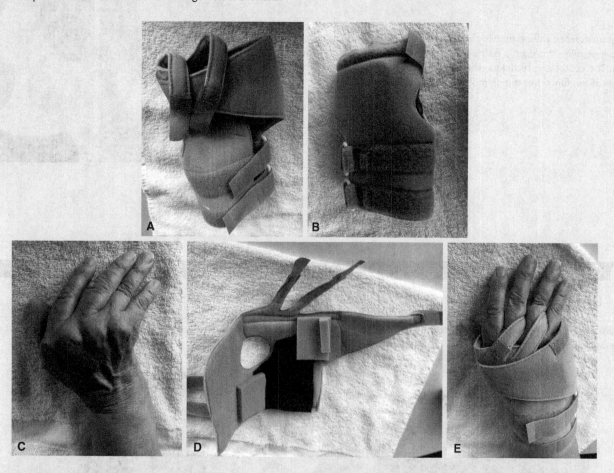

Orthosis - dorsal (**A**) and volar (**B**) view. **C,** Right hand long stand rheumatoid arthritis. Note the metacarpal radial deviation, MCP subluxation, and digit ulnar deviation posturing. **D,** The strategic placement of dense foam pads, and proper strap orientation, helps with gentle alignment of the hand and digits. **E,** Note the improved alignment with the orthoses after it has been modified.

Trigger Finger Orthosis: Ring Version

NIAMH MASTERSON, OT, HAND THERAPIST
Australia

Orficast is utilized to create a long tube first—heat fully and roll to create desired thickness. Smooth any rough edges using a heat gun and dry heat to further fuse and solidify the connected areas. Be sure to create opening large enough for patient to slide orthosis on/off without getting stuck at PIP joint (**A and B**).

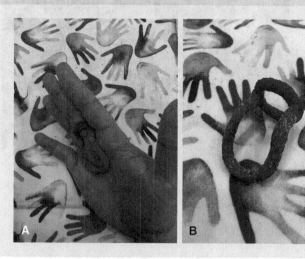

ULNAR MCP/PIP/DIP IMMOBILIZATION ORTHOSIS (HFO) (Fig. 1–11)

COMMON NAMES

- Hand-based ulnar gutter splint
- Hand-based ulnar fracture brace
- Metacarpal fracture brace
- Clamdigger splint

ALTERNATIVE OPTIONS

- Plaster cast

PRIMARY FUNCTIONS

- Immobilize proximal phalanxes and metacarpals of RF and SF to allow healing and/or protection of involved structure(s).

ADDITIONAL FUNCTIONS

- Restrict MCP joint extension secondary to low ulnar nerve injury (restriction).

Common Diagnoses	General Optimal Positions
Metacarpal head or neck fracture	MCP: 60°–90° flexion (may include PIP/DIP: 0°)
Proximal phalanx fracture	MCP: 60°–90° flexion; PIP/DIP: 0°
Complicated middle phalanx fracture	MCP: 60°–90° flexion; PIP/DIP: 0°
MCP capsulectomy	MCP: 60°–90° flexion; PIP/DIP: 0°
Digital ulnar nerve injury	MCP: 60°–90° flexion; PIP/DIP free (include fourth and fifth metacarpals)

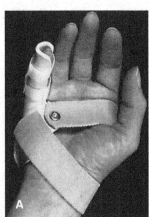
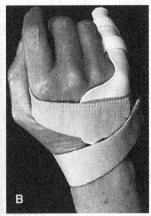

FIGURE 1–11

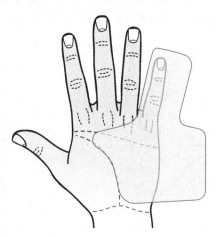

FIGURE 1–12

FABRICATION PROCESS

Pattern Creation (Fig. 1–12)

- Mark for proximal border at wrist crease, clearing ulnar styloid.
- Allow extra ½″ to 1″ of material distally to accommodate for flexion angle at MCP joints.

Refine Pattern

- Proximal border should allow full wrist motion.
- Radial border should allow full thumb, IF, and middle finger (MF) motion.
- Make sure pattern encompasses third metacarpal proximal to MCP joint. Remember, fourth and fifth metacarpals are relatively mobile compared to the radial side; thus, if goal is to immobilize a metacarpal fracture, orthosis must be anchored to stable third metacarpal.
- Allow unimpeded motion of MF by keeping pattern accurate.

Options for Materials

- Use drapable material to achieve intimate fit about MCP joints to prevent migration and improve comfort.
- Perforated thermoplastics may prevent skin maceration; consider using them for patients who require full-time use of orthosis.
- Materials that can be reheated and remolded several times are a good option if ongoing modifications become necessary to accommodate for fluctuations in edema and changes in MCP joint motion.

Cut and Heat

- Position patient's extremity with shoulder and elbow flexed with forearm pronation to achieve gravity-assisted position (ulnar border of hand should face upward).
- Place MCP joint in appropriate amount of flexion.
- If included, position PIP and/or DIP joints as per diagnosis.
- If using thin padding dorsally across MCP joints, apply to the area before heating material.

Evaluate Fit While Molding

- Place material on ulnar aspect of hand just distal to wrist.
- Gently stretch dorsal material over MCP joints while maintaining arches of hand.
- Allow gravity to assist while gently contouring and encompassing digits and MCP joints proximally.
- Incorporate natural descent of fifth MCP below fourth MCP.
- Be sure to maintain desired joint positions as material sets.
- Avoid applying direct pressure over dorsum of MCP and PIP joints while molding.
- Do not seal off distally; allow for ability to check for vascular compromise and provide some air exchange.
- Amount of MCP flexion requested may be difficult to achieve initially because of pain, stiffness, and/or dorsal edema; serial positioning into flexion may be necessary.

Strapping and Components

- Soft or elasticized straps work well around wrist to prevent migration.
- Consider a customized soft foam strap through first web space to improve comfort and prevent skin irritation caused by friction from traditional loop material.
- Consider using rivets to secure one end of proximal strap to minimize space needed for hook material.
- Traditional straps will suffice to secure digits; be sure to trim straps between digit web spaces to prevent skin irritation.

Survey Completed Orthosis

- Smooth material borders, making sure there are no sharp edges, especially at ulnar styloid.
- If PIP and DIP joints are included, trim excess material from distal end to allow for visualization of fingertips.
- Check clearance of wrist and MF, making sure there is no abutment with material.

PATTERN PEARLS 1–40 TO 1–42

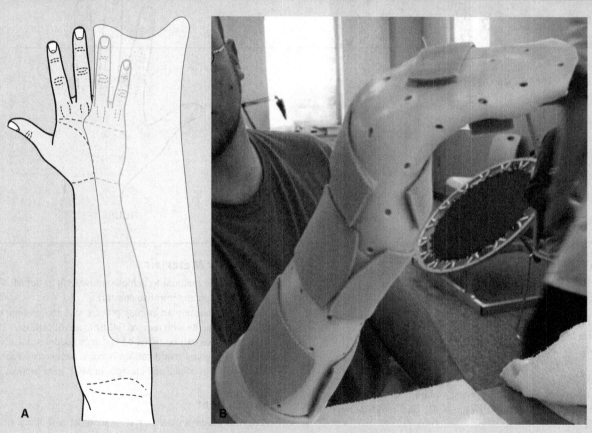

FIGURE PP1–40 **A and B,** Including the wrist in pattern.

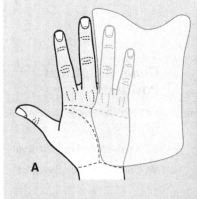
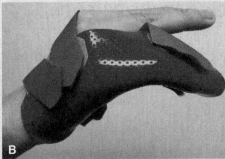

FIGURE PP1–41 A and B, Including RF and SF.

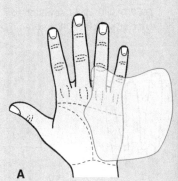
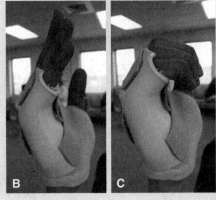

FIGURE PP1–42 A–C, IP joints free.

CLINICAL PEARL 1–19

Accommodation for Dorsal Pins

Using therapy putty (medium resistance) and sterile petroleum-impregnated gauze can be a way to safely make room and provide cover for dorsal protruding pins. Place gauze over pins. Then form a small ball of putty, partially flatten out, and gently rest over the pin(s), making sure to fully cover the pin and immediate surface area. Next, either place an additional piece of gauze over the putty prior to thermoplastic application or add a thin layer of lotion. This step is to prevent the thermoplastic material from "sticking" to the putty. Once molded and set, remove the thermoplastic material carefully from the hand. It should slide right off the putty without fear of pin extraction **(A-D)**. The putty and gauze can then be removed from the orthosis. The patient now has a well-molded orthosis with "bubbles" that protect the pin from external forces.

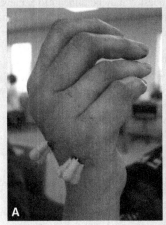
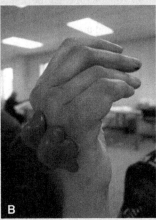
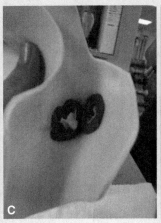
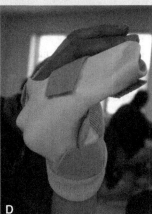

RADIAL MCP/PIP/DIP IMMOBILIZATION ORTHOSIS (HFO) (Fig. 1–13)

COMMON NAMES

- Hand-based radial gutter splint
- Hand-based radial fracture brace
- Metacarpal fracture brace
- Clamdigger splint

ALTERNATIVE OPTIONS

- Plaster cast

PRIMARY FUNCTIONS

- Immobilize proximal phalanxes and metacarpals of IF and MF to allow healing and/or protection of involved structure(s).

Common Diagnoses	General Optimal Positions
Metacarpal head or neck fracture	MCP: 60°–90° flexion (may include PIP/DIP: 0°)
Proximal phalanx fracture	MCP: 60°–90° flexion; PIP/DIP: 0°
Complicated middle phalanx fracture	MCP: 60°–90° flexion; PIP/DIP: 0°
MCP capsulectomy	MCP: 60°–90° flexion; PIP/DIP: 0°
Sagittal band injury or repair	MCP: 0° with slight deviation to affected side; PIP/DIP: free

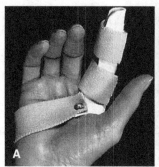
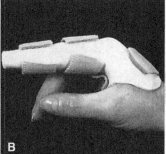

FIGURE 1–13

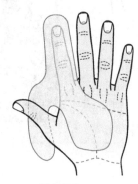

FIGURE 1–14

FABRICATION PROCESS

Pattern Creation (Fig. 1–14)

- Mark for proximal border at wrist crease.
- Allow extra ½" to 1" of material distally to accommodate for flexion angle at MCP joints.

Refine Pattern

- Proximal border should allow full wrist motion.
- Ulnar border should allow full MF motion.
- Make sure pattern encompasses third metacarpal dorsally for improved stability.

Options for Materials

- Use drapable material to achieve intimate fit about MCP joints to prevent migration and improve comfort.
- Perforated thermoplastics may prevent skin maceration; consider using them for patients who require full-time use of orthosis.
- Materials that can be reheated and remolded several times are a good option if ongoing modifications become necessary to accommodate for fluctuations in edema and changes in MCP joint motion.

Cut and Heat

- Position patient's forearm in neutral rotation to achieve gravity-assisted position.
- Place MCP joints in appropriate amount of flexion.
- Position PIP and DIP joints as per diagnosis; place thumb in palmar abduction and opposition.
- If using thin padding dorsally across MCP joints, apply to area before heating material.

Evaluate Fit While Molding

- Place material on radial aspect of hand just distal to wrist.
- Gently stretch dorsal material over MCP joint while maintaining arches of hand.
- Allow gravity to assist while gently contouring and encompassing IF/MF and MCP joints proximally.
- Be sure to maintain desired joint positions as material sets.
- Avoid applying direct pressure over dorsum of MCP and PIP joints while molding.
- Do not seal off distally; allow for ability to check for vascular compromise and provide some air exchange.
- Amount of MCP flexion requested may be difficult to achieve initially because of pain, dorsal edema, or stiffness; serial static positioning into flexion may be necessary.

Strapping and Components

- Soft or elasticized straps work well around wrist to prevent migration.
- Consider using rivets to secure one end of proximal strap to minimize space needed for hook material.
- Traditional straps suffice to secure digits; be sure to trim straps in between digit web spaces to prevent skin irritation.

Survey Completed Orthosis

- Smooth material borders, making sure there are no sharp edges, especially with thumb motion.
- If PIP and DIP joints are included, trim excess material distally to allow for visualization of fingertips.
- Check clearance of wrist and MF, making sure there is no abutment with material.

PATTERN PEARLS 1-43 TO 1-46

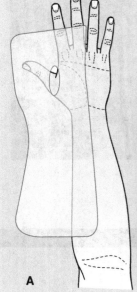
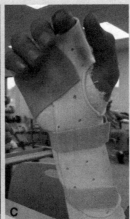
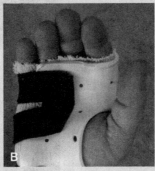

FIGURE PP1–43 A and B, Forearm based with IP joints free. **C,** Only DIP free.

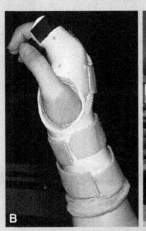
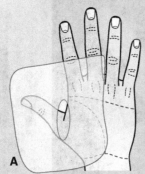

FIGURE PP1–44 A and B, IP joints free.

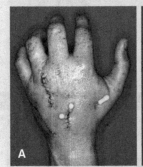
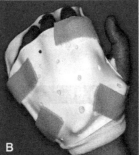
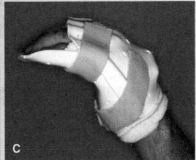

FIGURE PP1–45 A–C, Clamshell design to cover pins.

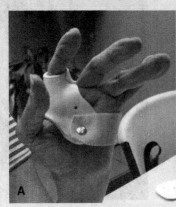
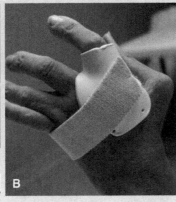

FIGURE PP1–46 A and B, IF MCP joint only.

CLINICAL PEARL 1–20

Pinch and Trim to Seal Distal Border

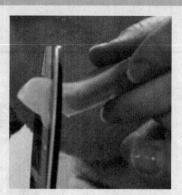

When an injury necessitates complete coverage of the distal digit(s), consider pinching excess material together and trimming with quality scissors. The trimming should be done when the material is still warm in order to form a seal. The material may still pop apart upon removal; however, hook-and-loop closures can be added.

CLINICAL PEARL 1–21

Clearing Thenar Region for Unrestricted Mobility

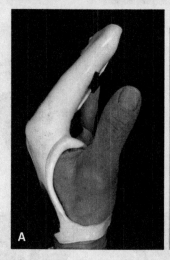

Careful attention should be taken when making an orthosis for the radial digits; the thumb is often left free (**A**). Material should be carefully molded about the thenar, leaving room for thumb mobility. Note: In this orthosis, the strapping system incorporates volar and dorsal adhesive hook in order to maximize surface area of strap application (**B**).

CLINICAL PEARL 1–22

MCP Flexion (Antideformity) Positioning

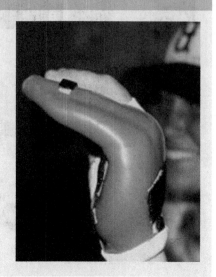

When molding about the MCP joints of the hand, meticulous attention should be given to proper angle measurements of not only the MCP but the IP joints as well. This orthosis holds the hand in the antideformity position. Note the clearance of the thumb.

THUMB MP IMMOBILIZATION ORTHOSIS (HFO) (Fig. 1–15)

COMMON NAMES

- Short opponens splint
- MP splint
- Basal joint splint
- First CMC splint
- Mickey Stanley (Detroit) splint
- Gamekeeper's thumb splint

ALTERNATIVE OPTIONS

- Prefabricated thumb supports
- Neoprene thumb and wrist wraps
- Ring design splints

PRIMARY FUNCTIONS

- Immobilize thumb MP joint to allow for healing of involved structure(s).
- Rest painful and/or inflamed MP joint.

ADDITIONAL FUNCTIONS

- Promote gliding of FPL tendon by restricting movement of MP joint during active thumb flexion exercises.

Common Diagnoses	General Optimal Positions
Ulnar collateral ligament (UCL) injury (grades 1–3)	Slight MP flexion with UD
Radial collateral ligament (RCL) injury (grades 1–3)	Slight MP flexion with RD
Trapeziometacarpal (TM or carpometacarpal [CMC]) joint arthritis	MP: slight flexion; CMC: neutral
MP joint arthritis	Position of comfort
MP joint arthroplasty	Near full extension
MP joint dorsal dislocation	20°–30° MP flexion

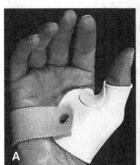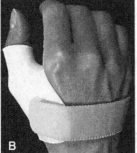

FIGURE 1–15

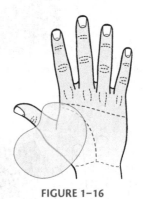

FIGURE 1–16

FABRICATION PROCESS

Pattern Creation (Fig. 1–16)

- Mark for proximal border just distal to wrist crease and distal border at IP joint.
- Mark for ulnar border at third metacarpal, which approximates the thenar crease.
- Pattern will resemble a symmetrical kidney bean with the dip in the bean at the IP joint.

Refine Pattern

- Proximal border should allow full wrist motion.
- Remember to allow unimpeded motion of wrist, IF MCP, and thumb IP joints by keeping pattern accurate.
- Volar ulnar border should allow full mobility of hypothenar area ending at thenar crease.
- May extend pattern distally to include IP joint if necessary.

Options for Materials

- Use drapable material to achieve intimate fit at MP joint, prevent migration, and improve comfort.
- Consider using coated material so circumferential thumb piece can be popped open without permanent bonding, providing an intimate contour at MP joint and proximal phalanx.

- Use thinnest material possible that provides necessary strength to decrease bulk.
- Remember that elastic materials tend to shrink around proximal phalanx of thumb (making it difficult to don and doff); do not remove until completely set.

Cut and Heat

- Position patient's forearm in slight supination for gravity-assisted molding.
- Place thumb in midpalmar-radial abduction and MP joint in slight flexion.
- Consider placing light layer of lotion on thumb before molding to ease removal.

Evaluate Fit While Molding

- Distally, place "dip of the bean" just proximal to IP joint on radial side of proximal phalanx.
- Mold material volarly to thenar crease and dorsally about proximal phalanx, being sure to extend to IP joint.
- Carefully tug and wrap material through first web space from volar to dorsal and overlap material onto itself by approximately 1″.
- After overlapping through thumb web space, have patient gently oppose to IF, which helps maintain desired thumb CMC and MP joint positions as material sets.
- Avoid applying direct pressure over dorsum of MP joint while molding.

Strapping and Components

- One 1″ strap around wrist provides secure fit. Place strap at base of hypothenar eminence to prevent migration.
- Elasticized straps are preferred to allow mobility of hypothenar muscles.
- If circumferential portion of orthosis needs to be popped apart for donning and doffing over IP joint, a small strap must be applied at this opening.

Survey Completed Orthosis

- Smooth distal and proximal borders.
- Gently flare proximal to thumb IP joint.
- Check clearance of wrist, thumb IP, and IF MCP joints, making sure there is no abutment with thermoplastic material.

PATTERN PEARLS 1–47 TO 1–53

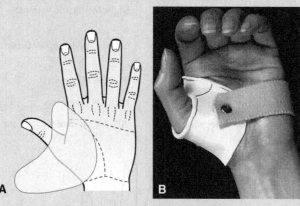

FIGURE PP1–47 A and B, MP joint left free.

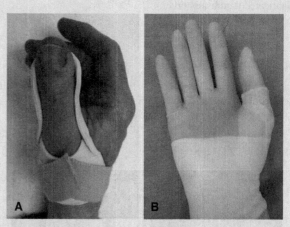

FIGURE PP1–48 Volar/dorsal design: **A,** IP included; **B,** IP free.

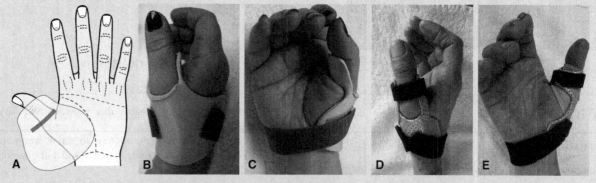

FIGURE PP1–49 A–C, Volar/dorsal design: IP free for trigger thumb hand based. **D and E,** Thumb based.

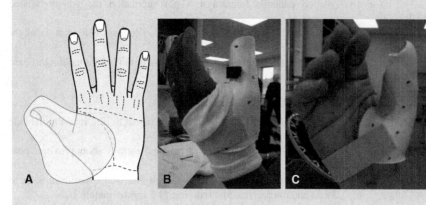

FIGURE PP1–50 A, IP joint included applied **(B)** dorsal and **(C)** volar.

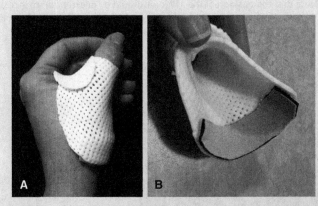

FIGURE PP1–51 **A and B,** Incorporated beneath orthosis at CMC region.

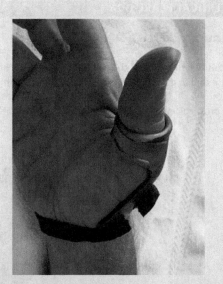

FIGURE PP1–52 "Ring" design: MP joint extension orthosis.

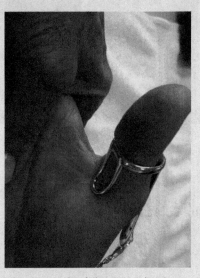

FIGURE PP1–53 Silver Ring™ Splint (Silver Ring Splint Company) to block MP joint motion.

CLINICAL PEARL 1–23

Easing Circumferential Thumb Orthosis Removal

If thumb orthosis needs to come off for exercise sessions, make sure the patient can indeed remove the orthosis. Often, the circumference of the IP joint is larger than that of the proximal phalanx **(A)**, making removal difficult or impossible. Wrapping tape or Coban™ around the proximal phalanx before molding can help to relatively build up the circumference of the phalanx region equaling the IP joint; once the material is set and cooled, the wrap can be pulled out **(B–E)**. One disadvantage is that this technique may cause some looseness in fit. Another method involves applying a thin layer of lotion to the thumb area before molding to ease removal. Consider using the trap door method as described elsewhere in this text.

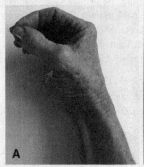
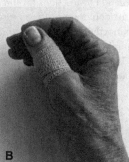
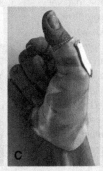
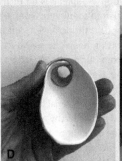
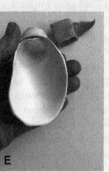

CLINICAL PEARL 1–24

Thumb Exercise Orthoses

A, An orthosis that immobilizes the thumb MP joint in extension can help direct the force of flexion to the IP joint during active exercises. This can be used as an exercise tool to increase active IP flexion and/or maximize FPL tendon glide. Note that the position of the MP joint should be in extension to increase tension on the FPL. **B,** A circumferential IP extension orthosis or plaster of paris cast can be used to isolate MP joint motion. Make sure that the orthosis has the longest proximal lever arm without interfering with volar MP flexion.

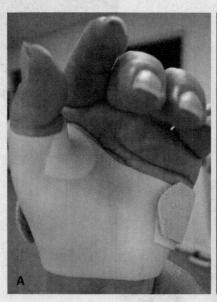
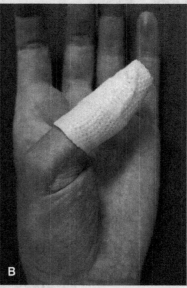

EXPERT PEARL 1–11

Neoprene: Sometimes the Unique Solution
HandLab: Clinical Pearls

JUDY C. COLDITZ, OT/L, CHT, FAOTA
North Carolina

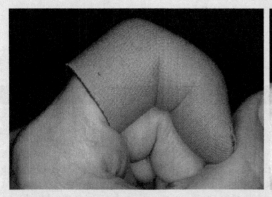
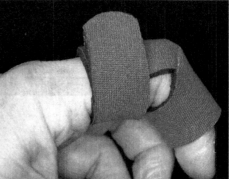
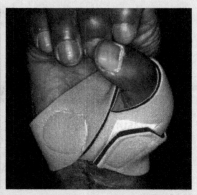

On occasion, therapists are faced with clinical challenges to which there is no readily available solution. Neoprene is an orthotic material which sometimes can provide a custom solution to a unique problem.

Perhaps the patient has a bulbous arthritic finger joint but wants to maintain some motion. A snug fitting neoprene sleeve can provide an external "ligament," diminishing pain during use. A sleeve can cover the entire finger to provide insulation against cold exposure, allowing the patient to return to work in a cold environment.

Neoprene is also an effective padding material, being especially effective at absorbing sheer force. The slightly stretchy and soft characteristics make it an ideal material for pressure distribution in some strapping applications. In our busy clinics, it is inefficient to construct a neoprene orthosis when there are many readily available commercial neoprene solutions. Constructing an orthosis of neoprene is best reserved for the one-of-a-kind problems for which you have nothing else to offer the patient.

This clinical pearl offers tips for working with neoprene and construction instructions for three specific orthoses: (1) A finger sleeve for insulation or for use as an external ligament, (2) a finger protector for a contracted finger with scleroderma, and (3) a soft orthosis to maintain thumb abduction in an insensate hand with median palsy.

These are only a few of the many ideas for the use of neoprene for unique clinical circumstances.

1. A neoprene-insulating finger sleeve
2. An easily removable neoprene protector for a contracted PIP joint resulting from scleroderma
3. A neoprene thumb support for median palsy

Disclaimer: HandLab Clinical Pearls are intended to be an informal sharing of practical clinical ideas; not formal evidence-based conclusions of fact.

Neoprene: Sometimes the Unique Solution (Continued)

Tips for Working With Neoprene

Uses for Neoprene

1. External Ligament: Elastic; allows motion while providing support
   a. Must be tight enough to provide support to joint but not constrict blood flow
2. Insulation; no water or air passes through
   a. Must be snug to block airflow but not constrict
3. Strapping; no sharp edges
   a. Distributes pressure over bony prominences
4. Padding; absorbs sheer force
   a. Small piece of adhesive hook can hold neoprene in place (if fabric cover is made of loop)
   b. Can be removable and washable

Working With Neoprene (Synthetic Rubber)

1. Choose material thickness
   a. Thickness measures neoprene (black core) only
   b. 3 mm (1/8") for most wrist/hand orthoses
   c. 1.5-2mm (1/16") for finger sleeves
   d. Type of fabric laminated to neoprene alters thickness
2. Determine stretch
   a. Amount of stretch varies based on fabric laminated to neoprene
   b. Directional stretch may vary greatly
3. Create pattern
   a. Make rough paper pattern (depending on direct of stretch)
   b. Cut pattern larger than needed (you can always make smaller!)
   c. Glue seams, evaluate fit, and adjust fit as needed by redoing seams
   d. Make fit snug; neoprene stretches with use

Technical Tips: Seaming Neoprene

1. Gluing seams (must use neoprene glue)
   a. Apply thin layer of glue to both sides (black edge only)
   b. Allow to dry until tacky
   c. Put edges together
   d. Avoid stress until glue cures 24 hrs.
2. Sewing seams
   a. Use largest needle possible
   b. Use longest stitch possible
   c. Place paper above and below neoprene for successful sewing
   d. Use stretch stitch (zig-zag)
3. Using heat-activated seam tape
   a. Place tape over seam, cover with paper, and apply heat from iron
   b. Hold iron in place until glue melts (this is longer than you think!)
   c. Tape best as reinforcement to glued seam; attach to one or both sides of seam
   d. Must cure 24 hours before stress

Creating Closures on Neoprene

1. Attaching neoprene to neoprene
   a. Use neoprene with UBL (unbroken loop: fuzzy material to which hook can be attached) on one side and a hook fastener on the other side. NOTE: The hook may appear to attach to some fabric covered neoprene, but unless it is UBL, it will not have useful durability
   b. Sew hook and/or loop fastener to neoprene in desired location/s
   c. Apply heat-activated hook and/or loop to neoprene
2. Attaching neoprene to thermoplastic materials
   a. Apply a small amount of adhesive hook closure to the inside of the thermoplastic and apply neoprene with UBL as strap
   b. Attach neoprene to noncoated (sticky) thermoplastic that has been heated (dry heat is best)
   c. Attach neoprene with rivets, making a large "washer" so the rivet does not pull out of the hole in stretchy neoprene

US Sources for Neoprene

- Seattle Fabrics; www.seattlefabrics.com
- Benik Corporation; www.benik.com
- Warm Belly Wetsuits (possibly for scraps of thin neoprene); www.warmbelly.com
- North Coast Medical; www.ncmedical.com
- Patterson Medical; www.pattersonmedical.com
- Your local dive shop

Reference

Colditz J. C. (1999). *Splinting With Neoprene*. North Coast Medical, Inc.

Neoprene Finger Sleeve (Insulation or Support)

Design & Instructions by Judy C. Colditz, OT/L, CHT, FAOTA.

NOTE: These instructions are for use with 1.5-2-mm (1/16")–thick neoprene with nylon knit fabric on both sides. If thicker material is used, width must be added to the pattern to accommodate the thicker material. For joint support of PIP, do not include fingertip.

STEP 1: Draw a straight line and place finger centered over line. Mark: (1) end of finger, (2) DIP joint, (3) PIP joint, and (4) base.

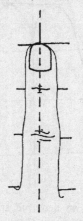

STEP 2: When the finger is removed, the drawing should look like this.

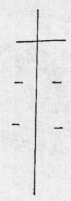

STEP 3: Connect the marks with straight horizontal lines.

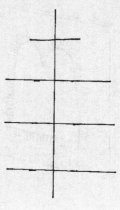

STEP 4: Measure circumference of DIP, PIP, and base. Center circumference measurement on center line and mark the length.

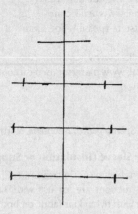

STEP 5: Connect the marked lines, curving both sides of the top as shown. Do not make tips too pointed. Cut out the pattern.

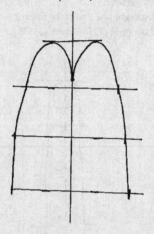

STEP 6: Place pattern on neoprene and mark edges with chalk. Maximum stretch across allows easiest flexion.

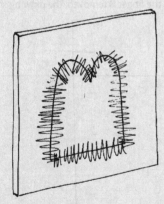

STEP 7: Cut outline created by chalk mark. Cut edges squarely.

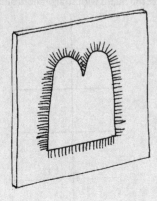

STEP 8: Apply glue on edges, starting in center. Dry until tacky.

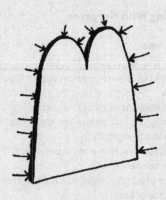

STEP 9: Start at center abutting the edges; cure 24 hours.

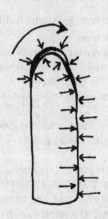

Finger Protector for Contracted Scleroderma PIP Joint

Design & Instructions by Judy C. Colditz, OT/L, CHT, FAOTA.

NOTE: These instructions are for use with 3-mm (1/8″)–thick neoprene with nylon knit fabric on both sides. This must be loose fitting; direction of stretch is not relevant.

STEP 1: Draw a pattern by taking measurements on the contracted finger. It is VERY IMPORTANT that this fits loosely so as not to constrict the already compromised blood flow; be generous; you can always make it smaller.

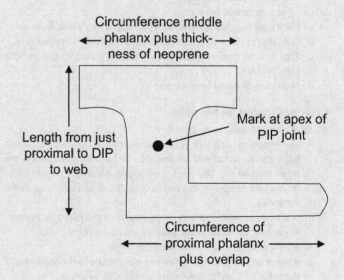

STEP 2: Cut out small triangles on each side of the PIP joint mark. The tips of the triangles almost meet in the middle.

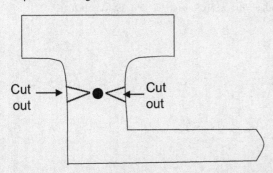

Cut out →   ← Cut out

STEP 3: Apply iron-on hook closure to the underside of the finger protector and iron-on loop closure to the outer side of the finger protector.

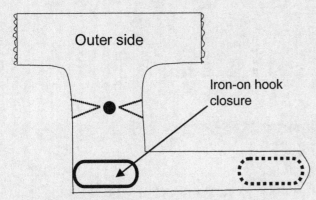

Outer side

Iron-on hook closure

STEP 4: Apply neoprene glue to the inside edges of the triangles and the edges of the closed loops. Edges to be glued marked are with: 〰️

STEP 5: Fit protector to patient, checking that the fit is LOOSE. If there is too much material over the PIP joint, cut larger triangles and reglue.

Neoprene Thumb Abduction Orthosis

Design & Instructions by Judy C. Colditz, OT/L, CHT, FAOTA.
   Use 3 mm (1/8″) thickness.
STEP 1: Cut an 18-inch length of 2-inch-wide Neoloop or neoprene with loop fabric on one side. Wrap around the thumb, overlapping as shown. Loop side should face outward.

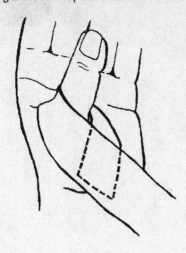

STEP 2: Mark the underneath strap where it is crossed over by the top strap. Also mark the top strap where the edges of the underlying strap meet it. Cut off the underlying strap at the angle marked.

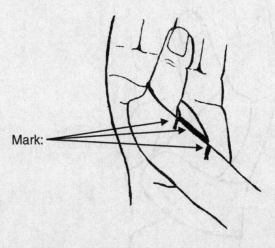

Mark:

STEP 3: Apply a thin layer of neoprene glue on the end of the strap you have just cut and on the edge of the strap between the marks. When the glue is tacky, place the two edges together to make the seam.

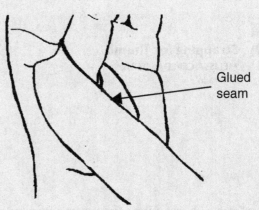

Glued seam

STEP 4: To reinforce the seam (optional), place a strip of seam tape with the glue side down over the seam. Apply heat from an iron directly to the seam tape until the glue melts. HINT: Use a piece of paper between the iron and tape and hold the iron. Do not move it back and forth. On this orthosis, you will be more successful applying the seam tape to the inside of the seam (nonloop side). Trim ends of tape if needed.

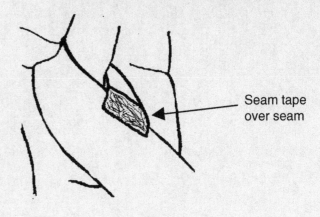

Seam tape over seam

STEP 5: Apply heat-sensitive hook closure on the inside of the overlapping strap where it overlaps the strap at the base of the thumb. Allow to set before pulling open and close.

Clinical Pearls reprinted with permission from Clinician's Classroom at BraceLab.com written by Judy Colditz OT/L CHT FAOTA, copyright HandLab/BraceLab, Raleigh NC. No. 39, March 2016.

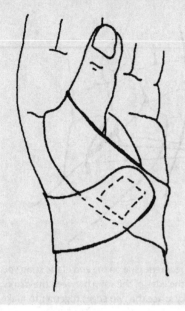

Finished orthosis

 EXPERT PEARL 1–12

Strapping for Thumb

MELISSA CEPEDA, OTR/L
Colorado

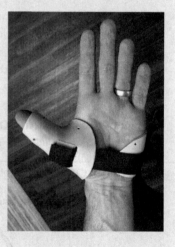

Strap pulled through slit in material creates more intimate fit. This technique can be utilized for creating an adjustable contoured fit of strap which is helpful to prevent orthosis migration during use of hand.

THUMB CMC IMMOBILIZATION ORTHOSIS (HFO) (Fig. 1–17)

COMMON NAMES

- CMC palmar abduction splint
- Short thumb spica splint
- Short opponens splint
- MP splint

ALTERNATIVE OPTIONS

- Prefabricated thumb support
- Comfort Cool® splint
- Push CMC brace
- Neoprene thumb and wrist wrap
- Plaster cast

PRIMARY FUNCTIONS

- Immobilize thumb CMC and MP joints to allow healing, rest, and/or protection of involved structure(s).

ADDITIONAL FUNCTIONS

- Improve functional use by positioning thumb in functional opposition.
- Promote gliding of FPL or extensor pollicis longus (EPL) tendon by restricting movement of MP and CMC joint during active flexion and extension exercises.

Common Diagnoses	General Optimal Positions
TM joint arthritis	Slight MP flexion with palm abduction and th opp
Lax or mildly subluxed TM joint	Slight MP flexion with palm abduction and th opp
UCL injury (grades 1–3)	Slight MP flexion with UD
RCL injury (grades 1–3)	Slight MP flexion with RD
Low median nerve injury	Slight MP flexion with palm abduction and th opp

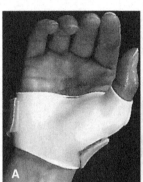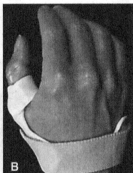

FIGURE 1–17

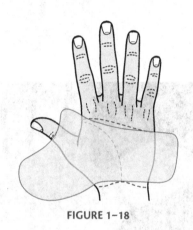

FIGURE 1–18

FABRICATION PROCESS

Pattern Creation (Fig. 1–18)

- Mark for proximal border just distal to wrist crease.
- Mark for distal border at thumb IP flexion crease and DPC.

Refine Pattern

- Allow unimpeded motion of wrist, thumb IP, and digit MCP joints by keeping pattern accurate.
- Provide ample material within web space to support palmar abduction position adequately.
- Allow enough material to mold around ulnar border without overlapping dorsally.
- May extend pattern distally to include IP joint or trim pattern to omit MP joint if necessary.

Options for Materials

- Use drapable material to achieve intimate fit about CMC and MP joints to prevent migration and improve comfort.
- Use coated material so circumferential thumb piece can be popped open without permanent sealing.
- Use thinnest material possible that provides necessary strength to minimize bulk.
- Remember that elastic materials tend to shrink around thumb (making it difficult to don and doff); do not remove until completely set.

Cut and Heat

- Position patient's forearm in slight supination to achieve gravity-assisted position.
- Place thumb MP joint in appropriate amount of flexion and CMC joint in desired amount of palmar abduction and opposition.
- Consider placing light layer of lotion on thumb before molding to ease removal.

Evaluate Fit While Molding

- Place material on volar aspect of hand and thumb while maintaining desired joint positions; at the same time, gently contour palmar arches.
- Carefully tug and wrap material through first web space from volar to dorsal; overlap material onto itself by approximately 1″.
- After overlapping through thumb web space, have patient gently oppose to IF, which helps maintain desired thumb CMC and MP joint positions as material sets.
- Avoid applying direct pressure over dorsum of MP joint while molding.
- Proximally, mold well around base of CMC joint.
- Ulnarly, wrap material around ulnar border to fourth metacarpal dorsally.
- Clear IP joint flexion crease.
- Avoid rolling material just proximal to the IP flexion crease (circumferentially) unless using a very thin material where light rolling may aid in strengthening this area.

Strapping and Components

- One 1″ strap attached dorsally to radial and ulnar segments suffices.
- Consider using rivets to secure dorsal strap.
- If circumferential portion needs to be popped apart for donning and doffing over IP joint, small strap must be applied at this opening.

Survey Completed Orthosis

- Smooth distal and proximal borders.
- Gently flare proximal to thumb IP joint.
- Check for clearance of wrist, thumb IP, and digit MCP joints. Make sure there is no abutment with thermoplastic material.

PATTERN PEARLS 1–54 TO 1–61

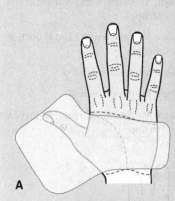
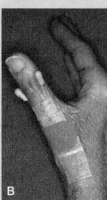
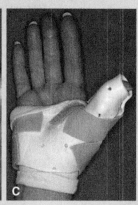

FIGURE PP1–54 **A–C,** IP joint included.

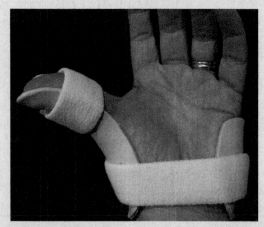

FIGURE PP1–55 IP joint included, molded dorsally.

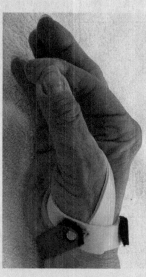

FIGURE PP1–56 Minimalist "strip" design to support CMC joint.

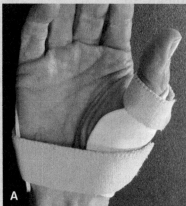
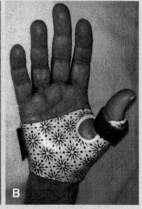

FIGURE PP1–57 **A,** Dorsal-based IP joint free. **B,** Thumb strap can be removed to allow full MP and IP motion; this design also prevents MP extension.

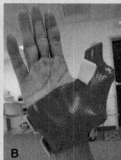
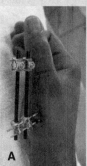
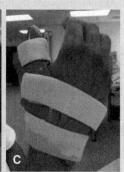

FIGURE PP1–58 **A–C,** Accommodation of external fixator.

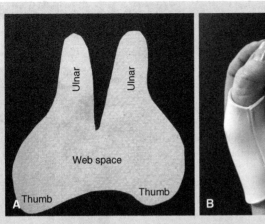

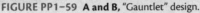

FIGURE PP1-59 **A and B,** "Gauntlet" design.

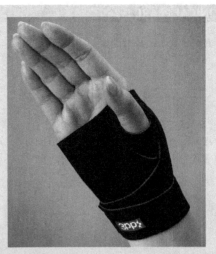

FIGURE PP1-60 3pp® ThumSling® NP prefabricated. (Photo courtesy of 3-Point Products, Stevensville, MD.)

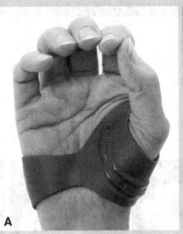

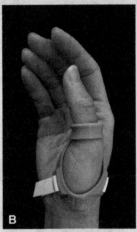

FIGURE PP1-61 **A,** The MetaGrip® (A, Photo courtesy of HandLab, Raleigh, NC.). **B,** Durathumb™ 3D-printed thumb stabilization splint (ZLNP Inc).

 CLINICAL PEARL 1–25

Trap Door for Circumferential Thumb Orthoses

A and B, To ease donning and doffing of a circumferential thumb orthosis, use a coated material (which will not adhere onto itself). Once the material is completely cool, pop apart the overlapped segment to create a trap door. Use a thin piece of loop material to "close" the door. This technique helps when there is an enlarged joint or potential fluctuating edema about the thumb MP or IP joint but still allows for complete immobilization of the MP joint. Permanently bonding this area may require enlarging the thumbhole to allow for donning/doffing, which can then allow MP motion, leading to possible areas of excess pressure. Note the rivet used to secure the strap. This is a small strap and can sometimes be lost or misplaced. Securing with a rivet allows for permanent placement. **C,** Use caution when "opening" or releasing the trap door. If the material has not completely cooled, the overlapping tab may stick to the material it was placed on and the top tab may loose its shape. This will then cause it to not sit flush once when trying to secure.

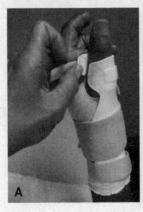

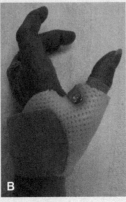

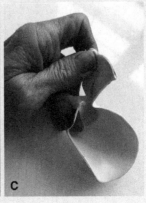

CLINICAL PEARL 1–26

IF MCP Joint Border

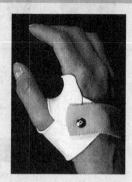

It is imperative when applying an orthosis around the first web space to be sure the index border is not too high. The orthosis shown here has an overgenerous border that impedes IF MCP joint motion; this may cause tissue irritation.

CLINICAL PEARL 1–27

Thumb Positioning

Always check thumb position before, during, and after the molding process. When positioning the thumb for function, the CMC joint should be placed midway between palmar **(A)** and radial **(B)** abduction, and the MP joint should be in slight flexion (20°–30°) **(C)**. This allows for effective pinch to the index and middle fingers. If the therapist is not careful, as the patient relaxes his or her hand during the molding process, the wrist will tend to flex, which promotes thumb extension and radial abduction. This places the thumb in a poor position for function.

In this exaggerated example, note the adduction posture of the first metacarpal and the hyperextension of the thumb MP joint **(D)**. Because the thumb was passively correctable, a custom orthosis was able to position the thumb to allow light opposition for daily activity **(E and F)**.

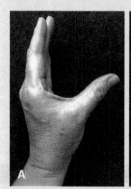
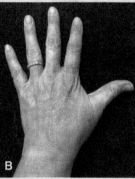
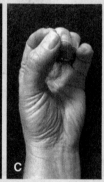
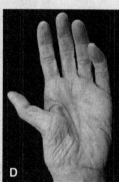
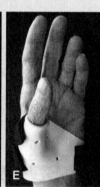
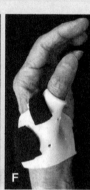

Modifying the Push® Metagrip® for Specific Patients
HandLab: Clinical Pearls

KAROL YOUNG, OTD, OTR/L, CHT
North Carolina

Therapists frequently stop by the BraceLab booth at conferences to offer positive feedback about the Push MetaGrip thumb CMC brace, often suggesting ways to modify the MetaGrip to suit their patients' individual needs. We believe "when you learn it, you should teach it," so we are passing along a few ideas therapists have "taught" us about MetaGrip modifications.

Strapping

Although the straps on the dorsum of the hand are a soft hook-and-loop fabric, they may cause pressure to those with fragile skin. This can be remedied by applying a piece of Velfoam® strapping material between the patient's skin and the straps **(A)**. Straps can be crossed before closing to get a more secure fit at the base of the brace **(B)**. Holes can be punched to enlarge the slits where the straps pass through, allowing individuals with a weaker pinch to more easily loosen or tighten the straps **(C)**.

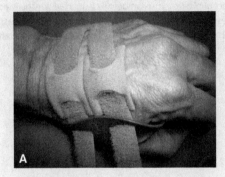

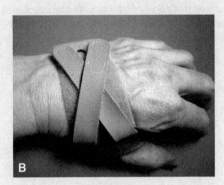

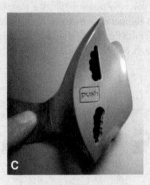

A. *Applying Velfoam strapping material*

B. *Crossing the straps*

C. *Widening the holes*

Boney Prominences

For individuals with a boney prominence on the dorsum of the CMC joint (shoulder sign), some therapists add a piece of adhesive gel on each side of the boney prominence to lift all pressure off. The photo shows the location of the gel on the patient's hand, but the gel is placed on the inside the MetaGrip at the corresponding location **(D)**. Adding padding directly over the boney area only adds pressure. Additionally, one can carefully dry heat and roll the edge at the base of the brace. Gently heat one small area at a time and be sure to protect your finger when pushing on the heated material, holding it until cooled **(E)**.

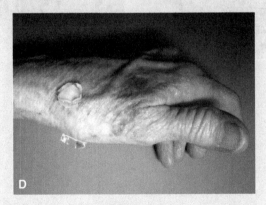

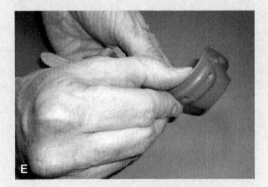

D. *Applying gel dots*

E. *Rolling the edge*

Thumb Web Space

One therapist explains, "The MetaGrip is like a pair of expensive leather shoes; it will soften with age, so expect the area in the thumb web space to soften with time." The MetaGrip web space can also be softened somewhat in the splint pan water and then pinched a few times to slightly recontour **(F)**. The high-temperature MetaGrip thermoplastic will not be as responsive as low-temperature thermoplastic materials.

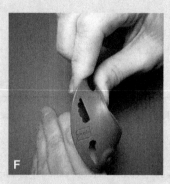

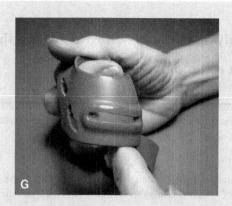

F. Pinching the web space

If the web space remains bothersome, sections can be heated with a heat gun and rolled **(G)**. **Important note:** Modifying the MetaGrip voids the manufacturer's warranty, so proceed carefully.

If you have never modified a MetaGrip, be assured that if you are familiar with handling low-temperature plastics, you can quickly gain a feel for the MetaGrip high-temperature material. If you have modified a MetaGrip with a technique you devised, please share with us so we can learn from one another and pass it on!

Clinical Pearls reprinted with permission from Clinician's Classroom at BraceLab.com written by Karol Young, OTD, OTR/L, CHT, copyright BraceLab/HandLab, Raleigh, NC. No. 60, January 2020.

 EXPERT PEARL 1–14

Thumb Positioning

BRUCE CURTIS, OT
Illinois

Use ¼″ wooden dowels of various lengths to place between the patient's thumb and a finger to hold the thumb in desired position **(A and B)**. The dowel will prevent the patient from moving from desired position; have them pinch the dowel lightly to prevent the thumb from collapsing.

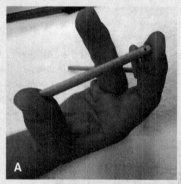

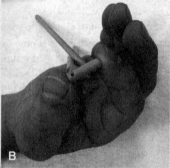

THUMB ABDUCTION IMMOBILIZATION ORTHOSIS (HFO) (Fig. 1–19)

COMMON NAMES

- CMC splint
- Web stretcher
- C-bar splint

ALTERNATIVE OPTIONS

- Plaster cast

PRIMARY FUNCTIONS

- Prevent soft tissue contracture of first web space as result of median nerve injury or disease.

ADDITIONAL FUNCTIONS

- Statically position first web space contracture at maximum palmar abduction to facilitate lengthening of tissue (mobilization).

Common Diagnoses	General Optimal Positions
Median nerve injury	Maximum palm and rad abduction
Postoperative contracture release	Maximum palm and rad abduction

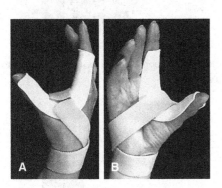

FIGURE 1–19

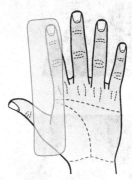

FIGURE 1–20

FABRICATION PROCESS

Pattern Creation (Fig. 1–20)

- Pattern is rectangular.
- Width is two-thirds circumference of the thumb.
- Length is measured from IF DIP joint to tip of thumb.

Refine Pattern

- Allow enough material to encompass two-thirds of thumb circumference ulnarly and two-thirds of IF radially.
- Provide ample material within web space to support palmar and radial abduction position adequately and to allow enough surface area for strap application.

Options for Materials

- Use ⅛″ thermoplastic material to provide rigidity needed to maintain position of tissue.
- Use highly drapable material to achieve intimate fit through web space to prevent migration and improve comfort.
- Consider perforated material when orthosis will be used in conjunction with scar management products such as elastomer or silicone gel.
- Materials that can be reheated and remolded several times are a good option if ongoing modifications become necessary to accommodate for changes in motion (a common issue because it is difficult to achieve desired joint position initially).

Cut and Heat

- Position patient with elbow resting on table and forearm in slight supination to achieve gravity-assisted position.
- Place thumb in appropriate amount of palmar and radial abduction.

Evaluate Fit While Molding

- Place warm material along thumb and IF while maintaining desired position.
- Mold with even pressure throughout length of orthosis, focusing on gentle abduction pressure to distal portions of first and second metacarpals. Avoid applying pressure at thumb distally, which can actually place undue tension on UCL, not first web space.
- Flare around thumb and IF MCP joints.
- Maintain desired thumb position as material sets.

Strapping and Components

- Apply one 1″ elasticized strap directed from volar web space around wrist 1½ times and attach to dorsal aspect.

Survey Completed Orthosis

- Smooth distal and proximal borders.
- Define consistent wearing schedule for patient. Many therapists suggest patients wear these orthoses at night only, allowing functional use during day.

PATTERN PEARLS 1–62 TO 1–66

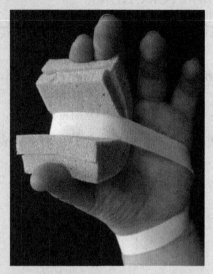

FIGURE PP1–62 Foam with strapping.

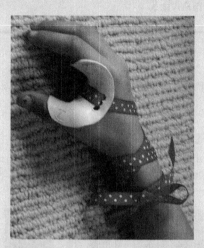

FIGURE PP1–63 Using ribbon as way to secure orthosis. (Photo courtesy of Jill Peck-Murray.)

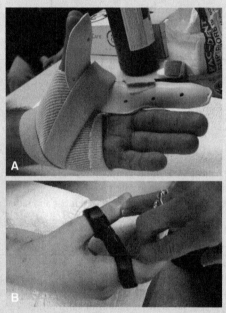

FIGURE PP1–64 **A,** Including full length of IF for better purchase; notice figure-of-8 strap around wrist. **B,** Another option for increased functional use while maintain "stretch" on the web space is this "ring-type" design. Note no strapping is necessary.

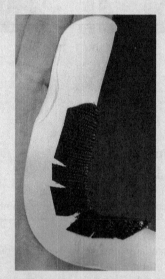

FIGURE PP1–65 Feathered hook in web space area to allow full contact.

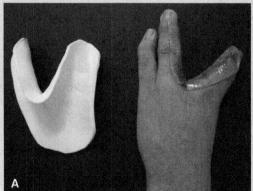 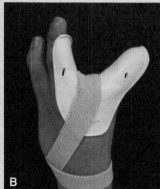 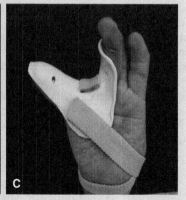

FIGURE PP1–66 **A–C,** Gel beneath orthosis used after web space reconstruction procedure. Note the widened middle portion of this pattern to achieve better purchase and stability on the hand.

CLINICAL PEARL 1–28

Thumb Post Orthosis

For patients without a thumb (congenital or traumatic), this design provides a functional pinch for light activities of daily living (ADLs) or may act as a temporary mold (pre-prosthesis) to allow the patient to adjust to the use of a prosthetic. This temporary mold may help determine the optimal length and position of a permanent prosthetic. The pattern depends on the level of the amputation or congenital anomaly **(A)**. Products such as elastomer or prosthetic foam instead of thermoplastic material can be used to fabricate the internal spacer **(B)**. The length and width of the post are determined by the amount of amputated thumb—use the unaffected side as a guide. Use ⅛″ material that has maximal rigidity and durability. Remember that this is a functional orthosis and must be able to withstand the rigors of ADLs **(C)**. While molding, maintain the desired thumb post position as the material sets to allow for effective three-point pinch. Because the prosthetic thumb has no sensation, tell the patient to use vision with all thumb activities.

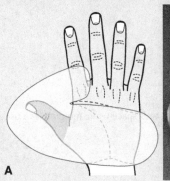
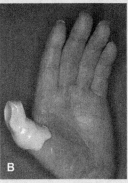
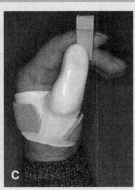

CLINICAL PEARL 1–29

Incorrect Pressure Application to Address First Web Tightness

If pressure is applied distal to the MP joint, stress is placed on the UCL instead of the intended first web space (as shown here). This force may eventually disrupt the UCL. Make sure pressure is applied to the most proximal ulnar portion of the first metacarpal and avoid applying pressure distal to the MP joint.

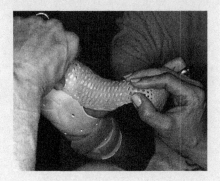

CLINICAL PEARL 1–30

Improving Pressure Distribution Beneath First Web Immobilization Orthosis

Gel products or open cell foams can be used under the orthosis for reducing scar sensitivity and improving pressure distribution **(A)**. Elastomer-type products can also be used to achieve better pressure distribution in such areas. Here, a previously molded 3/32″ perforated material is being applied over soft, curing elastomer **(B)**. Such curing materials can be made to seep through the holes in a perforated material, providing a way to secure the product onto the thermoplastic **(C)**. These products work well for patients who have undergone a first web space surgical release by incorporating the known benefits of scar management and maintaining the desired range of motion. **D,** A removable thermoplastic web "spacer" is applied over a thumb cast. Note the neoprene strapping which assists in adequately securing the web immobilization orthosis onto the cast.

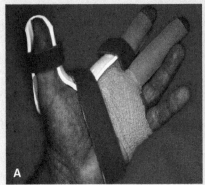
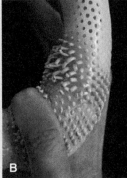
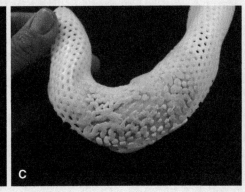
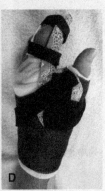

CLINICAL PEARL 1–31

First Web Space "Handshake Hold" Molding Technique

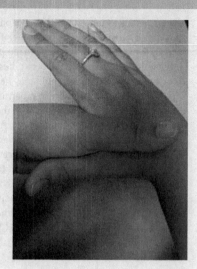

A great technique to maintain maximal stretch of the first web space while molding is to use a "handshake" hold (web space to web space) while applying the material.

3 Forearm-Based Orthoses

DORSAL WRIST IMMOBILIZATION ORTHOSIS (WHO) (Fig. 1–21)

COMMON NAMES

- Dorsal wrist cock-up splint
- Dorsal wrist support
- Wrist extension splint
- Static wrist splint
- Radial bar wrist splint

ALTERNATIVE OPTIONS

- Prefabricated wrist orthosis
- Cast
- Zipper design orthosis

PRIMARY FUNCTIONS

- Immobilize wrist joint to allow healing, rest, or protection of involved structures(s).

ADDITIONAL FUNCTIONS

- Substitute for weak or absent wrist extensor muscle function.
- Improve functional grasp and pinch by positioning wrist in extension and maximizing mechanical advantage of finger flexors.
- Provide base for outrigger attachment when fabricating digit extension mobilization orthoses.

Common Diagnoses	General Optimal Positions
Carpal tunnel syndrome	0°
Median and/or ulnar nerve repair	0°–15° flexion
Radial nerve palsy	20°–35° extension

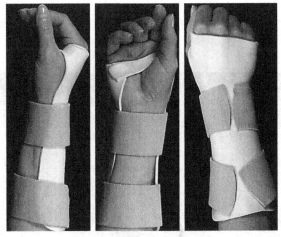

FIGURE 1–21

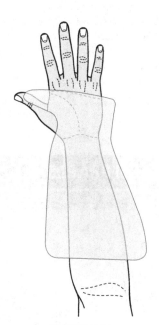

FIGURE 1–22

FABRICATION PROCESS

Pattern Creation (Fig. 1–22)

- Consider dorsal design for patients who are not comfortable in volar design.
- Dorsal design allows for better sensory input to palm than does volar design.
- Good design for patients with volar skin grafts, wounds, pins, or hypersensitive scars.
- Remember that this design may not provide necessary strength to immobilize wrist completely; volar thumbhole design is a better option for maximizing wrist immobilization.
- Mark for proximal border two-thirds length of forearm.
- Mark distal border just proximal to MCP joints.

- Distal radial tab (palmar bar) should be long enough (approximately 3″) to traverse through palm and secure on distal ulnar border.
- Tab should incorporate oblique angle from index to SF metacarpal heads.
- Mark thumb clearance by making arc from thumb MP to base of first CMC joint.
- Allow enough material to encompass two-thirds circumference of forearm, remembering that forearm tapers distally.

Refine Pattern

- Proximal border should allow full elbow motion.
- Distal border should allow unimpeded motion of digital MCP and thumb joints.
- Provide appropriate amount of material within palmar surface to support arches adequately.

Options for Materials

- Consider ⅛″ thermoplastic material to provide needed rigidity to maintain wrist position.
- If patient has difficulty maintaining wrist extension (e.g., secondary to radial nerve injury), consider uncoated materials or those that are slightly tacky to help prevent material from slipping and to make it easier to position patient and mold the orthosis.
- Gel- or foam-lined materials help provide dorsal wrist scar compression, decrease distal migration, and increase comfort.
- Consider perforated material when orthosis will be used during activity or in conjunction with scar-management products such as elastomer. Scar products seep through perforations, which helps anchor them into the orthosis.

Cut and Heat

- Position patient with elbow resting on table and forearm pronated for gravity-assisted molding. Position thumb in palmar abduction.
- Prepad ulnar styloid with adhesive-backed foam, putty, cotton ball, or silicone gel.

Evaluate Fit While Molding

- Position material on dorsum of involved hand and wrist just proximal to MCP joints.
- Place radial bar through thumb web and guide rest of bar along palmar surface just proximal to DPC, overlapping and securing on distal ulnar border (pull material if needed for increased length).
- Carefully incorporate arches of hand by using smooth, even strokes and constantly redirecting material into arches. Continual molding over volar bar is mandatory to prevent negative effects of gravity.

- Do not grab proximal region or try to secure with tight circumferential bandage. This may cause borders to irritate skin. Instead, allow gravity to assist in forming forearm trough.
- Make sure desired wrist position is maintained. Some patients tend to flex and deviate wrist while orthosis is being formed.

Strapping and Components

- Distal strap: 1″ strap connecting radial bar to distal ulnar border.
- Middle strap: (Key Strap!) 2″ strap just proximal to dorsal wrist crease; use piece of adhesive foam to further stabilize wrist and prevent migration. Foam should not overlap edges.
- Proximal strap: 2″ soft or elasticized strap is good choice, especially if patient will use orthosis for functional purposes. Such straps can better accommodate changes in forearm bulk during movement than traditional loop strap.

Survey Completed Orthosis

- Smooth and slightly flare borders.
- Gently flare around dorsal thumb region; avoid rolling, which can make future modifications difficult.
- Check clearance of elbow, radial and ulnar styloid processes, thumb, and MCP joints.
- Pay careful attention to index metacarpal, which frequently abuts radial tab as it traverses through first web space.
- Check for compression over radial and ulnar sensory nerve branches.

 PATTERN PEARLS 1-67 TO 1-70

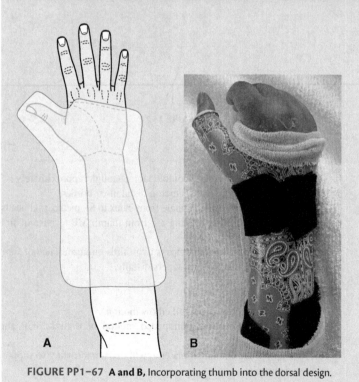

FIGURE PP1-67 A and B, Incorporating thumb into the dorsal design.

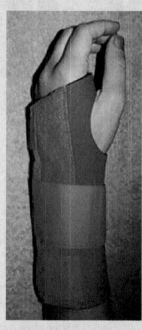

FIGURE PP1-68 Prefabricated wrist orthosis with dorsal stay as an alternative (Freedom® CTS Grip-Fit™ Splint by Alimed, Dedham, MA).

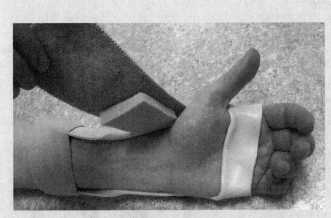

FIGURE PP1–69 Soft foam can assist in securing wrist position.

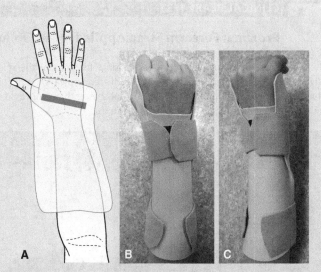

FIGURE PP1–70 **A–C,** A volar/dorsal design.

CLINICAL PEARL 1–32

Prepadding of the Ulnar Styloid

Adhesive foam can be used to prepad the ulnar styloid process before an orthosis is applied **(A)**. Dab the adhesive side of the foam a few times on a towel to decrease the tackiness and make removal more comfortable for the patient. Apply and gently mold the orthosis. Once the thermoplastic material has cooled, remove the padding from the skin and invert back onto the orthosis **(B)**. **C–F,** Alternative method that makes removal from thermoplastic in future easier if required.

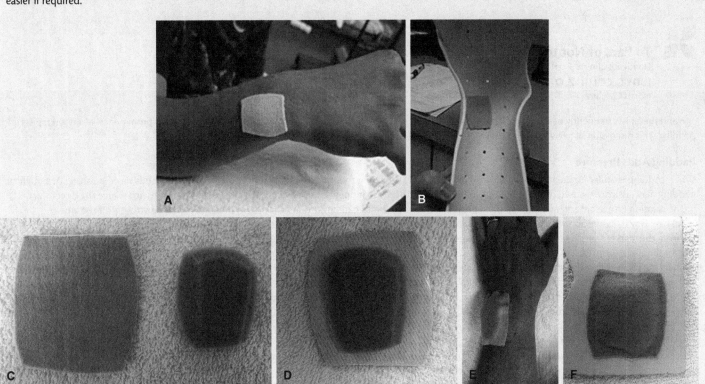

CLINICAL PEARL 1–33

Proximal Forearm Strap Applied on an Oblique Angle

To apply a strap appropriately around the proximal forearm, the therapist must appreciate the tapered shape of this region. Straps should be applied with a slight angle to avoid shear stress as shown by the red arrow **(A)** on the forearm tissue and achieve contour about the musculature. Soft or elasticized straps may contour and accommodate for forearm bulk better than more rigid straps **(B)**. **C,** Notice how adhesive hook is placed on angled strap in a "V" formation versus horizontally applied in circumferential strap.

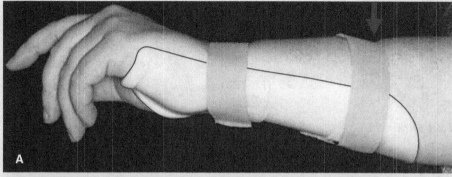

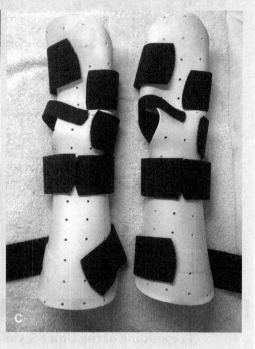

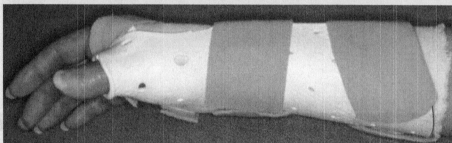

EXPERT PEARL 1–15

To Pad, or Not to Pad...That is the Question!
HandLab: Clinical Pearls
JUDY C. COLDITZ, OT/L, CHT, FAOTA
North Carolina

Hand therapists frequently need to modify orthoses to relieve pressure of an edge or pressure from an underlying bony prominence. Many therapists add padding. This discussion of a few basic principles may be of value to less experienced clinicians.

Padding Adds Pressure

When padding is added to an area of the orthosis that is already providing too much pressure, the additional padding adds more pressure! Although the padding may dissipate focused pressure (example: sharp edge of orthosis), it does not remove pressure and thus often does not relieve the discomfort.

The solution is to avoid adding padding to the pressure area; instead, add padding around the area of pressure to lift the orthosis off the area.

An easy way to assure accuracy is to mark the location of the pressure point on the patient's skin with a marker and then quickly apply the orthosis so the ink from the marker transfers to the inside of the orthosis. This mark defines the location around which padding should be added (or perhaps just proximally and/or distally).

There are many different types of padding, a discussion of which is beyond the scope of this Clinical Pearl. Suffice it to say that the padding must not be soft enough that it will compress so it no longer "lifts" the orthosis off the pressure point.

The ideal, however, is to heat the orthotic material and either slightly roll the edge or create a bubble shape over the bony prominence so the orthosis no longer touches the pressure area.

Padding Reduces Stability

The more intimately an orthosis fits the contours of the underlying body part, the greater the ability of the orthosis to stay in place. When padding is added, and especially when excessive padding is added, the orthosis is lifted away from the underlying contour and loses critical stability. For this reason, if padding is used at all, it should be the absolute minimal amount necessary. If extensive padding is required for comfort, a new orthosis is likely indicated.

(Continued)

Most Padding is Unhygienic and Difficult to Remove

Adding adhesive backed padding material to the interior of an orthosis is inviting moisture and germs. Removing and replacing adhesive backed padding is often unsuccessful and at best leaves a sticky residue.

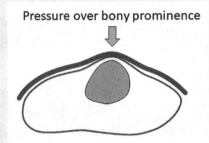

Pressure over bony prominence

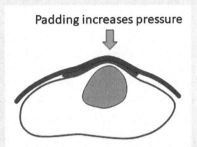

Padding increases pressure

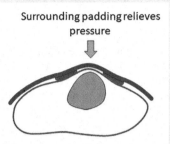

Surrounding padding relieves pressure

If the orthosis cannot be modified to relieve pressure and padding is indicated, the use of removable, washable padding may be the solution.

One method is to affix a narrow sliver of adhesive backed hook on the inside of the orthosis at the desired location of the padding and adhere the padding to the hook. One must use a padding material with a surface compatible with the adhesive hook. Neoprene materials that have a hook compatible side and some soft strapping materials can be used as removable padding.

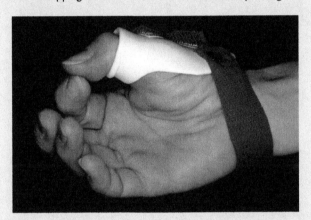

Orthosis to block thumb MP joint flexion creates pressure over the dorsum of the MP joint.

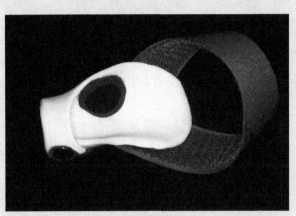

Small neoprene pad is positioned proximal to the MP joint and kept in place with a thin piece of adhesive hook. The pad is removable and washable.

The adhesive hook is kept to the absolute minimum amount to minimize bulk; all that is needed is enough to hold the padding in place. The patient can be given additional replacement pads, and/or the patient can remove, wash, and replace the pads.

Best Solution: No Padding

Of course, the ideal solution is to avoid the need for padding. One suggestion is to identify all potential areas of pressure and raise the contour of these areas before molding the orthosis. One technique is the use of relatively firm exercise putty. (Soft putty will not retain its shape when orthotic material is molded over it.)

Take a small amount of firm putty and roll it into a small ball (or a tube shape, if appropriate.) Place the shape over the prominence and gently smooth the putty so there is a soft transition. Place the warm orthotic material over the putty, molding the orthosis. When the orthosis has cooled, remove the putty so there is space between the material and the underlying contour.

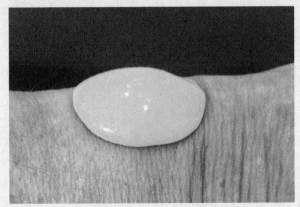

Smoothed putty over the distal ulna prominence creates extra space when the orthotic material is molded.

Clinical Pearls reprinted with permission from Clinician's Classroom at BraceLab.com written by Judy Colditz OT/L CHT FAOTA, copyright HandLab/BraceLab, Raleigh NC. No. 48, January 2018.

EXPERT PEARL 1–16

Carpal Tunnel Orthosis

DEBBIE FISHER, MS, OTR, CHT
Texas

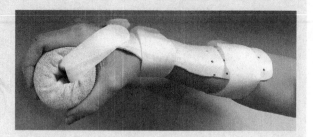

An inexpensive way to minimize lumbrical excursion for night orthosis to address carpal tunnel syndrome: cut swim noodle about the size of the palm of the hand and cover it with stockinette. Next, feed a piece of loop through the noodle and attach it to hook dorsally. This can be easily applied for night use or inconjunction with a prefabricate orthosis as well.

VOLAR WRIST IMMOBILIZATION ORTHOSIS (WHO) (Fig. 1–23)

COMMON NAMES

- Wrist cock-up splint
- Thumbhole wrist splint
- Wrist gauntlet splint
- Palmar wrist cock-up splint
- Static wrist splint
- Wrist drop splint

ALTERNATIVE OPTIONS

- Prefabricated wrist orthosis
- Cast
- Zipper design orthosis

PRIMARY FUNCTIONS

- Immobilize wrist joint to allow healing, rest, and/or protection of involved structures(s).

ADDITIONAL FUNCTIONS

- Statically position wrist flexion contracture at maximum extension to facilitate lengthening of tissue (mobilization).
- Substitute for weak or absent wrist extensor muscle function.
- Improve functional grasp and pinch by positioning wrist in extension and maximizing mechanical advantage of finger flexors.
- Provide base for outrigger attachment when fabricating mobilization orthoses.

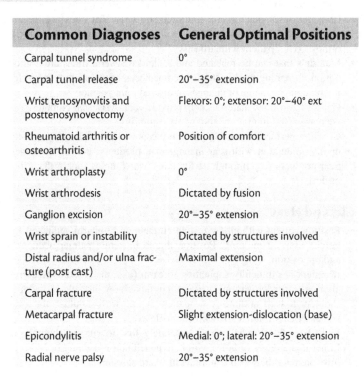

Common Diagnoses	General Optimal Positions
Carpal tunnel syndrome	0°
Carpal tunnel release	20°–35° extension
Wrist tenosynovitis and posttenosynovectomy	Flexors: 0°; extensor: 20°–40° ext
Rheumatoid arthritis or osteoarthritis	Position of comfort
Wrist arthroplasty	0°
Wrist arthrodesis	Dictated by fusion
Ganglion excision	20°–35° extension
Wrist sprain or instability	Dictated by structures involved
Distal radius and/or ulna fracture (post cast)	Maximal extension
Carpal fracture	Dictated by structures involved
Metacarpal fracture	Slight extension-dislocation (base)
Epicondylitis	Medial: 0°; lateral: 20°–35° extension
Radial nerve palsy	20°–35° extension

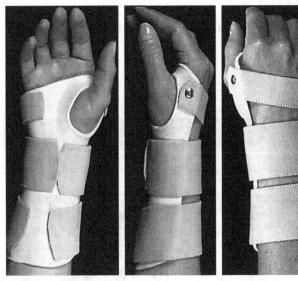

FIGURE 1–23

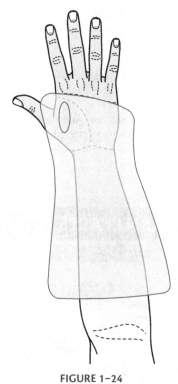

FIGURE 1–24

FABRICATION PROCESS

Pattern Creation (Fig. 1–24)

- Mark for proximal border two-thirds length of forearm.
- Mark for distal border at palmar crease.
- Incorporate oblique angle that traverses from index to small metacarpal heads.
- Mark for thumbhole in distal radial portion of pattern, approximately 1″ down and in.
- Allow enough material to encompass two-thirds circumference of forearm, remembering that forearm tapers distally.

Refine Pattern

- Proximal border should allow full elbow motion.
- To maximize leverage, distal border should end at DPC and thenar region should be cleared enough to allow opposition to index and MFs, clearing approximately two-thirds of thenar region.
- For average adult, thumbhole should be about the size of elongated half dollar. When measuring pattern on patient, hole should lie approximately over thumb MP joint.
- Provide appropriate width of material within first web space to support thumb position and provide adequate surface area for strap application dorsally.

Options for Materials

- Material selection depends on orthotic requirements.
- Consider ⅛″ thermoplastic material to provide needed rigidity to support an unstable ligamentous injury or postoperative repair.
- Consider 3/32″ material for immobilizing wrist that does not require rigid support or for patients who will not place high demands on the orthosis (e.g., patient with arthritis).
- Materials that can be reheated and remolded several times are a good option if ongoing modifications become necessary to accommodate for fluctuations in edema or changes in desired joint position.
- Gel- or foam-lined materials help provide volar wrist scar compression, decrease distal migration, and increase comfort.
- Consider perforated material when orthosis will be used during activity or in conjunction with scar management products such as elastomer. Scar products seep through perforations, which helps anchor them into orthosis.

Cut and Heat

- Position patient with elbow resting on table and forearm supinated for gravity-assisted molding. Position thumb in gentle palmar abduction and opposition.
- If patient has difficulty supinating forearm (e.g., distal radius fractures after cast immobilization), have patient flex elbow on table and adduct shoulder toward midline or lie patient supine with shoulder abducted and externally rotated 90° with elbow flexed.
- Fully heat distal/radial corner separately first to cut out thumbhole. Either make series of holes with hole punch before heating or by carefully piercing the warm material with sharp scissors.

Evaluate Fit While Molding

- Heat full pattern and lay warm material on towel, positioning thumbhole on correct side of material as if material were to be placed on supinated forearm.
- Using IFs, gently open hole, slightly enlarging and elongating it (making it egg shaped); avoid rolling. Use borders of thenar crease as landmarks for length and width of hole.
- Place thumbhole over thumb and guide rest of material evenly along volar wrist and forearm, keeping distal edge just proximal to DPC.

- Gravity tends to pull material away from hand dorsally (elongating thumbhole); continually reposition material as needed.
- Do not grab proximally or try to secure with tight circumferential bandage. This may cause borders to irritate skin. Instead, allow gravity to assist in forming forearm trough.
- Carefully incorporate arches of hand by using smooth, even strokes and constantly redirecting material into arches. Avoid strongly molding into arches, which may cause significant discomfort in palm once material has set.
- Rotate forearm into pronated position at end of molding to check for clearance of ulnar and radial styloid processes; flare about styloids as necessary.
- Make sure desired wrist position is maintained. Some patients tend to flex and ulnarly deviate wrist while orthosis is being formed.
- Caution should be taken when moving the forearm in order to correctly position the wrist. Occasionally, the forearm trough can get "twisted" through the distal molding process.

Strapping and Components

- Distal strap: 1″ strap directed from radial dorsal web area to distal ulnar border. Strip of adhesive foam can be used under strap to further stabilize metacarpals.
- Middle strap: (Key Strap!) 2″ strap just proximal to dorsal wrist crease; use piece of adhesive foam to further stabilize wrist and prevent migration. Foam should lie directly over ulnar styloid and should not overlap edges.
- Proximal strap: Depending on size of forearm, 1″ or 2″ strap may suffice; strap should have slight volar to dorsal angle.

Survey Completed Orthosis

- Smooth and slightly flare distal and proximal borders.
- Gently flare around thenar hole; avoid rolling, which can make future modifications difficult.
- Check clearance of elbow, radial and ulnar styloid processes, thumb, and finger MCP joints.
- Pay careful attention to index metacarpal, which frequently abuts radial portion as it traverses through first web space.

 PATTERN PEARLS 1–71 TO 1–74

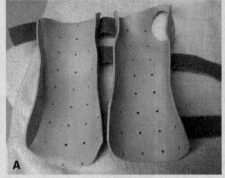 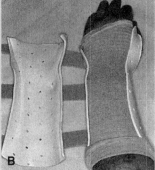 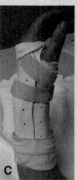 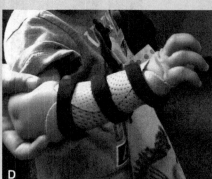

FIGURE PP1–71 A and B, Clamshell design: dorsal material applied to simulate a circumferential orthosis or cast. **C,** Secured wrist immobilization, clamshell design on this patient with a Barton fracture. **D,** A pediatric patient with a circumferential "clamshell-like" orthosis used to protect a greenstick fracture.

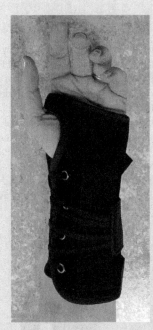

FIGURE PP1–72 Prefabricated wrist orthosis with hard stay (Suede Wrist Lacer Splint shown by Corflex, Manchester, NH).

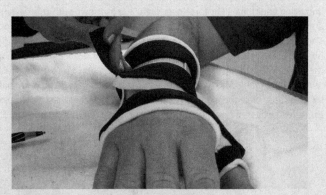

FIGURE PP1–73 Soft padding over the middle strap can assist in stabilization of wrist position.

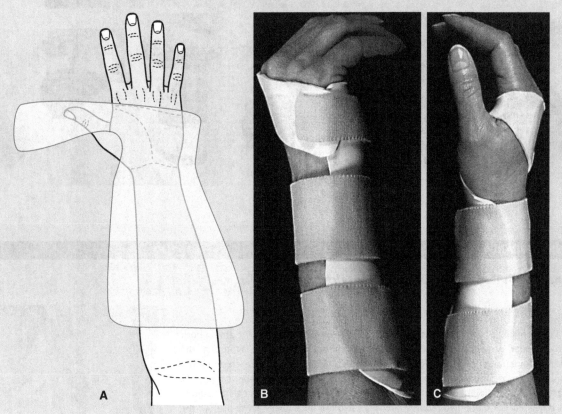

FIGURE PP1–74 **A–C,** Alternative pattern with wide dorsal segment to increase stability and pressure distribution.

CLINICAL PEARL 1–34

Alternative Methods for Securing Straps

A, Riveting straps helps secure and maintain the strap position and prevent the strap from falling off, especially in small areas where it may be difficult to adhere hook material. Always apply a thin lining material, such as Moleskin, on the underside of the rivet to avoid skin irritation (see Clinical Pearl 1–40 for further instruction). **B and C,** Alternatively, a strap can be riveted with the strapping material resting against the skin side. For many patients, this can be advantageous, imparting additional light force over the tissue as shown with this deviated rheumatoid wrist. **D and E,** Another method is to apply adhesive hook volar and dorsal on the radial web thumbhole segment. Direct the strap from the volar hook to the dorsal hook and then over to the ulnar border and rest the strap down. This method allows the clinician to use the full surface area about the thumbhole, which can often be challenging. Soft strapping material is recommended. **F,** A homemade rivet can also be made to secure strap. Fabricate out of thermoplastic material by heating a scrap piece of thermoplastic and forming into a small ball the size of a pea, and then hyperheat this over a heat gun. Prepare the attachment site surface for bonding by scratching the area and/or brushing with solvent to remove any coating. Make a hole through the strap and apply the warm ball through the hole and onto the orthosis. Be careful to correctly position and align the strap because once the material hardens, it is not easily adjusted. **G,** Note rivet and the dorsal wrist split strap with foam to add security to this orthosis. **H,** Note the adhesive backed hook that lies under the neoprene strap to further adhere and prevent migration of the neoprene material over the rivet.

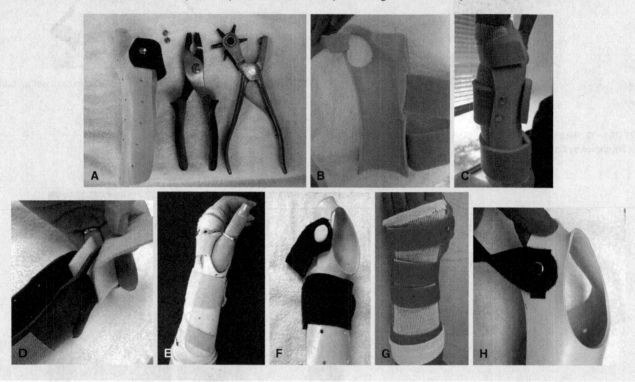

CLINICAL PEARL 1–35

Clearance of Radial and Ulnar Styloid Processes

Near the end of the molding process of an orthosis that includes the forearm, place the arm in both a pronated and supinated positions to check for clearance of the styloid processes. Note that the forearm muscle bulk orientation changes as the forearm rotates. Using IFs, gently reach under the slightly warm material and pull out or lift along the styloids **(A and B)**. When using elastic materials, constant redirecting or reminding the material is necessary. For plastic materials, one gentle adjustment is all that is needed. For more rigid rubber materials, a stronger lift is necessary to achieve the desired clearance.

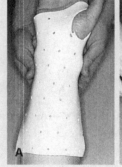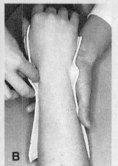

CLINICAL PEARL 1-36

Thumbhole Preparation Prior to Application

A, Heat radial-distal corner fully in preparation for cutting hole—this will prevent jagged edges and allow full control of material. **B,** Pierce material with quality scissors and use long and deep strokes as you cut out the thumb hole—rotating the material gently. **C,** Place material back in pan to uniformly heat and as soon as the material is removed from the water, place on smooth surface and gently elongate the hole into an oval shape oriented longitudinally (not in a circle, which is not the ideal shape to fit about the thenar region—this will get "stuck" at the MP joint). The therapist must take caution not to overstretch the material.

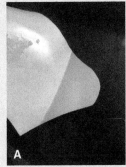 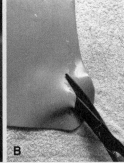 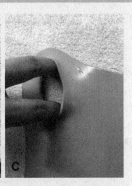

CLINICAL PEARL 1-37

Light Tip Pinch to Incorporate Palmar Arches

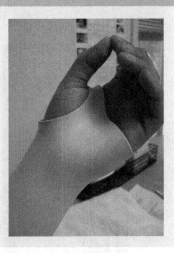

To improve incorporating the arches of the hand within an orthosis, have the patient very lightly oppose to their index finger or hold a piece of cotton (or like material). This technique can be used with many volar and circumferential orthoses to help achieve an intimate fit in the hand, improving comfort and maximizing functional use. Do not let patient pinch too hard because this may exaggerate thumb opposition, especially with thumb orthoses, because the "firing" of thenar muscles will make the orthosis too loose when the muscles are then relaxed.

CLINICAL PEARL 1-38

Preventing Buckling of Material About the Thumb

To prevent buckling radially **(A)** of material dorsally when fabricating the thumbhole wrist orthosis, consider the following points: (1) Do not overheat the thermoplastic material; (2) do not make the thumbhole too big; (3) when placing the heated material on the hand, think "distal and ulnar" and do not position the thumbhole too far radially (the hole should allow visualization of approximately two-thirds of thenar eminence) and should lie distally just under the distal palmar crease **(B)**; and (4) during the molding process, gently and continually reposition the dorsal piece against the skin to counteract the effects of gravity.

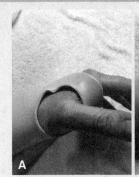 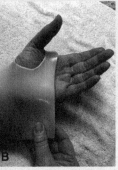

CLINICAL PEARL 1-39

Reinforcing Volar Portion of the Orthosis

A strip of thermoplastic material or thermoplastic tape can be used to reinforce potential areas of weakness within an orthosis. To reinforce an orthosis fabricated with a coated thermoplastic material, the therapist must first remove the coating with solvent or by vigorously scratching the surface.

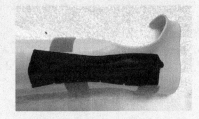

ULNAR WRIST IMMOBILIZATION ORTHOSIS (WHO) (Fig. 1–25)

COMMON NAMES

- Ulnar gutter splint

ALTERNATIVE OPTIONS

- Prefabricated wrist orthosis
- Cast

PRIMARY FUNCTIONS

- Immobilize wrist joint to allow healing of involved structure(s).

ADDITIONAL FUNCTIONS

- Maximize radial hand function while immobilizing ulnar side of hand.

Common Diagnoses	General Optimal Positions
RF or SF metacarpal fracture (base)	Wrist: 0°–20° extension; RD and UD: 0°
Lunate, triquetrum, or hamate	Wrist: 0°–20° extension; RD and UD: 0° instability or fracture
Triangular fibrocartilage	Wrist: 0°; RD and UD: 0° complex (TFCC) injury or repair
Extensor carpi ulnaris tenosynovitis	Wrist: 0°–20° extension with slight UD
Flexor carpi ulnaris tenosynovitis	Wrist: 0° with slight UD
Ulnar nerve compression at Guyon canal	Wrist: 0° with slight UD

FIGURE 1–25

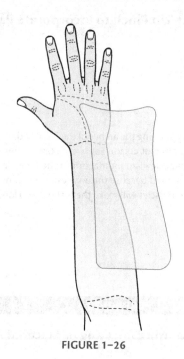

FIGURE 1–26

FABRICATION PROCESS

Pattern Creation (Fig. 1–26)

- Mark for proximal border two-thirds length of forearm.
- Mark distal border at DPC of MF to SF.
- Incorporate oblique angle that traverses from index to small metacarpal heads.
- Mark for thenar crease from MP flexion crease between IF and MF and base of CMC joint.
- Allow enough material to encompass two-thirds circumference of forearm, remembering that forearm tapers distally.

Refine Pattern

- Proximal border should allow full elbow motion.
- Distal border should allow unimpeded motion of MCP joints and full thumb mobility.

Options for Materials

- Consider ⅛″ thermoplastic material to provide needed rigidity to support unstable ligamentous injury or healing fracture.
- If patient has difficulty achieving gravity-assisted position, consider uncoated materials or those that are slightly tacky to help prevent material from slipping and to make it easier to position patient and mold orthosis.
- Gel- or foam-lined materials may help with molding over ulnar styloid and bony dorsum, decrease distal migration, and increase comfort.

Cut and Heat

- While material is heating, prepad ulnar styloid using self-adhesive padding or silicone gel.
- Position extremity with patient supine with shoulder and elbow flexed to 90° (ulnar aspect of hand facing ceiling) or with patient sitting with shoulder flexed to 90° and elbow flexed fully; radial side of hand (thumb) should be pointing toward floor.

Evaluate Fit While Molding

- Drape warm material centrally over ulnar border of forearm and hand, making sure palmar material lies along thenar crease and just proximal to DPC.
- Gently flare material along distal borders.
- If addressing RF or SF proximal metacarpal fracture, completely incorporate MF metacarpal to anchor orthosis and prevent mobility of ulnar two metacarpals.
- Do not grab proximally or try to secure with tight circumferential bandage. This may cause borders to irritate skin. Instead, allow gravity to assist in forming forearm trough.
- Carefully incorporate arches of hand by using smooth, even strokes and constantly redirecting material into arches.
- When material is almost set, gently rotate forearm to check for clearance of ulnar styloid. Styloid becomes more prominent with forearm rotation; if space is not incorporated when molding, ulnar styloid irritation may occur during functional use. If patient complains of abutment, carefully push out material, forming small bubble.
- Make sure desired wrist position is maintained. Some patients tend to flex and deviate wrist while orthosis is being formed.

Strapping and Components

- Distal strap: 1″ strap, trimmed to contour around first web space, is directed from volar radial to dorsal radial border. Consider riveting strap on volar surface to secure strap firmly and decrease bulk within palm.
- Middle strap: 2″ strap just proximal to dorsal wrist crease; use piece of adhesive foam to further stabilize wrist and prevent migration (avoid excessive compression over radial sensory nerve).
- Proximal strap: Depending on size of forearm, 1″ or 2″ strap may suffice; strap should have slight volar to dorsal angle.

Survey Completed Orthosis

- Smooth and slightly flare all borders.
- Check clearance of elbow, thumb, and MCP joints.

PATTERN PEARLS 1–75 AND 1–76

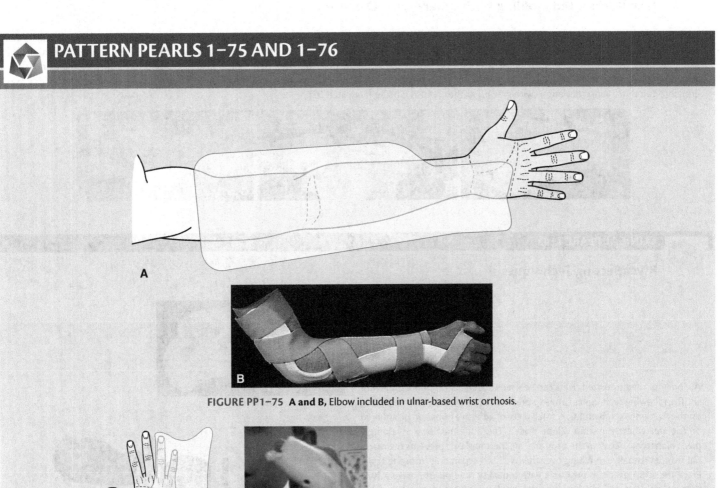

FIGURE PP1–75 **A and B,** Elbow included in ulnar-based wrist orthosis.

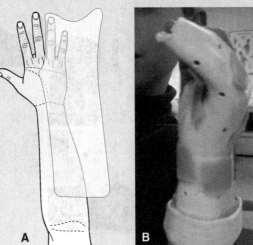

FIGURE PP1–76 **A and B,** RF and SF included in ulnar-based wrist orthosis.

CLINICAL PEARL 1–40

Ulnar Wrist Immobilization Orthosis for External Fixator

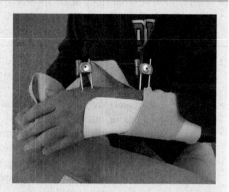

Commonly, patients are referred for a wrist orthosis to be worn in conjunction with an external fixator to provide added support to the wrist, improve comfort, and protect the arm from inadvertent external forces. Because the patient is unable to rotate the arm freely to achieve a gravity-assisted position, the therapist must use an alternative approach. Lay the patient supine with the elbow and shoulder flexed to achieve the desired gravity-assisted position for molding (see Clinical Pearl 1–39 for further instruction). Straps should be applied carefully and thoughtfully. Avoid strap contact with the pin sites, which can be sensitive and prone to skin irritation and infection. Be meticulous when trimming the straps to obtain a comfortable fit. As an alternative, circumferential wraps can be used to secure the orthosis on the arm; this is especially beneficial if edema is an issue.

CLINICAL PEARL 1–41

Gravity-Assisted Molding With Ulnar-Based Orthoses

When fabricating an ulnar-based orthosis, it can be quite helpful to have the patient place the arm in a gravity-assisted position with the ulnar side of the forearm facing upward parallel to the floor. This position can be achieved in several ways, but commonly it includes either a sitting or supine position. The patient or assistant can hold or rest the radial side of the forearm above or on the head, or the patient can be instructed to support the radial side of the arm out in front of him or her **(A and B)**. Whatever position is chosen when using gravity as an assist, the clinician must be acutely aware of not letting the wrist drop into too much radial deviation (with gravity) as the orthosis is being fabricated **(C)**.

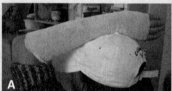
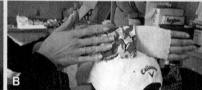
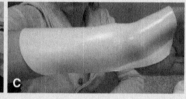

CLINICAL PEARL 1–42

Rivet Setting Techniques

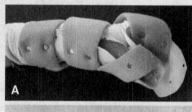

A, Small- or medium-sized rivets can be used to secure straps onto an orthosis. The following techniques can help prevent the loop material from pulling off the rivet once set. **B and C,** A small piece of adhesive hook can be adhered on the area where the strap will be placed. This additional step of adding a piece of material between the strap and the thermoplastic prevents the material from eventually stretching over the rivet and separating from the strap. Place the strap over this area and, with a quality hole punch, make a hole through all three pieces (thermoplastic, hook material, and strap), creating a clean small hole. Place the stem of the rivet on the skin side of the orthosis and push through all three layers. Apply the rivet cap and close together using blunt-nosed pliers. Remember to cover the surface of the rivet that contacts the skin with a thin adhesive lined material (such as Moleskin) to prevent skin irritation. **D,** Another technique to prevent the loop from pulling off includes using a homemade washer made out of thin thermoplastic material. This is placed between the rivet cap and the loop material as shown. This is especially helpful when using a stretchy strapping material.

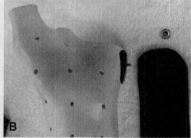
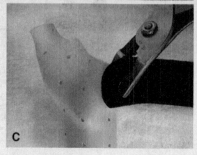
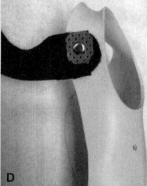

CLINICAL PEARL 1–43

Rivet Removal Techniques

Removal of rivets can be challenging but one needs to know how to get them off if needed. Careful planning of strapping systems is ideal to prevent this occurrence. There are a few techniques to remove rivets that are already fastened to the orthosis. **A,** Utilize pliers to bend the rivet "head" so that it pops off or **(B)** use cutting tool to remove the flat rivet "base."

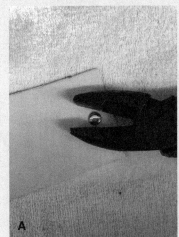
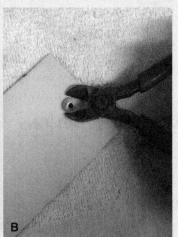

CLINICAL PEARL 1–44

Hole Punch Tips

Over time, hole punches can get dull making it difficult to cut through both thermoplastic and strapping. One trick is to utilize a scrap piece of plastic behind the material you are attempting to put a hole in—this consistently allows for the punch to cut through the top material.

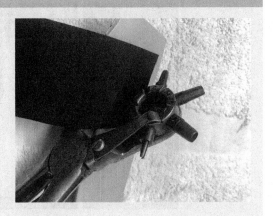

EXPERT PEARL 1–17

Edging Foam
ANNA OVSYANNIKOVA, MD, HAND THERAPY
Russia

A, Tilt the scissors to make the junction of foam padding and thermoplastic materials smoother. Creating an angled 'corner' in the foam; **(B)** Note placement of the foam on the orthosis and the angled edges. This technique allows for thin borders with gradual increase in thickness towards the middle of the pad.

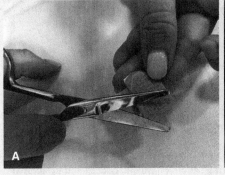
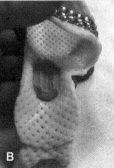

CIRCUMFERENTIAL WRIST IMMOBILIZATION ORTHOSIS (WHO) (Fig. 1–27)

COMMON NAMES

- Wrist fracture brace
- Circumferential wrist splint
- Circumferential wrist cock-up splint
- Circumferential thumbhole wrist splint
- Wrist gauntlet splint

ALTERNATIVE OPTIONS

- Clamshell wrist orthosis
- Cast
- Prefabricated orthosis

PRIMARY FUNCTIONS

- Immobilize wrist joint to allow healing, rest, and/or protection of involved structure(s).

ADDITIONAL FUNCTIONS

- Statically position wrist flexion or extension contracture at maximum length to facilitate lengthening of tissue (mobilization).
- Substitute for weak or absent wrist extensor muscle function.

- Improve functional grasp and pinch by positioning wrist in extension and maximizing mechanical advantage of finger flexors.
- Provide base for outrigger attachment when fabricating digital mobilization orthoses.

Common Diagnoses	General Optimal Positions
Wrist sprain or instability	Dictated by structures involved
Distal radius and/or ulna fracture (post cast)	Maximal extension
Carpal fracture	Dictated by structures involved
Metacarpal fracture or dislocation (base)	Slight extension

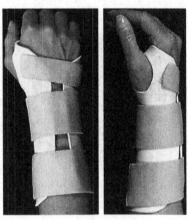

FIGURE 1–27

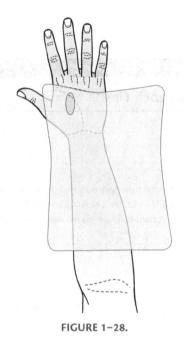

FIGURE 1–28.

FABRICATION PROCESS

Pattern Creation (Fig. 1–28)

- Alternative to clamshell wrist immobilization orthosis.
- Mark for proximal border two-thirds length of forearm.
- Mark for distal border just proximal to DPC.
- Widen pattern proximally, remembering that forearm tapers distally.
- Incorporate oblique angle that traverses from index to small metacarpal heads.
- Mark for thumbhole, located distally and approximately two-thirds from ulnar border; position hole down 1″ from this point.

Refine Pattern

- Proximal border should allow full elbow motion.
- Distal border should allow unimpeded motion of MCP joints and nearly full thumb mobility.
- For average adult, thumbhole should be about the size of elongated half dollar. When measuring pattern on patient, hole should lie approximately over thumb MP joint.

Options for Materials

- Elastic materials are an excellent choice because they tend to stretch easily when heated and provide an intimate fit. Remember that elastic materials tend to shrink around the body part; do not remove until it is completely set.
- Use 3/32″ material, which is adequate for stabilizing forearm; circumferential nature of this design makes it rigid.
- Although 1/8″ material can be used, its thickness increases the rigidity, making it difficult to remove.
- May use 1/16″ material for young children and older adults.
- Lightly perforated materials allow air exchange and increase flexibility, making donning and doffing easier.

Cut and Heat

- Position patient with elbow resting on table and forearm supinated for gravity-assisted molding. Position thumb in palmar abduction and opposition.
- If patient has difficulty supinating forearm, have the patient flex elbow on table and adduct shoulder toward midline or lay patient supine with shoulder abducted and externally rotated 90° with elbow flexed.

- Cut out thumbhole in material either by making a series of holes with hole punch before heating or by carefully piercing the slightly warm material with sharp scissors.
- Prepad ulnar styloid (and radial styloid, if necessary) with adhesive-backed padding or gel.

Evaluate Fit While Molding

- Lay warm material on towel, positioning thumbhole on correct side of material as if it were to be placed on forearm.
- Using IFs, gently open hole, slightly enlarging and elongating it.
- Place thumbhole over thumb (using thenar crease as guide) and gently stretch and guide rest of material evenly.
- Do not grab proximal portion or try to secure with tight circumferential bandage.
- Gently redirect dorsal surface by applying smooth strokes over area.
- Carefully incorporate arches of hand by using smooth, even strokes and constantly redirecting material into arches. Avoid strongly molding into arches, which may cause significant discomfort in palm once material has set.

- Rotate forearm into pronated position at end of molding to check for clearance of ulnar and radial styloid processes.
- Make sure desired wrist position is maintained. Some patients tend to flex and deviate wrist while orthosis is being formed.

Strapping and Components

- Self-adhesive D-ring straps: 1″ strap distally and 2″ straps proximally work well because they allow firm and easy closure. Patient can make adjustments according to comfort.

Survey Completed Orthosis

- Smooth and slightly flare distal and proximal borders as well as thenar hole.
- Check clearance of elbow, radial and ulnar styloid processes, thumb, and finger MCP joints.
- Pay careful attention to index metacarpal, which frequently abuts radial portion as it traverses through first web space.

 PATTERN PEARLS 1–77 TO 1–79

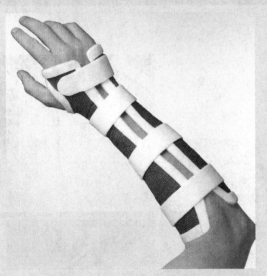

FIGURE PP1–77 Delta-Cast® material used as an alternative. (Photo courtesy of Essity, Charlotte, NC.)

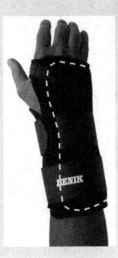

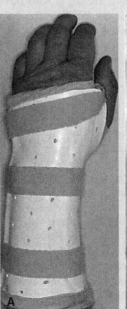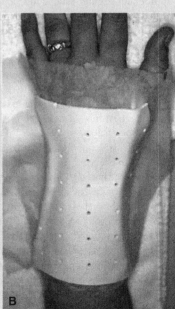

FIGURE PP1–78 A and B, A simple "clamshell" design.

FIGURE PP1–79 Prefabricated wrist orthosis with moldable thermoplastic stay (dotted yellow line). (W-310 Wrist Support shown. Photo courtesy of Benik Corp, Silverdale, WA.)

CLINICAL PEARL 1–45

Circumferential Orthosis as a Base for Mobilization Components

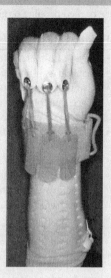

Circumferential designs provide a stable base for attaching mobilization components to address distal issues. Because of the intimate fit provided with this all-encompassing circumferential design, migration can be minimized. Flexion glove used over a Rolyan® Aquaform™ Zippered Wrist Splint to provide a flexion mobilization force to the digits while the wrist is stabilized in extension. This prevents the common compensation problem of the wrist flexing to reduce the stretch on tight digits caused by the flexion force. Component systems, both homemade and commercially available, can also be attached directly to this orthosis.

CLINICAL PEARL 1–46

Zippered Circumferential Wrist Orthosis

A, The Rolyan® AquaForm™ Zippered Wrist Splint (Performance Health) provides another option for a circumferential design. Choose the appropriate size per catalog instructions, keeping in mind that these tend to run large; so, when in doubt, opt for the smaller size because this elastic material stretches. Position the patient with the elbow resting on a table and forearm in neutral. Fully heat and apply the warmed orthosis (material should be completely clear or opaque) with the zippered edge along the dorsal ulnar border, zip it down while keeping the distal border at the DPC—this can be challenging to get the zipper started so if the material starts to set, immediately remove and reheat fully. Because this is elastic material, it will shrink back to the original shape. The distal edge needs to stay as distal as possible, allowing full MCP motion, but do not overclear for the DPC, which can affect the mechanical advantage and allow for wrist motion within the final orthosis. Once zippered, gently place the wrist in desired position by having patient assume a gently opposed posture to capture the arches in the hand. Remember to use the stretch in this material to your advantage; the "shrinking" will provide for a well-contoured final product. While the material sets, gently rotate the forearm from midpronation to midsupination to allow for a small hollowed area to form for the ulnar styloid process. This orthosis is an excellent option for patients who require continued immobilization (e.g., fractures, wrist fusion) yet need to remove the orthosis for protected exercises and hygiene. This is not appropriate for patients presenting with significant or fluctuating edema because of potential circulation issues. This can be tricky to don and doff; be sure to educate the patient and or caregiver on how best to apply. If required, this device can be remolded as needed by reheating the whole orthosis fully; avoid partially heating a small area because the elasticized nature of this material will cause localized shrinkage and possible fit issues. **B–D,** The length can be cut down as needed and a homemade zipper stop fabricated from scrap thermoplastic to prevent the zipper from falling off. Be sure to prepare the proximal on the orthosis with solvent and heat briefly with heat gun to ensure a strong bond.

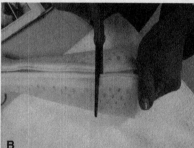

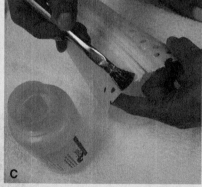

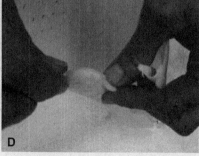

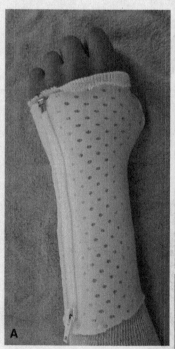

CLINICAL PEARL 1-47

Material With Memory: Using Stretch, Pinch, and Cut Technique

Thin perforated materials with memory and a protective coating have minimal resistance to stretch and can be used for making lightweight circumferential orthoses. Most of these materials can be reheated as often as needed to achieve optimal positioning. Once the material is heated and applied to the hand/forearm, the therapist can gently stretch and pinch the borders together. Once sealed but still warm, the material can be trimmed to form a seam **(A)**. The therapist can leave this sealed or can snap the borders apart (once the material has cooled) and apply straps for closure **(B and C)**. If straps are applied, the borders may be lined with a material such as Moleskin or a stockinette can be applied prior to orthosis application.

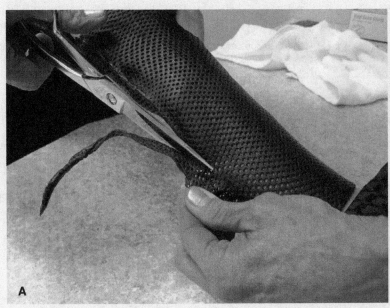
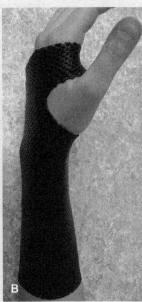
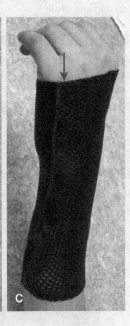

RADIAL WRIST/THUMB IMMOBILIZATION ORTHOSIS (WHFO) (Fig. 1–29)

COMMON NAMES

- Radial gutter splint
- Radial gutter thumb spica splint
- Thumb gauntlet splint
- Radial wrist support
- Long opponens splint

ALTERNATIVE OPTIONS

- Prefabricated wrist and thumb orthosis
- Cast

PRIMARY FUNCTIONS

- Immobilize wrist and thumb joint(s) to allow healing, rest, and/or protection of involved structure(s).

ADDITIONAL FUNCTIONS

- Improve functional pinch by positioning wrist and thumb in optimal positions.

Common Diagnoses	General Optimal Positions
deQuervain tenosynovitis	Wrist: 20° extension; th CMC: between rad and palm abduction; MP: slight flex; IP: included or free, depending on severity
Th UCL reconstruction	Wrist: 20° extension; th CMC: palm abduction; MP: 5° flexion and slight UD
Th RCL reconstruction	Wrist: 20° extension; th CMC: palm abduction; MP: 5° flexion and slight RD
Th scaphotrapeziotrapezoid (STT) or CMC joint arthritis	Wrist: 0°–20° extension; th CMC: between rad and palm abduction; MP: 5°–10° flexion
EPL repair	Wrist: 25°–30° extension; th CMC: rad abduction; MP: extension; IP: slight hyperextension
Tendon transfers for th extension	Wrist: 25°–30° extension; th CMC: rad abduction; IP: slight hyperextension

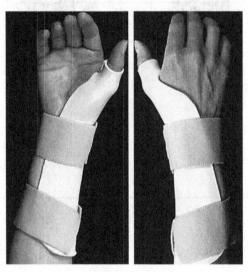

FIGURE 1–29

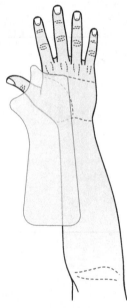

FIGURE 1–30

FABRICATION PROCESS

Pattern Creation (Fig. 1–30)

- Mark proximal border two-thirds length of forearm.
- Mark distal border at IF and MF proximal palmar crease.
- Mark ulnar and radial sides of thumb IP joint.
- Allow enough material to encompass one-half circumference of forearm, remembering that forearm tapers distally.

Refine Pattern

- Proximal border should allow full elbow motion.
- Distal border should allow unimpeded motion of MCP joints and thumb IP flexion.

- Circumferential thumb portion should allow enough material to overlap ½″ to 1″.
- Provide an appropriate amount of material within and dorsal to web space to support thumb position adequately and provide surface area for strap application dorsally.

Options for Materials

- Remember that materials with memory tend to shrink around proximal phalanx; do not remove until completely set.
- Use coated material so material will pop apart once completely cooled, forming trap door to allow for easy donning and doffing.
- Use 1/16″ or 3/32″ material for immobilizing patients with arthritis; this makes for lightweight orthosis with adequate rigidity.
- Gel- or foam-lined materials may help provide radial styloid scar compression, decrease distal migration, and increase comfort.

Cut and Heat

- While material is heating, prepad (with soft adhesive foam, silicone gels) at first dorsal compartment if tender.
- Consider placing light layer of lotion on thumb before molding to ease removal.
- Position patient with elbow resting on table with forearm slightly supinated for gravity-assisted molding.
- Thumb should be positioned per diagnosis. Commonly, position of function is palmar abduction and opposition.

Evaluate Fit While Molding

- Place thumb portion of material on radial proximal phalanx and guide rest of material evenly along radial forearm.
- Carefully contour dorsal section of distal thumb material through web space.
- Gently pull and overlap dorsal thumb material through web space to support proximal phalanx and lightly overlap onto volar piece.
- Avoid direct pressure over radial styloid, STT joint, and dorsal MP joint.

- Do not grab proximally or try to secure with tight circumferential bandage. This may cause borders to irritate skin. Instead, allow gravity to assist in forming forearm trough.
- Carefully incorporate arches of hand by using smooth, even strokes and constantly redirecting material into arches.
- Make sure desired wrist position is maintained. Some patients tend to flex and deviate wrist while orthosis is being formed.

Strapping and Components

- Distal strap: 1″ strap directed from dorsal web area to volar ulnar border.
- Middle strap: 2″ strap just proximal to dorsal wrist crease; use piece of adhesive foam to further stabilize wrist and prevent migration. Foam should lie directly over ulnar styloid and should not overlap edges.
- Proximal strap: Depending on size of forearm, 1″ or 2″ strap may suffice; strap should have slight volar to dorsal angle.

Survey Completed Orthosis

- Smooth and slightly flare all borders and around thumb opening.
- Check clearance of elbow, thumb IP joint, and IF MCP joint flexion.

 PATTERN PEARLS 1–80 TO 1–82

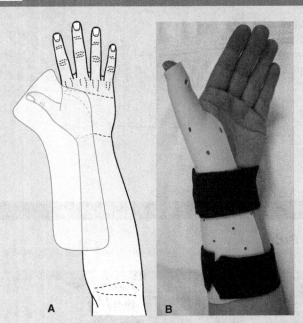

FIGURE PP1–80 **A and B,** IP joint included.

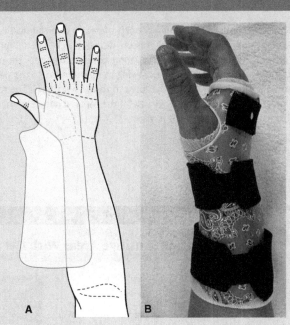

FIGURE PP1–81 **A and B,** MP joint free.

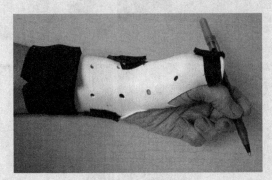

FIGURE PP1–82 Thumb MP and IP joints can be released for light functional use.

CLINICAL PEARL 1–48

Contouring About Wrist

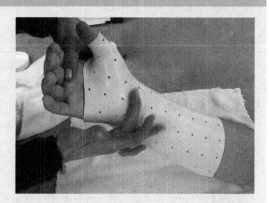

Gentle contouring about the pisiform/ulnar wrist will assist in better orthosis purchase and assist in decreasing distal migration. Choosing a material that drapes well and being sure to heat it fully is key to successfully obtaining this desired contour.

CLINICAL PEARL 1–49

Estimating Material Required to Obtaining Two-Thirds Forearm Circumference

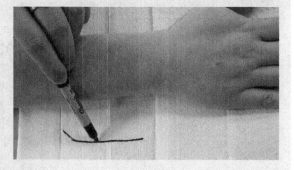

Including two-thirds the circumference of the forearm when fabricating forearm-based orthoses not only provides for maximal pressure distribution but also improves the rigidity of the final orthosis. This generally results in a more comfortable fit for the patient. To estimate the amount of material needed while drawing the pattern, angle the pen at 45° on the dorsal forearm and draw both side of the forearm to the wrist level. The resulting pattern should have more material proximally because of the tapered nature of the musculature, covering approximately two-thirds of the forearm.

CLINICAL PEARL 1–50

Accommodating Sensitive Areas With Gel and Foam Padding

A thin layer of silicone gel can be placed directly over **(A)** or around **(B)** the radial sensory nerve to prevent pressure on a hypersensitive area/scar either postinjury or surgery. This collegiate volleyball player had a custom orthosis fabricated that incorporated the silicone gel (over the radial sensory nerve) and foam padding (over the ulnar styloid) to protect her during play **(B and C)**. Strapping systems can also be modified by cutting out a protective "donut" with adhesive padding to improve comfort as they traverse bony and sensitive areas. Shown is a patient with a hypersensitive scar post–open reduction and internal fixation (ORIF) for a distal ulnar fracture **(D)**. As another alternative, therapy putty can be used to create a "bubble" over the sensitive area or bony prominence. To prevent the putty from sticking to the thermoplastic, apply a thin layer of lotion prior to molding. After the orthosis has set, remove the putty to form the protective bubble.

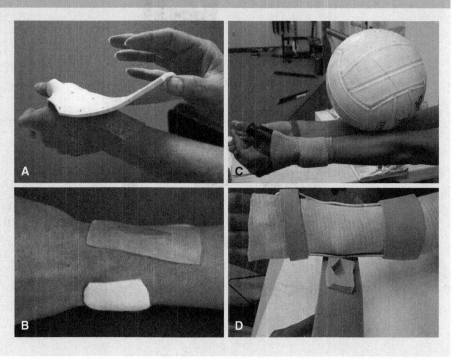

EXPERT PEARL. 1–18

Decorating Orthoses

ANNA OVSYANNIKOVA, MD, HAND THERAPY
Russia

Use dry heat to make the thermoplastic material sticky. Put stickers and scraps of thermoplastic materials to create unique designs for your patient **(A-D)**.

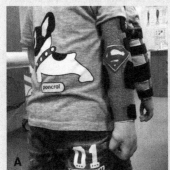
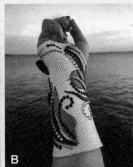
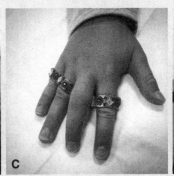
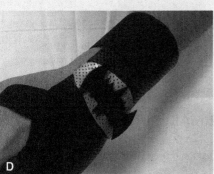

EXPERT PEARL 1–19

Muenster: Ulnar-Based Design Using Woodcast

NIAMH MASTERSON, OT, HAND THERAPIST
Australia

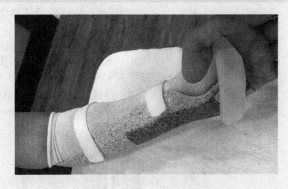

Woodcast is an environmentally friendly product manufactured from wood and biodegradable plastic that can be molded directly to a patient without water or gloves (currently not available in the United States). Additional Woodcast strips can be secured to the base to increase strength over joints such as the wrist and can also help to seal edges and areas where the material has been joined together.

VOLAR WRIST/THUMB IMMOBILIZATION ORTHOSIS (WHFO) (Fig. 1–31)

COMMON NAMES

- Thumb spica splint
- Long opponens splint

ALTERNATIVE OPTIONS

- Prefabricated wrist and thumb orthosis
- Zipper design thumb and wrist orthosis
- Cast
- Silicone rubber orthosis

PRIMARY FUNCTIONS

- Immobilize wrist and thumb joint(s) to allow healing, rest, and/or protection of involved structure(s).

ADDITIONAL FUNCTIONS

- Improve functional pinch by positioning wrist and thumb in optimal positions.

Common Diagnoses	General Optimal Positions
Scaphoid fracture (after cast immobilization)	Wrist: 0°–20° extension; RD and UD: 0°; th: between rad and palm abduction; MP: 10° flexion; IP: free
Bennett fracture (after cast immobilization)	Wrist: 0°–20° extension; RD: 5°; th: 45° rad abduction; MP: 5°–10° flexion
deQuervain tenosynovitis	Wrist: 20° extension; th CMC: between rad and palm abduction; MP: slight flexion; IP: included or free (depends on severity)
Intersection syndrome	Wrist: 20° extension; RD and UD: 0°; th CMC: rad abduction; MP: 5°–10° flexion

Common Diagnoses	General Optimal Positions
Th STT or CMC joint arthritis	Wrist: 0°–20° extension; th CMC: between rad and palm abduction; MP: 5°–10° flexion
STT or CMC/TM arthroplasty	Wrist: 20° extension; RD and UD: 0°; th: between rad and palm abduction; MP: 5°–10° flexion
Lax or mildly subluxed STT joint	Wrist: 0°–20° extension; th CMC: medium palm abduction; MP: slight flexion
EPL repair (th CMC: slight rad abduction)	Wrist: 20°–40° extension; MP: 0°; IP: 0°–5° extension
Extensor pollicis brevis (EPB)	Wrist: 20°–40° extension; thor abductor pollicis CMC: slight rad abduction; MP: 0°longus (APL) repair
Tendon transfers (opponensplasty)	Wrist: 0°; th CMC: medium palm abduction; MP: 5°–10° flexion
Th UCL reconstruction	Wrist: 20° extension; th CMC: palm abduction; MP: 5° flexion with slight UD
Th RCL reconstruction palm	Wrist: 20° extension; th CMC: abduction; MP: 5° flexion with slight RD

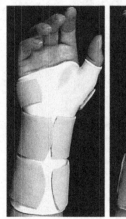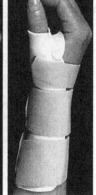

FIGURE 1–31

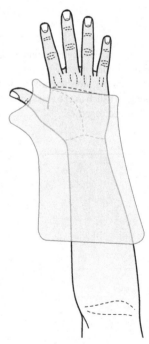

FIGURE 1–32

FABRICATION PROCESS

Pattern Creation (Fig. 1–32)

- Mark proximal border two-thirds length of forearm.
- Mark distal border at thumb IP flexion crease and DPC.
- Allow enough material to encompass one-half to two-thirds circumference of forearm, remembering that forearm tapers distally.

Refine Pattern

- Proximal border should allow full elbow motion.
- Distal border should allow unimpeded motion of IF to SF MCP and thumb IP joint.
- Provide an appropriate amount of material within and dorsal to web space to support thumb position adequately and provide surface area for strap application dorsally.

Options for Materials

- Use drapable material to achieve intimate fit about thumb STT and MP joints to prevent migration and improve comfort.
- Remember that elastic materials tend to shrink around proximal phalanx; do not remove until orthosis is completely set.
- Consider placing light layer of lotion on thumb before molding to ease removal.
- Use coated material to allow material to pop apart once completely cool. This forms trap door for easy donning and doffing.
- Use 1/16″ or 3/32″ material for immobilizing patients with arthritis; this makes for lightweight orthosis with adequate rigidity.
- Consider perforated material when orthosis will be used during activity.

Cut and Heat

- Position patient with elbow resting on table and forearm slightly supinated for gravity-assisted molding.
- Position thumb per diagnosis. Commonly, position of function is gentle palmar abduction and opposition.
- If patient has difficulty supinating forearm (e.g., after cast immobilization), have the patient flex elbow on table and adduct and externally rotate shoulder toward midline.
- Consider prepadding of radial or ulnar styloid if prominent.

Evaluate Fit While Molding

- Lay warm material on towel, positioning thumb portion on correct side of material as if it were going to be placed on supinated forearm.
- Place thumb portion centrally over thumb and guide rest of material evenly along arm.
- Gently pull and overlap volar thumb material through web space to support proximal phalanx and lightly overlap onto dorsal piece. It is important for material to mold through web space to radial side of second metacarpal to provide adequate immobilization.
- Avoid direct pressure over radial styloid, STT joint, and dorsal MP joint.

- Do not grab proximally or try to secure with tight circumferential bandage. This may cause borders to irritate skin. Instead, allow gravity to assist in forming forearm trough.
- While molding, place thumb joints in appropriate position. Have patient gently oppose to IF during the molding process.
- Carefully incorporate arches of hand by using smooth, even strokes and constantly redirecting material into arches.
- Make sure desired wrist position is maintained. Some patients tend to flex and deviate wrist while orthosis is being formed.
- Clear for radial and ulnar styloid, avoiding pressure over radial sensory nerve.
- Once material has cooled completely, pop apart overlapped thumb piece if concerned about doffing difficulty.

Strapping and Components

- Distal strap: 1″ strap directed from radial dorsal web area to volar ulnar border. Use piece of adhesive foam under strap to further stabilize metacarpals if needed.
- Middle strap: 2″ strap just proximal to dorsal wrist crease; use piece of adhesive foam to further stabilize wrist and prevent migration. Foam should lie directly over ulnar styloid and should not overlap edges.
- Proximal strap: Depending on size of forearm, 1″ or 2″ strap may suffice; strap should have slight volar to dorsal angle.
- Apply small ½″ strap across trap door.

Survey Completed Orthosis

- Smooth and slightly flare all borders.
- Check for clearance of radial and ulnar styloids, elbow, thumb IP joint, and finger MCP joints.
- Pay careful attention to IF MCP, which frequently abuts radial portion as it traverses through first web space. If orthosis is to be functional, check that patient can at least touch thumb to index fingertip.
- Make sure that patient does not experience pinching under overlapped thumb portion.

 PATTERN PEARLS 1–83 TO 1–86

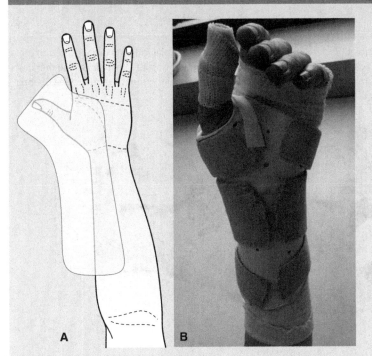

FIGURE PP1–83 A and B, Thumb MP joint free, often used post–scaphoid fracture (note the IP orthosis used for concomitant distal phalanx fracture).

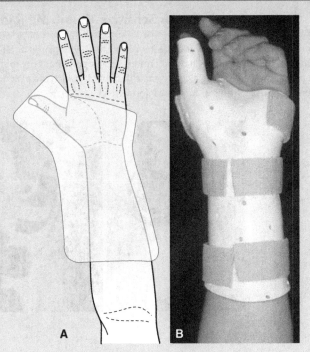

FIGURE PP1–84 A and B, IP joint included.

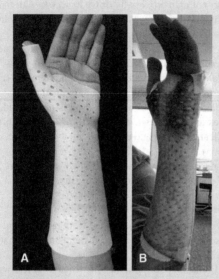
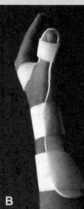

FIGURE PP1–85 Rolyan® AquaForm™ Zippered Wrist and Thumb Splint Zipper with IP included **(A)** and free **(B)** (Performance Health).

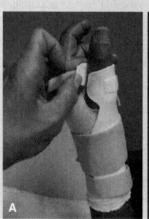
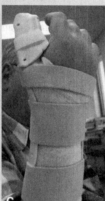
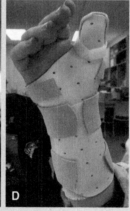

FIGURE PP1–86 A, Trap door for easy donning/doffing and **(B)** optional "open" design to accommodate for edema or healing wounds. **C and D,** Clamshell design for protection of pin and easy access to clean the sites.

 CLINICAL PEARL 1–51

Neoprene Strap for Sensitive Thumb MP Joint

Commonly, there can be irritation of the skin at the thermoplastic distal MP joint border. Alternatively, a soft neoprene volar sling can be fabricated to substitute for a circumferential "hard" thermoplastic support about the thumb column. Neoprene will adhere to warm thermoplastic material so the therapist can be creative in designing a comfortable thumbhole, which the patient can slip on and off with ease and use functionally without irritation. (See Chapter 14 on "Neoprene Orthoses" for more information.)

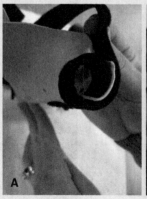
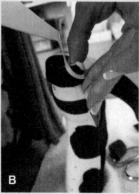
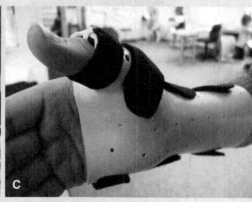

CLINICAL PEARL 1–52

Gentle Traction on Thumb During Molding Process

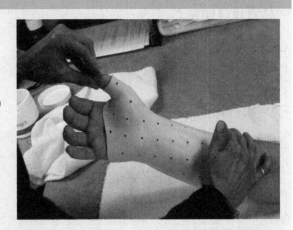

Applying gentle traction distally in the desired direction/position of the thumb will assist in proper molding and minimize undesired "excessive" thumb MP flexion.

EXPERT PEARL 1–20

deQuervain Orthosis
JOANNA JOURDAN, OT
Germany

Allows flexion and extension of the wrist. This limits prolonged thumb and wrist abduction/ulnar deviation and therefore can be used as a conservative solution for this overuse problem **(A and B)**. Utilize thumb nuts to create moveable hinge and uncoated thermoplastic to allow for easy bonding.

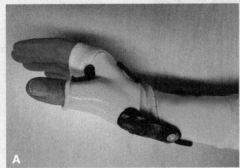

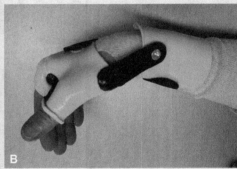

DORSAL WRIST/HAND (OPTIONAL THUMB) IMMOBILIZATION ORTHOSIS (WHFO) (Fig. 1–33)

COMMON NAMES

- Dorsal protective splint
- Dorsal blocking splint
- Extension block splint
- Dorsal shell

ALTERNATIVE OPTIONS

- Cast

PRIMARY FUNCTIONS

- Immobilize wrist, MCP, PIP, and DIP joints in flexion to allow healing of involved structures(s).

ADDITIONAL FUNCTIONS

- Promote early protected active and/or passive motion of repaired tendons to facilitate healing and prevent adherence to surrounding structures (mobilization or restriction).

Common Diagnoses	General Optimal Positions
Optimal positions for tendon and nerve injuries depend on the severity of the injury, the integrity of repaired structures (tendon, nerve, vascular structures, pulleys, and bone), and the physician's rehabilitation protocol. Chapter 19 provides details.	
FDS or FDP tendon repair	Wrist: 0°–45° flexion; MCP: 30°–60° flexion; IP: 0°–30° extension (depending on nerve status)
FPL tendon repair	Wrist: 0°–45° flexion; th CMC: 0°–45° palm abduction; MP: 20°–40° flexion; IP: 0°–20°

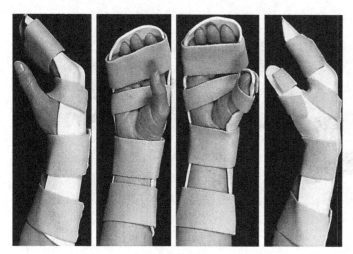

FIGURE 1–33

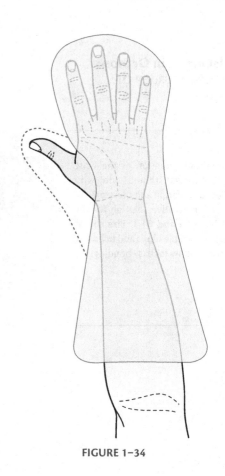

FIGURE 1–34

FABRICATION PROCESS

Pattern Creation (Fig. 1–34)

- Note: Because unimpeded active motion is contraindicated, draw pattern on uninjured hand if possible.
- Mark for proximal border two-thirds length of forearm.
- Mark distal border approximately 1″ distal to fingertips; this additional material is necessary to compensate for flexed position of wrist and MCP joints.
- If thumb is not involved, mark thumb clearance by making an arc from thumb MP to base of first STT joint (using thenar crease as landmark).

- If thumb is involved, mark 1″ distally and allow enough material around borders to support thumb and allow for strap application (dotted line on pattern).
- Allow enough material to encompass two-thirds circumference of forearm, remembering that forearm tapers distally.

Refine Pattern

- Proximal border should allow full elbow motion.
- Distal border should completely protect and cover fingertips (and thumb, if applicable).
- If thumb is not involved, full mobility should be available.

Options for Materials

- Use ⅛″ thermoplastic material to provide needed rigidity to maintain joint positions.
- If patient has significant pain and swelling, the fabrication process may be quite difficult. Consider uncoated materials or those that are slightly tacky and drapable to help prevent material from slipping and to make it easier to position patient and mold the orthosis.
- Materials that can be reheated and remolded several times are a good option if ongoing modifications become necessary to accommodate for fluctuations in edema or changes in desired joint position.
- Consider ⅛″ perforated material because orthosis will likely be worn continuously for several weeks.

Cut and Heat

- Position patient with elbow resting on table and forearm pronated for gravity-assisted molding. If involved, position thumb in gentle palmar abduction and opposition.
- If wound dressings are necessary, they must be incorporated into the design. Place stockinette over dressing to prevent thermoplastic material from sticking. This can be easily cut away when molding process is complete.
- Consider using palmar support to rest hand on; this helps control of positioning wrist and MCP joints during fabrication.
- Prepad ulnar/radial styloids and Lister tubercle with adhesive foam or silicone gel if appropriate.

Evaluate Fit While Molding

- Lay warm material on towel, positioning thumb cut out or thumb piece, if involved, on correct side of material as if it were going to be placed on pronated forearm.
- Position material on dorsum of involved hand, wrist, and forearm. Be sure to cover fingertips adequately. Allow gravity to aid in contouring about metacarpal heads and styloids.
- Depending on material chosen, molding around IF and SF metacarpal borders may be difficult; buckling of material may occur.

- Do not grab proximally or try to secure with tight circumferential bandage. This may cause borders to irritate skin. Instead, allow gravity to assist in forming forearm and hand trough.
- Digits often want to assume flexed posture secondary to edema, pain, and postsurgical complications, making molding of dorsal hood in 0° of IP extension a challenge. Gently lift material and approximate optimal position. Volarly applied soft strap progressively extends digits to reach dorsal hood.
- Make sure desired wrist and digit positions are maintained. It is crucial to use goniometer to ensure accurate positioning. Be careful of joint position during removal of orthosis.

Strapping and Components

- Distal strap: 2″ soft strap running slightly oblique from radial distal border to ulnar distal border. Strap should traverse and support all fingertips against dorsal hood. Use adhesive foam on straps to support digits in position.
- Volar MCP strap: 1″ to 2″ (trimmed) strap provides support volarly to MCP joints; use piece of adhesive foam to further stabilize wrist and prevent migration. Foam should not overlap edges.
- Wrist strap: 2″ soft strap with adhesive foam to further stabilize joints and prevent migration.
- Proximal strap: 2″ soft or elasticized strap.
- Thumb strap: 1″ strap traversing on oblique angle to incorporate thumb IP and proximal phalanx.

Survey Completed Orthosis

- Smooth and slightly flare all borders.
- Gently flare around dorsal thumb and lateral MP regions; do not roll, which makes future modifications difficult and makes it unnecessarily bulky.
- Check clearance of elbow and thumb (if applicable).
- Check for compression stress at radial and ulnar styloid processes and over dorsal MCP joints.
- Check for compression over radial and ulnar sensory nerves.

 PATTERN PEARLS 1–87 AND 1–88

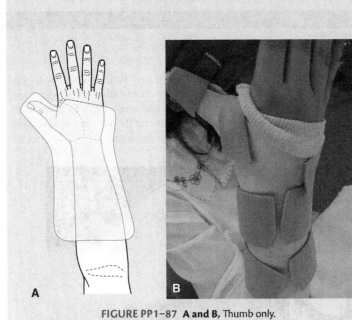

FIGURE PP1–87 **A and B,** Thumb only.

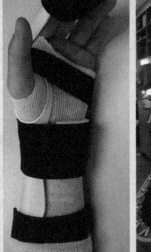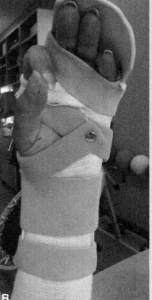

FIGURE PP1–88 **A,** Radial digits only. **B,** Ulnar digits only.

Use of Hand Rest for Joint Positioning

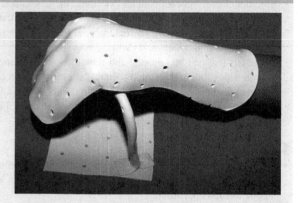

A rest for the palmar surface of the hand can aid considerably when fabricating a dorsal wrist and hand immobilization orthosis. This device, consisting of a platform and rolled palmar support, can be constructed from thermoplastic material. The raised palmar support should be oblique in form to support distal transverse arch. The rest should also be high enough to allow the fingers and thumb to drape over it without touching the table and keeping the wrist in the desired amount of flexion.

Techniques for Accommodating MCP Flexion Angle

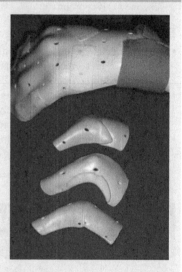

When molding material dorsally over flexed MCP joints, it can be challenging to accommodate for the flexion angle. Consider the following techniques (shown here from top to bottom): (1) Cut just enough material to support the area. If using a material with some drapability, with a small tug distally, the material will fall into place without overlapping. This is an advanced technique that takes much practice but provides the most cosmetically pleasing look. Be careful not to pull the material too much or the material will thin out and weaken the area. (2) Dog-ear the material by first snipping in approximately ½″ at the MCP joints and then overlapping it. The material must be treated with solvent to remove any coating and heated with a heat gun to ensure a strong bond. This technique makes future modifications of the MCP flexion angle difficult. (3) Gently stretch and overlap the material dorsally at the MCP joints to take up the excess. Note that the material is not rolled. This technique also makes future changes a challenge. (4) Pinch the excess material together when warm and snip it off. May need to reinforce this seam with additional thermoplastic material or a thermoplastic tape in order to prevent the seam from popping apart.

Strapping Techniques to Prevent Distal Migration

Orthoses may shift in position if not secured adequately. This can adversely alter joint angles and place the repaired or healing structures at risk for attenuation. To help prevent this occurrence, the following strapping techniques can be employed. **A,** Apply an adhesive foam to the 2″ strap just proximal to the distal wrist crease (arrow depicts placement). **B,** Split the 2″ strap in half at the thenar crease. **C,** Utilize a rivet by adding an additional 1″ strap to the MCP joint strap at the midthenar crease to anchor the orthosis about the base of the thumb. **D and E,** Mold a thermoplastic palmar bar from the radial or ulnar dorsal aspect of the MCP area. In fabricating the palmar bar, carefully incorporate the arches of the hand by using smooth, even strokes, constantly redirecting the material into the arches.

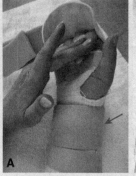
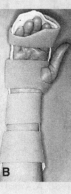
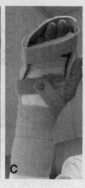
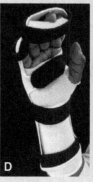
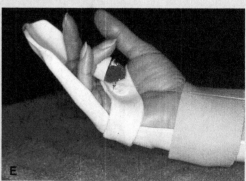

EXPERT PEARL 1–21

Molding Orthosis
NGAIRE TURNBULL, OT, HAND THERAPIST
Australia

Cling wrap (or similar) can be used to create a layer between compression/dressings and the warm thermoplastic while molding to prevent the thermoplastic from sticking to the layers underneath.

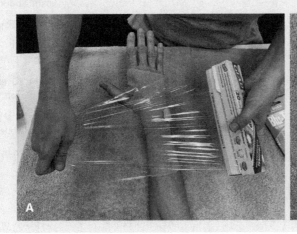

EXPERT PEARL 1–22

Putty for Bony Regions
NGAIRE TURNBULL, OT, HAND THERAPIST
Australia

As an alternative to foam, try using Blu-Tack (adhesive reusable putty) to protect bony prominences. This contours really well and leaves breathing space around prominences leading to a more comfortable orthosis.

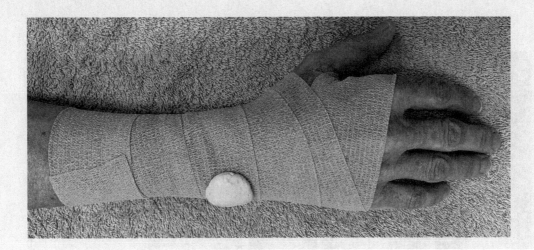

VOLAR WRIST/HAND (OPTIONAL THUMB) IMMOBILIZATION ORTHOSIS (Fig. 1–35)

COMMON NAMES

- Resting hand splint
- Resting pan splint

ALTERNATIVE ORTHOSIS OPTIONS

- Prefabricated orthosis
- Cast

PRIMARY FUNCTIONS

- Immobilize wrist and hand (and thumb) joints to allow healing or rest of involved structure(s).

ADDITIONAL FUNCTIONS

- Statically position tight flexor tendons at maximum extension to facilitate lengthening of tissue (mobilization orthosis).
- Prevent or minimize joint contractures of wrist, fingers, and thumb.
- Prevent overstretching of weak or absent wrist and digit muscle-tendon units.
- Aid in reducing muscle tone in wrist and digits.

Common Diagnoses	General Optimal Positions
Burn injury	Wrist: 30° extension (volar or circumferential burns), 0° (dorsal burns); MCP: 60°–90° flexion; IP: 0°; th: between palm abduction and th opp
Rheumatoid	Wrist: 30° extension; MCP: slight arthritis flex; IP: comfortable flexion; th: abduction and th opp (Note: If patient has carpal tunnel symptoms, decrease wrist extension)

Common Diagnoses	General Optimal Positions
Crush injuries	Wrist: 30° extension; MCP: 60° flexion; IP: 0°; th: palm abduction
Tendon transfers	Dictated by structures involved
Extensor tendon repairs (zones V to VI)	Wrist: 40°–45° extension; MCP: 0°–20° flexion; IP: 0°
Radial nerve injury or repair	Wrist: 30° extension; MCP: 30°–40° flexion; PIP: 40° flexion; DIP: 20° flexion; th: rad abduction
Infection or cellulitis	Functional position or intrinsic plus position; include one joint higher than infection
Replantation or transplantation	Dictated by structures involved
MCP capsulectomy	Wrist: 10°–30° extension; MCP: 75°–90° flexion; IP: 0°
Abnormal tone	Depends on therapist and physician rationale

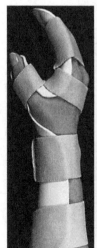
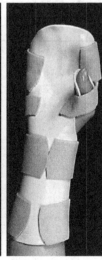
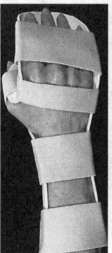
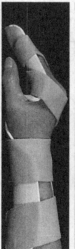
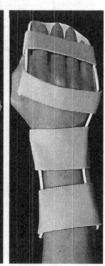

FIGURE 1–35

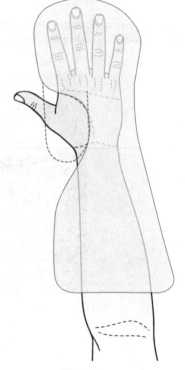

FIGURE 1–36

FABRICATION PROCESS

Pattern Creation (Fig. 1–36)

- Mark for proximal border two-thirds length of forearm.
- Allow enough material to encompass one-half to two-thirds circumference of forearm, remembering that forearm tapers distally.
- Mark width of hand plus ¼″ to ½″ on each side to allow for hand trough.
- Mark distal border, approximately 1″ distal to fingertips.
- Mark for thumb only if included in orthosis.
- Radial aspect of thumb: From distal border (approximately 1″ radial to index fingertip), draw line through center of thumb IP joint proximally toward thumb MP joint, ending just proximal to CMC joint.
- Proximal and medial aspect: Curve proximal and medial to CMC joint along palmar edge of thenar eminence. Curved thumb pattern should end at midthenar mass (along thenar crease), in line with third metacarpals.

Refine Pattern

- Proximal border should allow full elbow motion.
- If thumb is free, check for nearly full motion.
- If thumb is included, thumb piece should be wide and deep enough to encompass thumb.

Options for Materials

- Material selection depends on requirements.
- Consider ⅛″ thermoplastic material to provide needed rigidity to maintain stretch on tight tissue or support painful edematous hand.
- Materials with moderate stretch properties can be difficult to handle when fabricating this orthosis, especially if patient has increased tone.
- If patient has difficulty achieving supinated gravity-assisted position, consider uncoated materials or those that are slightly tacky to help prevent material from slipping and to make it easier to position patient and mold orthosis.
- Materials that can be reheated and remolded several times are a good option if ongoing orthosis modifications become necessary to accommodate for fluctuations in edema or changes in desired joint position.
- Gel- or foam-lined materials help provide volar wrist scar compression, decrease distal migration, and increase comfort.
- Consider perforated material when orthosis will be worn continually or in conjunction with scar management products such as elastomer. Scar products seep through perforations, which helps anchor them into orthosis.

Cut and Heat

- Position patient with elbow resting on table with forearm supinated for gravity-assisted molding.
- Position thumb or leave free per diagnosis.
- If patient has difficulty supinating forearm (e.g., pain extremity), have the patient flex elbow on table and adduct shoulder toward midline or lie supine with shoulder abducted and externally rotated 90° with elbow flexed.
- When cutting thumb area of orthosis, leave small space (make notch) between proximal thumb piece and radial forearm trough to keep material ends from touching and adhering during molding process.

Evaluate Fit While Molding

- Lay warm material on towel, positioning thumb piece on correct side of material as if it were going to be placed on supinated forearm.
- Position material on volar aspect of involved hand and wrist, with thumb component applied within index and thumb web space (commonly referred to as C-bar). Material must be stretched slightly to achieve even contouring along dorsal web and within palm.

- Lift thumb trough and place it centrally over thumb's medial/ulnar border. Once positioned, carefully stretch outer border to form a C-shape. Medial portion (snipped section) should adequately cover wrist and partially cover thenar eminence. Pay close attention to thumb joint positions.
- Use palmar aspect of hand to help support volar arches and first web space, simulating handshake hold.
- Position digits in slight abduction with MCP, PIP, and DIP joints positioned per diagnosis.
- Guide rest of material evenly along arm.
- Borders of orthosis should be curved to form hand trough (¼″ to ½″ at hand and thumb). These curved sides keep fingers from falling off orthosis border.
- Gravity tends to pull material away from thumb and toward IF; continually reposition material as needed.
- Do not grab proximal orthosis or try to secure with tight circumferential bandage. This may cause borders of orthosis to irritate skin. Instead, allow gravity to assist in forming forearm trough.
- Check for pressure areas at ulnar aspect of thumb MP and IF and SF MCP joints.
- Check for compression of dorsal sensory branches of radial and ulnar nerves.
- Rotate forearm into pronated position at end of molding to check for clearance of ulnar and radial styloid processes; flare around styloids as necessary.
- Make sure desired wrist position is maintained. Some patients tend to flex and deviate wrist while orthosis is being formed. May use goniometer to ensure correct positioning; this is especially important for diagnoses requiring specific positioning (e.g., tendon repairs and transfers).
- Do not stress UCL of thumb MP joint when attempting to palmarly abduct thumb.
- When fabricating an orthosis for increased tone or for use with serial static designs, it may be necessary to reinforce wrist portion with another strip of thermoplastic material or consider different design, such as a dorsally based orthosis.

Strapping and Components

- Distal strap: 1″ to 2″ strap directed from radial border of proximal IF to ulnar border of proximal SF. Strip of adhesive foam can be used under strap to stabilize and contour about proximal phalanxes.
- Metacarpal strap: 1″ strap directed from radial web space to midulnar border.
- Wrist strap: 2″ strap just proximal to dorsal wrist crease; use piece of adhesive foam to further stabilize wrist in orthosis and prevent migration. Foam should lie directly over ulnar styloid and should not overlap orthosis edges.
- Proximal strap: Depending on size of forearm, 1″ or 2″ strap may suffice; strap should have slight volar to dorsal angle.
- Thumb strap: 1″ strap across proximal phalanx.
- In some cases (e.g., with severe edema), traditional strapping may not be appropriate; cotton wrap or elasticized bandage may be better option.
- Some conditions of arthritis may require straps or finger separators to aid in positioning deviating joints.
- Patients with an increase in tone may need additional straps to maintain joint position.

Survey Completed Orthosis

- Smooth and slightly flare distal and proximal borders.
- Gently flare around thenar segment; avoid rolling, which makes future orthosis modifications difficult and leads to unnecessarily bulky orthosis.
- Check clearance of elbow, styloid processes, thumb, and IF to SF joints.

PATTERN PEARLS 1–89 TO 1–93

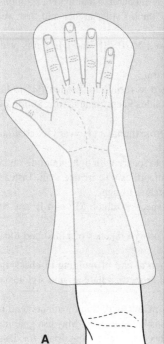

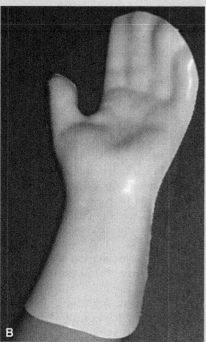

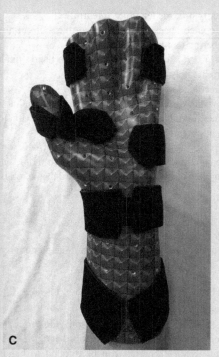

FIGURE PP1–89 A–C, "Mitt" design: wrist/hand/thumb immobilization orthosis. Note the intimate contouring made utilizing a plastic based material (low resistance to stretch) **(B)**.

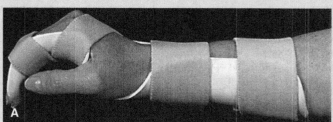

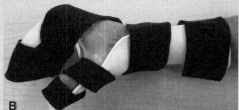

FIGURE PP1–90 A, Position of function. **B,** Antideformity position.

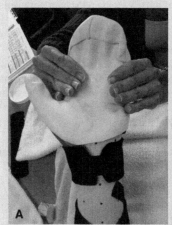

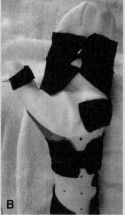

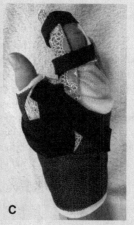

FIGURE PP1–91 A–C, Addition of material to create a volar wrist/hand orthosis. Volar hand segment added over the cast for finger positioning.

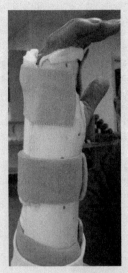

FIGURE PP1–92 Digit IP joints free to promote tendon gliding.

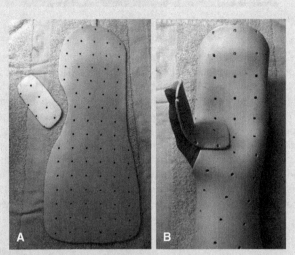

FIGURE PP1–93 **A and B,** When faced with a challenging patient to position all the involved joints, consider this optional method to add thumb component to the base orthotic design. This allows for positioning the wrist/hand separately and provides the ability to focus on thumb position in isolation. Be sure to utilize a material without a coating—or remove the coating to be sure the thumb segment fully adheres to the base. Heating both regions with a heat gun prior to pressing together will maximize adherence.

CLINICAL PEARL 1–56

Dacron Batting to Absorb Perspiration

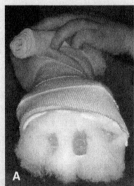

Patients who have to wear an orthosis for extended periods of time (e.g., after surgery), especially in warmer months, tend to perspire within the orthosis, which may lead to skin maceration and an unpleasant odor. Polyester batting **(A)** (used for quilting), applied between the digits and lightly about the hand and forearm, wicks away moisture from the skin, promoting a dry environment. The batting, readily available at most fabric stores, should be changed daily. Note the bias cut material used to secure the orthosis **(B)**. This nonelastic wrap applies gentle circumferential pressure to aid in reducing edema. It is applied with gentle tension in much the same manner as an elasticized wrap. This technique of securing the orthosis can be used temporarily during the initial days postinjury/surgery followed by a transition to traditional strapping.

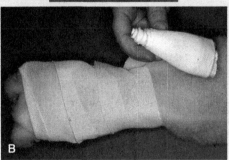

CLINICAL PEARL 1–57

Finger Separators

There are several creative ways to position deviating (or potentially deviating) joints of patients with rheumatoid arthritis. Finger spacers are often necessary for correct positioning and comfort. Thermoplastic separators can be formed using scissors, bandage applicator, pencil or a similar object. When designing the pattern, allow extra material at the hand and digit width. While the material is still warm, gently take the edge of a pair of closed scissors (tip pointing into the web) or another similarly shaped object and apply pressure volar to dorsal to create a trough for each digit that is approximately ½" deep. Lightly pinch together and move on to the next digit **(A and B)**. Foam finger separators can be constructed using an adhesive-backed product such as 3/8" Rolyan® Temper® Foam (Performance Health) or ¼" Rolyan® Polycushion® Padding (Performance Health) **(C and D)**. These do not need to extend completely into the web to provide slight abduction. **E and F,** Another option is to use Rolyan® 50/50 Mix™ Elastomer Putty (Performance Health) to create an insert for the hand to rest within. They are very comfortable and easy to apply. For patients with dense scar between the digits, a mold can be used to aid in scar remodeling. **G and H,** Make slits in the material and weave soft **(G)** strapping or thin strapping **(H)** about the middle phalanx portion of the orthosis to form individual "tunnels" for each digit. **I,** Fabricate soft strap separators from about 12" strip of 2" soft strapping. Apply adhesive hook to the volar portion of the orthosis and form gullies or troughs with the soft strap. This technique works well for patients with arthritis or fragile skin.

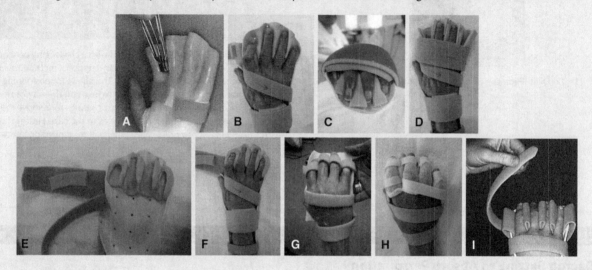

CLINICAL PEARL 1–58

Strap Placement to Facilitate Digit Joint Alignment

Strapping techniques can be the key to improving positioning of the distal joints. **A,** Riveting the radial end of the MCP strap within the orthosis can help guide the IF metacarpal head ulnarward while the distal straps can be directed radially (see arrow). **B,** The placement of the distal strap can aid in aligning the proximal structures as well. **C,** Post–extensor tendon realignment: The distally placed straps and the proximal wrist strap help prevent recurrent ulnar deviation and maintain neutral alignment of the wrist and digits; notice strategically placed blue foam within the strapping system. **D and E,** Strap weaving techniques work well to encourage proper digit alignment. Soft straps can be incorporated into a night resting orthosis for maintaining and correcting the digit position for diagnoses such as rheumatoid arthritis and Dupuytren release. The slits can be made with a hole punch, drill (Dremel), or heated awl. Adhesive hook is applied to the surface of the orthosis material corresponding to each involved digit. The loop material for each finger attaches first to the hook and then is directed about the digit and through the appropriate web space slit, terminating back on the hook.

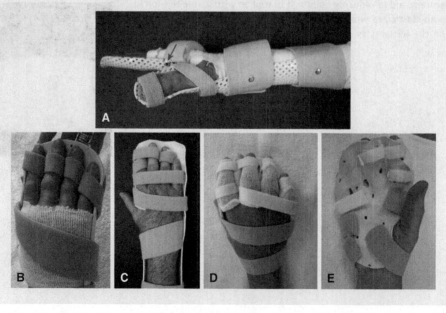

CLINICAL PEARL 1–59

Hints for Molding First Web Space

The "handshake hold" technique helps control the thermoplastic material while maintaining the first web space. Use a light grasp distally while working proximally. Stretch and contour the material between the IF and thumb to create a "C" (similar to a thumb abduction orthosis) for the thumb and IF to rest in. Be careful not to dig the fingertips into the warm material, creating a potential pressure area.

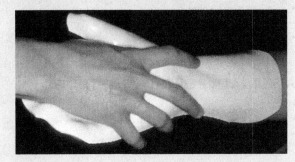

VOLAR/DORSAL WRIST/HAND IMMOBILIZATION ORTHOSIS (WHFO) (Fig. 1–37)

COMMON NAMES

- Antispasticity splint
- Bisurfaced forearm-based static wrist hand orthosis
- Dorsal platform splint
- Dorsal resting splint

ALTERNATIVE ORTHOSIS OPTIONS

- Cast
- Prefabricated antispasticity orthosis
- SaeboStretch® orthosis

PRIMARY FUNCTIONS

- Immobilize wrist and hand joints to allow healing, rest, or proper positioning of involved structure(s).

ADDITIONAL FUNCTIONS

- Statically position tight flexor tendons at maximum extension to facilitate lengthening of tissue and lessen joint contractures (mobilization orthosis).
- Aid in reducing muscle tone in wrist and digits.

Common Diagnoses	General Optimal Positions
General hand trauma	Wrist: 30° extension; MCP: 60° flexion; IP: 0°
Burn injuries	Wrist: 30° extension; MCP: 60°–90° flexion; IP: 0°
Rheumatoid arthritis	Wrist: 30° extension; MCP: slight flexion; IP: comfortable flexion (Note: If patient has carpal tunnel symptoms, decrease wrist extension)
Abnormal tone	Depends on therapist and physician rationale

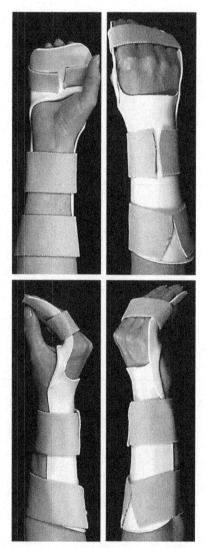

FIGURE 1–37

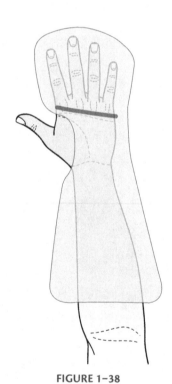

FIGURE 1–38

FABRICATION PROCESS

Pattern Creation (Fig. 1–38)

- Can be an alternative pattern to volar or dorsal wrist and hand immobilization orthosis; may be used when it is necessary to avoid fabricating an orthosis over fragile or grafted dorsal or volar surfaces (burns, skin grafts, pins, open wounds).
- Positions depend on injury and structures involved.
- Mark for proximal border two-thirds length of forearm.

- Allow enough material to encompass one-half to two-thirds circumference of forearm, remembering that forearm tapers distally.
- Mark distal border approximately 1″ distal to fingertips; this additional material may be necessary to compensate for material consumed by positions of joints.
- Mark thumb clearance by making an arc from thumb MP to base of first CMC joint.
- Opening for digits should be marked at mid-IF MCP joint and run slightly oblique to SF MCP joint.

Refine Pattern

- Proximal border should allow full elbow motion.
- Distal border should protect fingertips.
- Make sure that opening for digits is wide enough to accommodate width of MCPs, allowing approximately ½″ material on sides.
- To aid in tone inhibition, incorporate finger separators into volar pan.

Options for Materials

- Use ⅛″ material because strength and rigidity are important characteristics for this device, especially because of potentially weak and narrow area at junction of MCPs.
- Materials with high resistance to stretch may offer more control for therapist; highly conforming materials may be difficult to control against gravity.
- Increase strength at borders of slotted piece by overlapping edges.
- If patient has significant pain and swelling, fabricating an orthosis with this design may be quite awkward and difficult; consider materials that are slightly tacky and drapable to help prevent material from slipping and to make it easier to position patient and mold orthosis.

Cut and Heat

- Before fabrication, use a technique to reduce tone in extremity if needed (see Chapter 23).
- Ideally, position forearm and hand in pronation; forearm can rest on elevated platform with MCPs over edge.
- Prepad ulnar/radial styloids and Lister tubercle with adhesive foam or silicone gel if appropriate.

Evaluate Fit While Molding

- Lay warm material on towel and position MCP slot on correct side of material as if it were going to be placed on pronated forearm. (The MCP slot should be more distal on radial side.)

- Slide digits through slot, then carefully lay proximal portion on dorsal forearm and allow gravity to assist.
- One hand should simultaneously support volar piece at MCPs and digits, incorporating arches.
- Fold MCP flaps over onto material and flatten out to add strength to this potentially weak section.
- Do not grab proximal orthosis or try to secure with tight circumferential bandage. This may cause borders of orthosis to irritate skin. Instead, allow gravity to assist in forming forearm trough.
- Make sure desired wrist and digit positions are maintained.

Strapping and Components

- If orthosis is to be used for burn injury management, consider circumferential bandages to avoid localized pressure caused by straps on fragile healing skin or grafts.
- Distal strap: 1″ or 2″ strap to traverse across PIP joints. May use foam to improve extension positioning of digits.
- Wrist and proximal strap: 2″ strap of soft, elasticized, or traditional loop.
- If adhesive foam is used to pad ulnar styloid during fabrication, carefully lift it off patient's skin and place it back into orthosis.

Survey Completed Orthosis

- Check that opening for digits is wide enough for easy donning and doffing of orthosis.
- Make sure that sides of IF and SF MCPs are strong enough to support weight of digits. If not, an additional strip of thermoplastic material may be added for support.
- May need to apply piece of thermoplastic material volarly to reinforce wrist position.

PATTERN PEARLS 1-94 TO 1-98

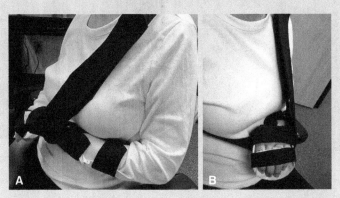

FIGURE PP1-94 **A and B,** Application of shoulder strap to control elbow flexion and forearm rotation.

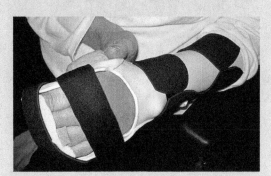

FIGURE PP1-95 Adhesive foam on distal straps can assist in positioning digits in extension to manage flexion contractures.

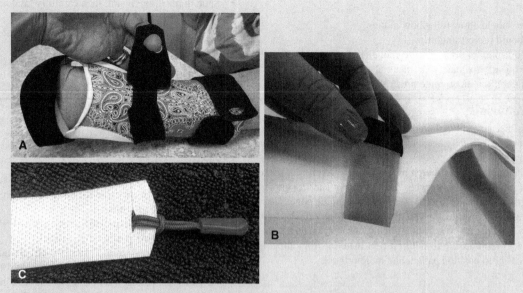

FIGURE PP1–96 A, Loops incorporated into strapping system can make application and removal easier for specific patient populations. **B,** Thermoplastic adhered to end of strapping, and **(C)** coat pull attached to hole in strapping to ease removal for patient.

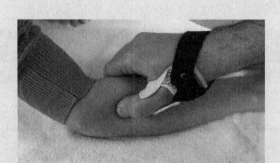

FIGURE PP1–97 Alteration of design used to stabilize the thumb MP and CMC joints for a massage therapist.

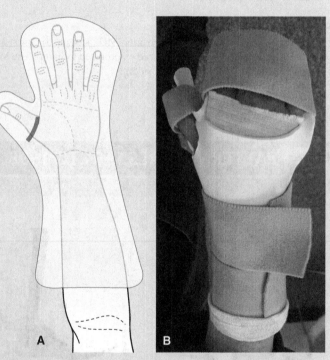

FIGURE PP1–98 A and B, Addition of thumb into design.

ANTISPASTICITY CONE ORTHOSIS (Fig. 1–39)

COMMON NAMES

- Antispasticity splint
- Forearm-based ulnar cone-style splint

ALTERNATIVE ORTHOSIS OPTIONS

- Cast
- SaeboStretch® orthosis
- Prefabricated antispasticity orthosis

PRIMARY FUNCTIONS

- Immobilize wrist, digits, and thumb for individuals with moderate to severe spasticity.
- Help decrease tone and reduce risk of joint and soft tissue contracture.

ADDITIONAL FUNCTIONS

- Statically position tight flexor tendons at maximum extension to facilitate lengthening of tissue and reduce or prevent contractures (mobilization orthosis).

Common Diagnoses	General Optimal Positions
Abnormal tone	Depends on therapist and physician rationale
Joint contractures and muscle	Functional position shortening

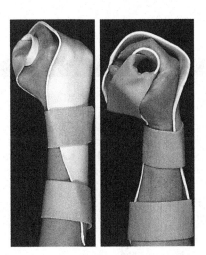

FIGURE 1–39

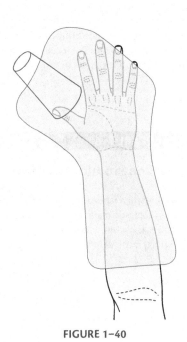

FIGURE 1–40

FABRICATION PROCESS

Pattern Creation (Fig. 1–40)

- Note: Because of increased tone, positioning extremity for creating this pattern may be quite difficult; draw pattern on contralateral extremity or estimate size.
- Mark for proximal border two-thirds length of forearm.
- Allow enough material to encompass one-half to two-thirds circumference of forearm, remembering that forearm tapers distally.
- Mark distal border using pattern illustration for an example. Material distally follows contour of digits.
- From MF distal phalanx tip radially, pattern extends beyond thumb approximately 2″.
- Pattern follows contour of thumb proximally, leaving 1½″ to 2″ border radially. At this point, pattern comes in toward proximal thumb MP 1″ then continues proximally.

Refine Pattern

- Proximal border should allow full elbow motion.
- Distal border should protect digits.

- To prevent adherence, line cone (fabricated from thermoplastic or commercial) with light layer of lotion before placing on material.
- Make sure that pattern material for cone portion is generous and wide enough to accommodate hand size. Patients with tight, contracted hands may need to start with smaller cone that can be progressively enlarged as tissue elongates.

Options for Materials

- Use ⅛″ material because strength and rigidity are important characteristics for this orthosis.
- Consider perforated materials, which allow air exchange between skin and orthosis, especially for patients who are cognitively impaired or who lack full sensation.
- Skin breakdown and maceration can become problems under these orthoses. Do not line orthosis with Moleskin or similar padding because they tend to absorb moisture and are difficult to clean. Closed cell foam that can be readily washed may work well.
- If patient has significant tone, fabricating an orthosis with this design may be quite awkward and difficult. Consider materials that are less conforming and more rigid to make it easier to position patient and mold orthosis.

Cut and Heat

- Before fabrication, use a technique to reduce tone in extremity (see Chapter 23).
- While material is heating, prepad ulnar styloid using self-adhesive padding or silicone gel.
- Ideally, position extremity with shoulder and elbow flexed and forearm neutral to achieve gravity-assisted position.
- Make sure desired position is maintained.

Evaluate Fit While Molding

Note: The fabrication of this orthosis may warrant an "extra set of hands" to assist during the molding process.

- Lay warm material on towel, positioning large radial section on correct side of material as if it were going to be placed on extremity.
- Place warm material on proximal forearm and allow gravity to hold it in place.
- Working distally, lay material into palm and place cone on material. Wide end of cone is on ulnar border pointing through web space.
- Wrap thumb portion over cone, then bring distal straight border over this material to forming cone. (While this occurs, ulnar aspect of orthosis should form an ulnar trough for digits to rest in.)

- Keep redirecting wrist into appropriate position. If there is considerable tone in hand, then orthosis can be made in sections. After molding forearm and wrist portions, cone section can be made while the orthosis is off patient.
- Do not grab proximal portion of the orthosis or try to secure with tight circumferential bandage. This may cause borders of the orthosis to irritate skin. Instead, allow gravity to assist in forming forearm trough.

Strapping and Components

- Digits: Often not necessary.
- Cone straps: Straps originating from top of cone can be quite effective for keeping hand correctly positioned. Soft 1″ straps traversing just proximal to MCP, PIP, DIP, thumb MP, and IP joint(s) are appropriate.
- Wrist and proximal strap: 2″ strap of soft, elasticized, or traditional loop.
- If 3/8″ adhesive foam or silicone was used to pad ulnar styloid during fabrication, carefully lift it off patient's skin and place it back into orthosis to cushion styloid.

Survey Completed Orthosis

- Smooth and slightly flare borders.
- Check that cone is of adequate width to position digits properly.
- Check clearance of elbow.

CLINICAL PEARL 1–60

Therapy Cone to Aid Fabrication of Antispasticity Orthoses

A, Using a therapy cone when fabricating the central portion of this orthosis can be extremely helpful. If an appropriately sized cone is not available, fabricate one out of scrap thermoplastic material. If there is a chance that the materials may stick to each other during the fabrication process, simply wrap the cone with a wet paper towel, layer with lotion, or cover with a stockinette. **B–D,** A cone made out of thermoplastic material and covered in neoprene **(B and C)** (removable for washing) is useful to keep the digits as open as possible while the fabrication of a neoprene-based orthosis is applied **(D).**

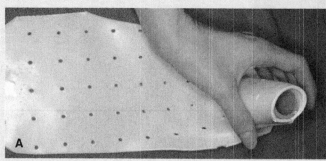

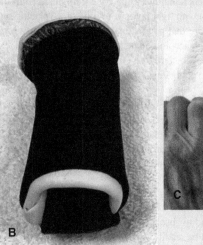

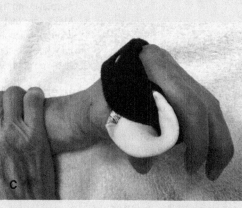

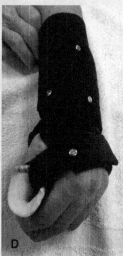

ANTISPASTICITY BALL ORTHOSIS (WHFO) (Fig. 1–41)

COMMON NAMES

- Antispasticity splint

ALTERNATIVE ORTHOSIS OPTIONS

- Prefabricated antispasticity orthosis
- SaeboStretch® orthosis

PRIMARY FUNCTIONS

- Immobilize wrist, digits, and thumb for individuals with moderate to severe spasticity.
- Aid in decreasing tone and reducing risk of tissue contracture.

ADDITIONAL FUNCTIONS

- Statically position tight flexor tendons at maximum extension to facilitate lengthening of tissue and to reduce or prevent contractures (mobilization orthosis).

Common Diagnoses	General Optimal Positions
Abnormal tone	Depends on therapist and physician rationale
Joint contractures and muscle shortening	Functional position

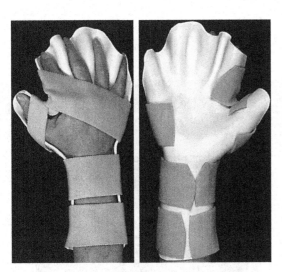

FIGURE 1–41

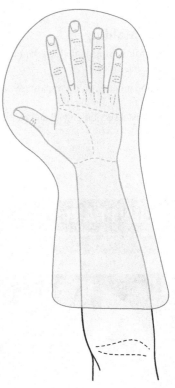

FIGURE 1–42

FABRICATION PROCESS

Pattern Creation (Fig. 1–42)

- Note: Because of increased tone, positioning extremity for creating this pattern may be quite difficult; draw pattern on contralateral extremity or estimate size.
- Mark for proximal border two-thirds length of forearm.
- Allow enough material to encompass one-half to two-thirds circumference of forearm, remembering that forearm tapers distally.
- Mark distal border, approximately 1″ beyond fingertips, using pattern illustration for an example.
- Radially, follow contour of first web space along distal and radial thumb borders, meeting at thumb base. Allow ½″ distally and 1″ radially for sufficient troughing and strap application.

Refine Pattern

- Proximal border should allow full elbow motion.
- Distal border should extend just distal to fingertips.
- Make sure that digit and thumb material is generous and wide enough to accommodate web spacers.

Options for Materials

- Use ⅛″ material because strength and rigidity are important characteristics for this orthosis.
- Consider perforated materials, which allow air exchange between skin and orthosis, especially for patients who are cognitively impaired or who lack full sensation.
- Skin breakdown and maceration can become problems under these devices. Do not line orthosis with Moleskin or similar padding because they tend to absorb moisture and are difficult to clean.

- Consider material with no memory, because maintenance of web spacers after material has been stretched is key to this design.
- If patient has significant tone, fabricating an orthosis with this design may be quite awkward and difficult. Consider materials that are less conforming and more rigid to make it easier to position patient and mold orthosis.

Cut and Heat

- Before fabrication, use a technique to reduce tone in extremity (see Chapter 23 for specific information).
- Consider placing light layer of lotion on ball before molding to prevent thermoplastic from adhering.
- Consider fabricating forearm trough first and then making hand component as described in the following text. This will allow more control over an already hard-to-control extremity.
- Prepare to pronate hand on medium-sized ball (large enough to encompass entire hand).

Evaluate Fit While Molding

Note: The fabrication of this orthosis may warrant an "extra set of hands" to assist during the molding process.

- To simplify fabrication process, warm forearm section first and carefully mold to achieve good fit.
- Next, place warmed distal section on ball and rest patient's hand over it.

- Make sure that digits and thumb are fully abducted.
- Use pair of closed scissors, small dowel, or bandage applicator to pull material up between fingers and thumb (see Clinical Pearl 1–57).
- During this process, it helps to have an assistant maintain wrist and forearm position.

Strapping and Components

- Digits and thumb: 2″ soft strap just distal to MCP joints is sufficient. Some patients with severe flexor tone need straps threaded over proximal and distal phalanges.
- To prevent digits from lifting off palmar piece, 1″ soft foam strap can be woven through web spacers.
- Wrist and proximal strap: 2″ strap of soft, elasticized, or traditional hook can be used.

Survey Completed Orthosis

- Smooth and slightly flare borders.
- Check that palmar section is of adequate width to properly position digits and allow easy donning and doffing of orthosis.
- Check clearance of elbow.

 PATTERN PEARLS 1–99 AND 1–100

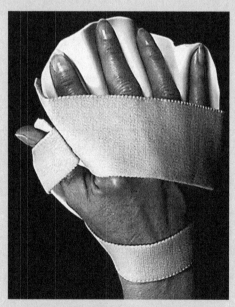

FIGURE PP1–99 Hand-based design.

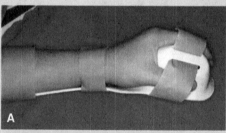

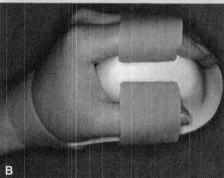

FIGURE PP1–100 A, Rolyan® Preformed Neutral Position Splint. **B,** Hand-based design (Performance Health).

4 Arm-Based Orthoses

POSTERIOR ELBOW IMMOBILIZATION ORTHOSIS (EO) (Fig. 1–43)

COMMON NAMES

- Posterior elbow splint

ALTERNATIVE ORTHOSIS OPTIONS

- Cast
- Prefabricated orthosis

PRIMARY FUNCTIONS

- Immobilize elbow joint and surrounding soft tissues to allow healing, rest, and/or protection of involved structures(s).

ADDITIONAL FUNCTIONS

- Limit or prevent forearm rotation.
- Statically position an elbow extension contracture at maximum flexion to facilitate lengthening of tissue (mobilization orthosis).
- Restrict specific degree of elbow extension (restriction orthosis).

Common Diagnoses	General Optimal Positions
Rheumatoid arthritis	Position of comfort
Elbow arthroplasty	Dictated by structures involved
Ulnar nerve compression at cubital tunnel	Elbow: 30°–45° flexion; forearm: neutral
Ulnar nerve transposition:	Elbow: 70°–90° flexion; forearm: neutral to 30° pronation; wrist: 0°
Nerve repairs (high lesions)	Elbow: 30°–45° flexion (depends on repair); forearm: neutral; wrist: 0° to slight extension; digits free
Tendon transfers for wrist and digit extensors	Elbow: 90°; forearm: pronated; wrist: 30°–45° extension; MCP and th: extended
Biceps tendon repair	Depends on physician and status of tendon repair; generally, start elbow 45° active extension to 90° passive flexion

Common Diagnoses	General Optimal Positions
Posterior or anterior dislocation	Elbow: 90°; forearm: neutral
Collateral ligament repair (medial or lateral)	Elbow: 90°; forearm: supinated with 10° deviation to side of repair
Proximal radius dislocation	Elbow: 90°; forearm: supinated
Medial epicondyle fracture	Elbow: 90°–110°; forearm: pronated
Lateral epicondyle fracture	Elbow: 90°–110°; forearm: supinated
Olecranon fracture	Elbow: 20°–35° flexion; forearm: neutral
Acute lateral epicondylitis	Elbow: 90°; forearm: neutral; wrist: 30°–45° extension
Acute medial epicondylitis	Elbow: 90°; forearm: neutral; wrist: 0°

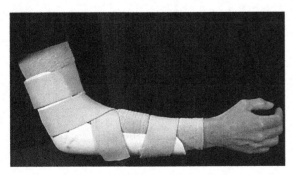

FIGURE 1–43

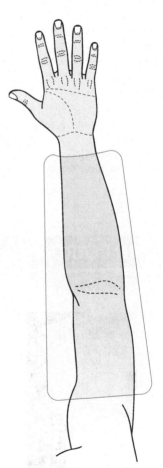

FIGURE 1–44

FABRICATION PROCESS

Pattern Creation (Fig. 1–44)

- Posterior design is better for positioning elbow at greater than 45° of flexion. Volar design is more appropriate for positioning elbow at less than 45°.
- Mark for proximal border two-thirds length of humerus.
- Mark for distal border just proximal to ulnar styloid.
- Allow enough material to encompass one-half to two-thirds circumference of upper arm and forearm.
- Remember that the longer and wider the orthosis, the more comfortable it is to wear.

Refine Pattern

- Proximal border should allow unimpeded shoulder motion and not irritate axillary region with arm positioned at side of body.
- Distal border should allow full wrist motion.
- Note that pattern should be wider proximally because circumference of upper arm is greater than that of forearm.
- Make sure there is enough material to encompass elbow posteriorly. Insufficient material in this area requires stretching of material, which weakens the orthosis' support.

Options for Materials

- Use ⅛″ material because strength is necessary for this orthosis.
- Consider rubber-based material to have more control and to minimize stretching.
- Gel- or foam-lined materials help provide scar compression, decrease distal migration, and increase comfort.
- Consider perforated thermoplastics for patients who require full-time orthosis use.

Cut and Heat

- While material is heating, consider prepadding medial and lateral epicondyles and olecranon process.
- Position patient to allow for gravity-assisted molding: prone with shoulder neutral; supine with shoulder flexed 90°; or standing while leaning on table, forward flexed at waist, and shoulder extended (upper arm parallel to floor).
- If possible, have an assistant help support proper elbow and forearm positions.

Evaluate Fit While Molding

- Drape warm material centrally over posterior aspect of upper arm and forearm, allowing gravity to assist. Be sure to position material proximal enough to support upper arm.
- Gently stretch and flare material around epicondyles and distal and proximal borders.
- Depending on desired degree of elbow flexion, excess material at elbow flexion crease may require attention.
- Techniques such as pinching, snipping, and folding material over to make the complete corner may be useful.
- Do not grab the orthosis or try to secure with tight circumferential bandage. This may cause borders of orthosis to irritate skin. Instead, allow gravity to assist in forming upper arm and forearm troughs.
- Check for clearance of ulnar styloid distally.
- Make sure desired elbow flexion and forearm rotation positions are maintained. Some patients tend to flex their elbows excessively while orthosis is being formed.

Strapping and Components

- Use stockinette or elasticized sleeve (if edema is present) to eliminate pinching of skin against orthosis borders once straps are applied.
- Proximal strap: 2″ soft strap applied at most proximal portion of orthosis to anchor orthosis adequately to upper arm.
- Middle straps: Crisscross design directly over anterior elbow to maintain elbow position.
- Distal strap: 1″ or 2″ soft strap.
- Consider securing orthosis with elasticized wrap if edema is problematic.

Survey Completed Orthosis

- Smooth and slightly flare all distal and proximal borders.
- Check for clearance and/or irritation at axilla, ulnar styloid, epicondyles, and olecranon process.
- Check for compression of ulnar nerve at cubital tunnel area and of superficial sensory branch of radial nerve.

 PATTERN PEARLS 1–101 TO 1–103

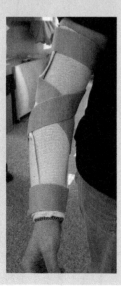

FIGURE PP1–101 Crossing straps on anteriorly to increase purchase.

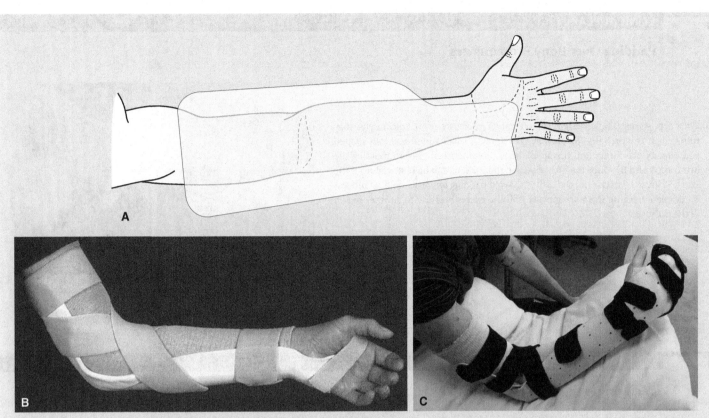

FIGURE PP1–102 A and B, Posterior elbow orthosis including wrist, commonly with forearm in neutral rotation. **C,** Including dorsal wrist and hand for concomitant flexor tendon injury.

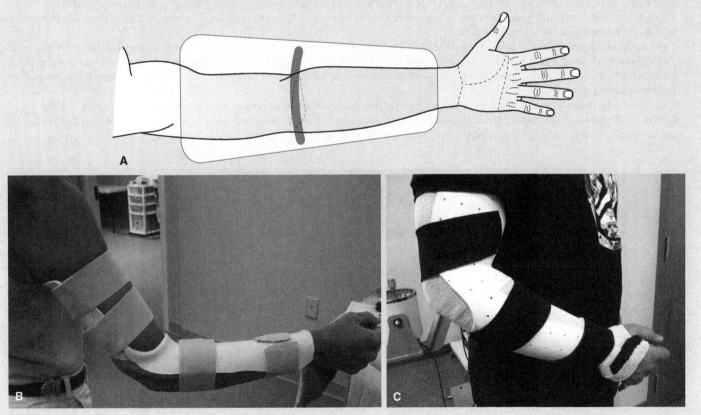

FIGURE PP1–103 A–C, Anterior/posterior design: two options.

CLINICAL PEARL 1–61

Padding Over Bony Prominences

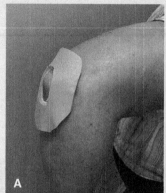

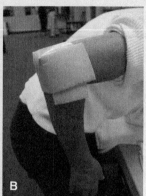

With a posterior elbow design, the olecranon process and/or epicondyles may rub against the orthosis. To prevent this, apply a small adhesive donut-shaped pad directly over or around the at-risk bony prominence(s) *prior* to molding the orthosis **(A and B)**. Once the orthosis is set, the padding can be removed from the skin and inverted back onto the orthosis. Avoid padding *after* the molding process is complete because this may actually shift the excess pressure to another region of the orthosis.

CLINICAL PEARL 1–62

Techniques to Accommodate Elbow Flexion Angle

A common problem occurs when fabricating an orthosis for the elbow in a flexed position (similar to molding over the flexed MCP joints dorsally): managing the excess material at the elbow flexion crease. There are several techniques that can be used to accommodate for this angle.

A, Carefully take up material medially and laterally and then overlap it onto itself, as shown. Make sure not to inadvertently apply excess pressure onto the bony areas. This technique adds strength and support to the curved area of the orthosis. However, making adjustments later may be difficult.

B, Gently stretch and contour the material to provide a seamless, streamlined trough. This can be challenging for less experienced therapists and works best for angles of flexion that are less than 90°, as shown.

C and D, The excess material can be pinched together rather aggressively (to ensure the material coating has been disrupted) and then cut to form a seam. This technique is the most cosmetically appealing and readily allows for orthosis adjustments. However, the orthosis is less stable and more susceptible to breaking at this seam. Treat the seam with solvent, cut a strip of scrap thermoplastic, and heat both regions until tacky. Attach strip onto seam to prevent area from cracking open.

E, Take the excess material, pinch it, and then overlap it onto itself. This method is simple but can be bulky and future modifications are difficult.

F, Make small transverse snips medially and laterally and dog-ear the material onto itself. Use solvent and a heat gun to create a strong bond between the two surfaces. This method makes future orthosis adjustments difficult, and the orthosis may look bulky and thick.

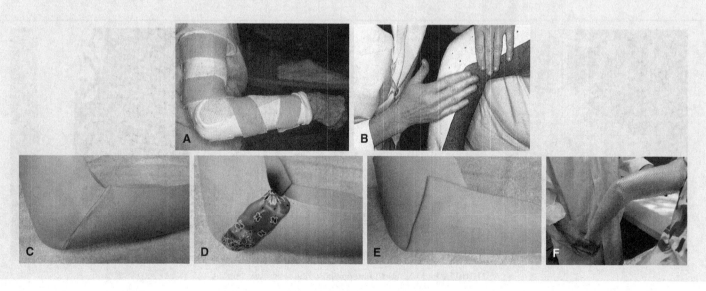

ANTERIOR ELBOW IMMOBILIZATION ORTHOSIS (EO) (Fig. 1–45)

COMMON NAMES

- Anterior elbow splint

ALTERNATIVE ORTHOSIS OPTIONS

- Cast
- Prefabricated orthosis

PRIMARY FUNCTIONS

- Immobilize elbow joint and surrounding soft tissues to allow healing of involved structures(s).

ADDITIONAL FUNCTIONS

- Limit or prevent forearm rotation.
- Statically position elbow flexion contracture at maximum extension to facilitate lengthening of tissue (mobilization orthosis).
- Restrict specific degree of elbow flexion (restriction orthosis).

Common Diagnoses	General Optimal Positions
Rheumatoid arthritis	Position of comfort
Ulnar nerve compression at cubital tunnel	Elbow: 30°–45° flexion; forearm: neutral
Nerve repairs (high lesions)	Elbow: 30°–45° flexion (depends on repair); forearm: neutral; wrist: 0° to slight extension; digits free
Olecranon fracture	Elbow: 20°–35° flexion; forearm: neutral

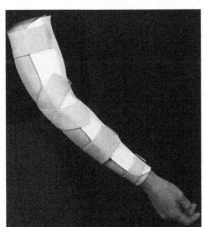

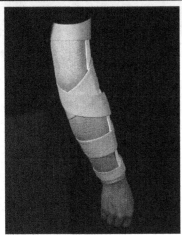

FIGURE 1–45

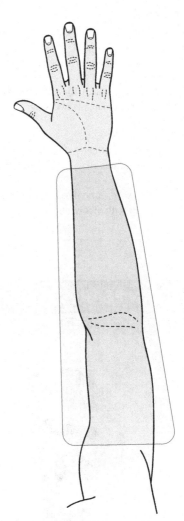

FIGURE 1–46

FABRICATION PROCESS

Pattern Creation (Fig. 1–46)

- Anterior design is best used for positioning elbow in less than 45° of flexion. Posterior design is more appropriate for positioning elbow greater than 45°.
- Mark for proximal border two-thirds length of humerus.
- Mark for distal border just proximal to ulnar styloid.
- Allow enough material to encompass one-half to two-thirds circumference of upper arm and lower forearm.
- Remember that the longer and wider the orthosis, the more comfortable it is to wear.

Refine Pattern

- Proximal border should allow unimpeded shoulder motion and not irritate axillary region with arm positioned at side of body.
- Distal border should allow full wrist motion.
- Note that pattern should be wider proximally because circumference of upper arm is greater than that of forearm.
- Make sure there is enough material to encompass elbow posteriorly. Insufficient material in this area requires stretching of material, which weakens orthosis' support.

Options for Materials

- Use either 3/32″ or ⅛″ thermoplastic material, depending on patient's arm size and desired orthosis strength.
- Gel- or foam-lined materials help provide scar compression, decrease distal migration, and increase comfort.
- Consider perforated thermoplastics for patients who require full-time orthosis use and when air exchange is necessary.

Cut and Heat

- While material is heating, consider prepadding medial and lateral epicondyles if needed; remember that a well-formed orthosis does not require padding.
- Position patient to allow for gravity-assisted molding: supine with shoulder neutral or seated with elbow resting on table.

Evaluate Fit While Molding

- Drape warm material centrally over volar aspect of upper arm and forearm, allowing gravity to assist. Be sure to position material proximal enough to support upper arm.
- Gently flare material around epicondyles, distal, and proximal borders.
- Do not grab orthosis or try to secure with tight circumferential bandage. This may cause borders of orthosis to irritate skin. Instead, allow gravity to assist in forming upper arm and forearm troughs.
- Check for clearance of wrist distally.
- Make sure desired elbow extension and forearm rotation positions are maintained. Some patients tend to flex their elbows excessively while orthosis is being formed. Gently support patient's arm in correct position by supporting at wrist.

Strapping and Components

- Use stockinette or elasticized sleeve if edema is present to eliminate pinching of skin against orthosis borders once straps are applied.
- Proximal strap: 2″ soft strap applied at most proximal portion of orthosis to anchor orthosis adequately to upper arm and to prevent rocking.
- Middle straps: 2″ straps to hold elbow adequately in orthosis.
- Distal strap: 1″ or 2″ soft strap.
- Consider securing orthosis with elasticized wrap if edema is problematic.

Survey Completed Orthosis

- Smooth and slightly flare all distal and proximal borders.
- Check for clearance and/or irritation at axilla and epicondyles.
- Check for compression of ulnar nerve at cubital tunnel area and of superficial sensory branch of radial nerve.

PATTERN PEARLS 1–104 TO 1–107

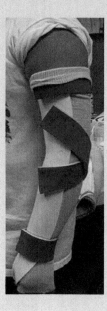

FIGURE PP1–104 Crossing straps on posteriorly to increase purchase.

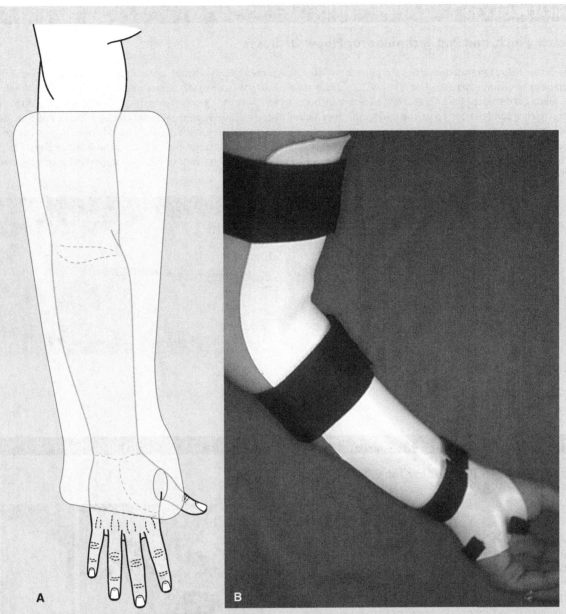

FIGURE PP1–105 **A and B,** Anterior elbow orthosis including wrist, commonly with forearm in neutral to full supination.

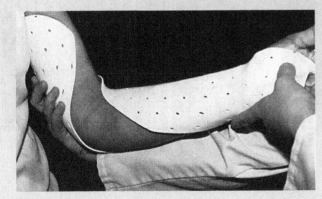

FIGURE PP1–106 Spiral design to avoid pressure on sensitive scar area medially.

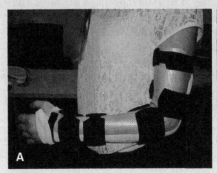
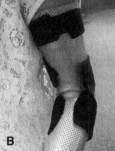

FIGURE PP1–107 **A and B,** Anterior elbow orthosis with seam to accommodate for 90° flexion angle.

CLINICAL PEARL 1-63

Stretch, Pinch, and Pop Technique for Elbow Orthoses

This technique can be helpful in situations when the patient is unable to assume a gravity-assisted position or when the therapist is challenged managing a large pattern of orthotic material. Use ⅛" or 3/32" coated elastic material (such as Aquaplast®; Performance Health). When the material is stretched, the coating is disrupted partially to allow a temporary bond where pieces are gently pinched together. Keep in mind that the farther the material has to stretch around the body part, the thinner the material will become, possibly weakening the overall orthosis. Position the patient in the desired position. After heating fully, the material can be applied to the body parts desired surface and then quickly stretched and pinched segmentally along the opposite surface **(A)**. Be sure to maintain the desired positions while the material cools. Once the orthosis is completely set, pop the seams apart. Neatly trim and smooth any rough edges **(B)**. This technique can be used about joints or to fabricate nonarticular arm (humerus) or forearm orthoses (as shown in A).

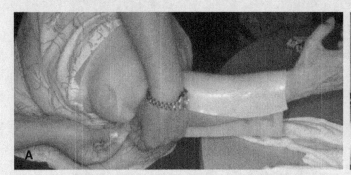

CLINICAL PEARL 1-64

Gravity-Assisted Positioning for Elbow Orthoses

When fabricating an elbow orthosis (anterior or posterior), it can be quite helpful to have the patient place the arm in a gravity-assisted position to ease the molding process. This position can be achieved in several ways, but common to all is the goal of having the area to be covered with the thermoplastic facing the ceiling. **A,** For an anterior orthosis, simply lean the olecranon on a table and control the amount of extension by placing appropriately sized towel rolls at upper arm and wrist. For posterior designs, the patient or assistant can hold the various positions as shown: **(B)** prone on plinth, **(C)** flexed at hips with upper arm parallel to floor (good position to control amount of forearm rotation distally), and **(D)** shoulder abducted with hand resting on head. Whatever position is chosen when using gravity as an assist, the clinician must be acutely aware of not letting the elbow drop into too much flexion with posterior orthoses or too much extension (with anterior designs) as the orthosis is being fabricated.

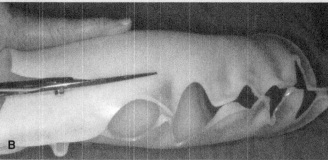

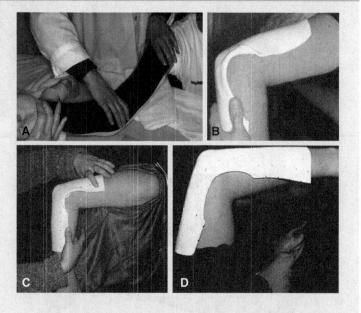

SHOULDER ABDUCTION (OR ADDUCTION) IMMOBILIZATION ORTHOSIS (SO/SEO) (Fig. 1–47)

COMMON NAMES
- Gunslinger splint
- Airplane splint

ALTERNATIVE ORTHOSIS OPTIONS
- Prefabricated orthosis

PRIMARY FUNCTIONS
- Immobilize shoulder joint to allow healing of involved structure(s).

Common Diagnoses	Optimal Positions
Brachial plexus injury	Shoulder: 30° abduction, 30°–45° flexion, slight ER; elbow: 90° flexion; forearm: neutral rotation
Tendon transfers for plexus injury	Shoulder: adduction, 30°–45° flexion, slight ER; elbow: 90° flexion; forearm: neutral rotation
Shoulder and humeral arthroplasty	Shoulder: 30° abduction and flexion; 15° ER; elbow: 90° flexion; forearm: neutral rotation

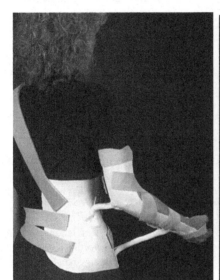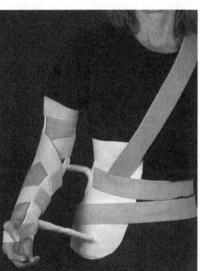

FIGURE 1–47

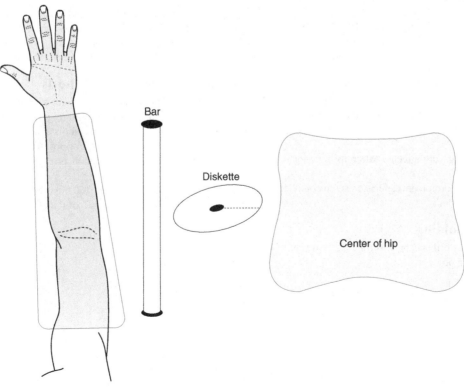

Bar

Diskette

Center of hip

FIGURE 1–48

FABRICATION PROCESS

Pattern Creation (Fig. 1–48)

- Correct positions of shoulder and elbow depend on injury and/or surgical procedure. Communicate with physician before orthosis application.
- Pattern should be made with patient's clothing on. If possible, fabricate trunk orthosis before surgical procedure; posterior elbow orthosis may also be fabricated before surgery. But remember that postoperative edema may alter fit, and accommodation may be needed.
- Posterior elbow component
  - Follow directions for posterior elbow immobilization orthosis, making certain that there is adequate troughing to accommodate connector bars.
- Trunk component
  - Take measurements on affected side with patient standing.
  - Mark distal border from midsternum to vertebral border dorsally.
  - Mark proximal border from naval to vertebral border dorsally.
  - Connect to form lateral borders (should somewhat rectangular).
- Connector component
  - Length of connector bars determined by desired shoulder position: the more elevation, the longer the bars.
  - Measure 1½″ to 2″ for width. This material will be rolled onto itself for added strength.
  - Four 2″ in diameter disks of thermoplastic material help secure connector bars onto trunk and elbow portions.

Refine Pattern

- Wrist inclusion is optional, depending on diagnosis and patient comfort.
- After determining length of connector bars, allow extra 1″ on each end for application onto trunk orthosis.
- To provide added strength, include 3/32″ aluminum wire within thermoplastic roll. This is especially helpful for maintaining shoulder elevation, owing to potential high force delivered to connector bars.

Options for Materials

- Use uncoated thermoplastic material to aid in bonding of connector bars. If uncoated materials are not available, then disrupt coating on all connected surfaces before adhering.
- Posterior elbow component: use ⅛″ uncoated perforated plastic or elastic-based material. Choose elastic material if patient has pain and/or cannot assist in shoulder positioning because tackiness may aid during molding process.
- Trunk component: consider ⅛″ solid, rubber-based, uncoated material for its strength and stability.
- Connector component: use ⅛″ solid, rubber-based, uncoated material for bars and disks.

Cut and Heat

- Use plinth where there is full access to involved extremity to increase ease of molding process. Have assistant support arm in appropriate position.
- Position patient side lying with affected extremity superior to achieve gravity assistance.
- If necessary, prepad bony prominences: iliac crest, epicondyles, olecranon process, and ulnar styloid.

Evaluate Fit While Molding

Note: The fabrication of this orthosis may warrant an "extra set of hands" to assist during the molding process.

- Posterior elbow component
  - Carefully mold as described for posterior elbow immobilization orthosis.
  - Allow enough material for connector bar application.

- Trunk component
  - Remove warm material from heating pan and support with both hands. Carefully place along trunk, as shown.
  - Mold well about waist and over iliac crest to prevent orthosis from sliding off hip.
- Connector component
  - Remove warm material and place on flat surface. Position wire in center of material and roll onto itself, forming thick bar. Repeat process for the other bar.
  - Apply strapping before adhering components together.

Strapping and Components

- Posterior elbow component
  - Use stockinette or elasticized sleeve if edema is present before orthosis application to eliminate pinching of skin once straps are applied.
  - Apply 2″ soft straps to proximal and distal portions of orthosis.
  - Proximal strap should be wide and applied at most proximal portion of orthosis to prevent rocking.
  - Crisscross design directly over anterior elbow helps maintain elbow securely in orthosis.
  - Consider using an Ace™ wrap or 3″ Coban™ to secure if edema is an issue.
- Trunk component
  - Apply one 3″ to 6″ soft strap or two 2″ straps with D-ring closure about waist (width and number of straps depend on patient's trunk size).
  - Apply 2″ soft strap directed from sternum, across uninvolved shoulder, to posterior vertebral border. D-ring attachment is recommended for ease of adjustment.
  - Pad portion of strap that traverses opposite shoulder to maximize comfort.
- Connector components
  - Disks act as reinforcements and should be applied once bars are attached.
  - While an assistant maintains desired position of shoulder, apply trunk and elbow orthosis.
  - Mark for upper and lower bar placements on both orthosis components.
  - Prepare all surfaces for bonding.
  - Heat 1″ of both ends of two connector bars and secure to premarked areas.
  - Throughout process, check that correct shoulder position is maintained; making adjustments can be difficult.
  - Heat disk thoroughly; make slit halfway through disk; open; and wrap about bar and orthosis base, molding firmly into place.

Survey Completed Orthosis

- Trunk orthosis can be lined with Microfoam™ tape or padding material (gel or foam) to help prevent migration and rotation.
- Smooth and slightly flare all distal and proximal borders.
- Check for clearance and/or irritation of trunk, axilla, ulnar styloid, epicondyles, and olecranon process (thumb and MCP joints, if wrist included).
- Check for compression of ulnar nerve at cubital tunnel area and of superficial sensory branch of radial nerve.

CHAPTER 1: IMMOBILIZATION ORTHOSES DISCUSSION POINTS

1. What types of injuries are most appropriate for an Immobilization orthosis?
2. What stage of wound healing is most often treated with immobilization?
3. Give two examples of immobilization orthosis for a wrist fracture. Include
   - the proper positioning of the joints involved;
   - proper placement of straps and foam'
   - what are the most important considerations during fabrication?
4. Give an example of an immobilization orthosis that would allow increased functional use of the hand.
5. Explain the importance strapping proper strapping plays in the fabrication of an orthosis.

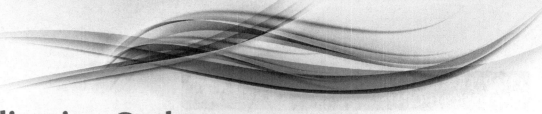

2 Mobilization Orthoses

MaryLynn A. Jacobs, MBA, MS, OTR/L, CHT
Noelle M. Austin, MS, PT, CHT

GENERAL CLINICAL PEARLS RELATED TO MOBILIZATION ORTHOSES

CLINICAL PEARL 2–X1

Fingernail Attachments

A, Hook material. A small piece of hook strapping material (size should accommodate the length and width of the nail) can be glued to the fingernail using a gel-based glue. Once set, a strip of ½" loop (preferably soft material such as Rolyan® SoftStrap®, Performance Health) can be added to the hook with the line attached and pulling proximally. This technique may work well for patients who have a large nail surface area.

B, Dress hooks. A dress hook can be glued to the nail using a gel-based glue. Bend the hook slightly to provide optimal contour with the nail (contoured hooks can be purchased). Take care to place the hook as proximal on the nail as possible. If the hook is placed too far distally, the force may apply undue pressure on the nail bed. The line is either applied directly to the hook or attached first to a small piece of loop that has been attached to the dress hook. Some clinicians prefer this loop method because it prevents the line from digging into the skin as it traverses over the fingertip.

C, Commercially available devices. Prefabricated devices are available lines with nonskid material to prevent slippage. 3pp® Finger Trapper™ (IF) and Rolyan® Wrap-On™ Finger Hooks offer an alternative to using glue on the nail (both available through Performance Health).

D–G, Therapeutic tape. Custom trim a piece of therapeutic tape and attach directly to the fingertip as shown.

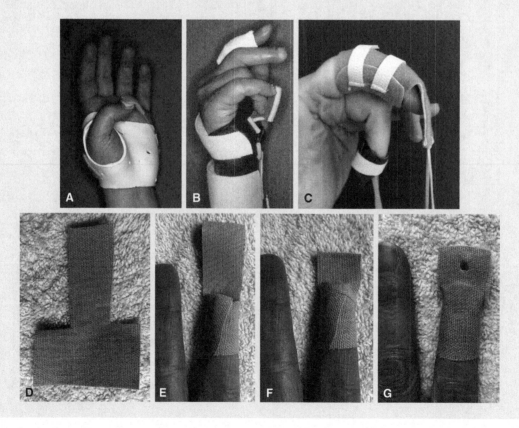

CLINICAL PEARL 2–X2

Static Line

Fishing line was traditionally used by therapists **(A)**, shown with this MCP mobilization orthosis. However, this product can be challenging to visualize, manage, and keep knots tied because of its smooth texture. **B and C,** Nymo Cord (Performance Health) offers a superior option that is easier to handle when knotting and guiding through pulley systems. The knots stay intact, and the color white is easy to visualize.

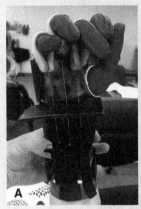
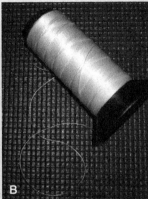
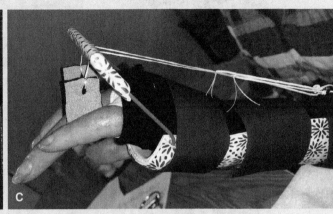

CLINICAL PEARL 2–X3

Wrapped Elastic Cord

Wrapped elastic cord is a latex-free option allowing for easy modification of force applied and does not degrade as traditional elastics do over time. May also bypass the need for using static line since the cord can pass through pulley systems with larger holes. Shown here with an ulnar boost and thumb mobilization orthosis.

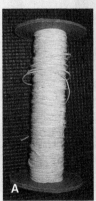
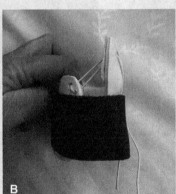
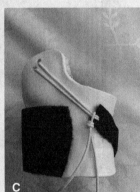
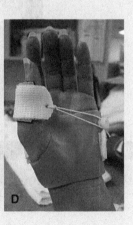

CLINICAL PEARL 2–X4

Digit Slings

A, Commercially available devices. Several styles of slings are commercially available in a multitude of materials with various thicknesses. Care should be taken with slings that converge into one line (also known as a loop—shown here on small finger). This design allows little accommodation for fluctuations in edema, potentially causing compressive forces about the lateral aspects of the digit, which may lead to neurovascular compromise. Note the difference of the loop that is joined at the top of the small finger versus the sling on the index finger (two lines pulling up). The index finger has no pressure along the lateral borders. **B–E, Homemade.** Consider utilizing scraps of thermoplastic **(B)**, loop material **(C)**, neoprene **(D)** or rubber tubing which adds the benefit of nonskid to prevent migration **(E)**.

F–I, Thermoplastic. Mold 1/16″ material to the volar **(F)** or dorsal **(G)** aspect of a digit to function as a sling. The material should extend the full length of the segment being mobilized (clearing the creases) and encompass half to two-thirds the circumference of the segment. The thermoplastic sling maximally distributes pressure and prevents excessive compressive forces, which are sometimes caused by constrictive soft slings (refer to Chapter 4 for greater detail). A small strip of adhesive hook is placed on the middorsal or volar portion of the sling. The midpoint of a 1″ by 3″ strip of loop material is placed over the adhesive hook. One hole is punched on both distal ends of the loop material. Monofilament line or elastic force is then attached at both ends of the loop and fed through the line guide and pulley to the proximal attachment device **(F and G)**. A thin layer of foam can be added beneath the thermoplastic sling to increase comfort, if necessary. Another option is using neoprene or foam material on the digit, then forming a more rigid sling over the material with a thermoplastic tape such as QuickCast 2 shown (Performance Health) **(H)**. Thermoplastic tape can be used as a circumferential immobilization orthosis under a sling to provide a dual purpose. In this case, the thumb IP is held in extension to direct all forces of flexion to the thumb MP joint **(I)**.

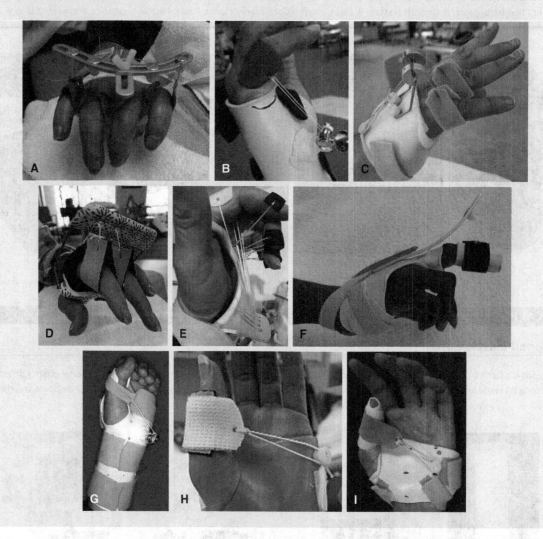

CLINICAL PEARL 2–X5

Custom-Bent Aluminum Wire Outrigger

Occasionally, commercial outriggers are not adequate to accommodate for the correct angle of application; therefore, a therapist can choose to create a custom outrigger by carefully bending aluminum wire. The wire can be purchased, or a wire clothes hanger can do the trick! Note the severe PIP flexion contracture of the RF **(A)**. The outrigger has to be extended far enough distally to be able to create a 90° angle of application **(B and C)**. Shown here is a custom-bent wire with a piece of thermoplastic connecting the distal portion. Holes have been added, via hole punch, to the material so that the correct angle of application can gently draw the PIP joints into extension **(D)**.

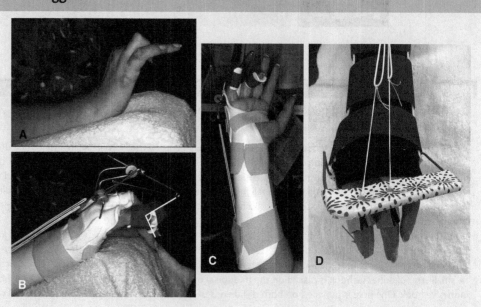

CLINICAL PEARL 2–X6

Line Guides

A, Safety pin. A safety pin is a cost-effective way to provide a smooth and simple guide for a monofilament line. Shown is a small finger PIP extension (dynamic via rubber band and Phoenix Outrigger System; Performance Health) mobilization orthosis. Note how the placement of the safety pin lifts the monofilament line off the dorsum of the MCP joint, preventing the line from dragging across the orthosis base. To apply, bend and flatten the wide end of the safety pin. Scratch the application surface and use solvent over this area. Next, holding the "eye" end of the safety pin with flat nose pliers, heat the flattened end with a heat gun and embed it into the desired area of the orthosis. This step should be completed with the orthosis off the patient's hand. Secure the safety pin by adding a scrap piece of thermoplastic material over the union. Allow the area to set before feeding the line through the hole.

B and C, Thermoplastic. Scrap pieces of thermoplastic material can be used to create a line guide in many orthoses. **B,** In this case, an MCP flexion mobilization orthosis. The length and width of the line guide depends on the location and severity of the contracture(s). Secure the thermoplastic line guide to the orthosis base by scraping the attachment site and using solvent to remove any protective coating. Heat the section of material that will be attached, dry off water, and then embed that section into the prepared base. Hold the nonheated section in a perpendicular fashion, maintaining a 90° angle with the segment that is to be mobilized (in this case, the proximal phalanges). Once set, use a hole punch to create holes at the appropriate area to form a 90° angle of force application. As ROM increases, create a new hole to maintain the optimal angle of pull; the material can also be cut down. Highly perforated material provides many holes to choose from, eliminating the need for a hole punch. Note the two homemade proximal attachment devices. **C,** For an MCP extension mobilization orthosis, a scrap piece of thermoplastic material can be rolled and formed into an outrigger. Adhesive hook material can be applied dorsally to guide the lines. Use a strip of loop on top to keep lines in place.

D, Custom-bent outrigger and perforated thermoplastic. An outrigger can be created by bending 3/32" aluminum wire to form a dorsal segment. Cover it with perforated material, slightly overlap the material at the wire's edge, and then pinch and seal it. The slings are placed on the digits, and the line is threaded through the appropriate hole in the thermoplastic material to produce a 90° angle of pull. The elastic force is then attached to the line and directed to the proximal attachment device. **E,** Bent coat hanger with solid thermoplastic piece molded over edge with holes formed using hole punch to allow line to pass through.

F–I, Commercially available devices. Commercially available guides are simple to attach, remove, and reuse. However, some of these devices do not provide the extended length and adjustability many orthoses require to maintain the desired 90° angle of force application. If the angle is not close to 90°, the line may drag through an edge of the line guide, creating increased frictional force. **F,** The Phoenix Single-Digit Outrigger (Performance Health); **G,** Rolyan® Individual Line Guides (Performance Health); **H,** Base 2™ Outrigger System (North Coast Medical) and commercially available line guides; and **I,** Orfitube™ System (North Coast Medical) with cap ends to prevent elastic from fraying.

J–L, Aquatubes®. Used as line guides, Aquatubes® (Performance Health) can prevent the lines from getting caught on an adjacent digit's line or on clothing and bed linens. **J,** Cut the Aquatubes® into ¼" disks, spot heat, and attach to a thermoplastic outrigger to create a line guide. **K,** Aquatubes® can be cut into small tubes (1" to 2"), and the pieces can be used to create a low-profile design. **L,** The Aquatube® was heated and formed into this line guide to maintain optimal line of force application. **L,** Aquatube was adhered to the base and prior to setting was pinched to flatten out where the monofilament line was desired to pass. Then a hole punch was used to "punch out" a smooth hole. **M,** In this IP flexion mobilization orthosis (static progressive approach), a small section of the distal border of the thermoplastic was spot heated and punctured to create a guide for the monofilament line. The hole was placed in alignment with the longitudinal axis of the middle finger.

N, Orthosis base. Utilize this technique to create a streamlined line guide that you do not have to worry about any parts of orthosis falling off. Create small holes with hole punch, heat area with heat gun, and utilize a paper clip to gently "lift" the region between the holes to form the line guide.

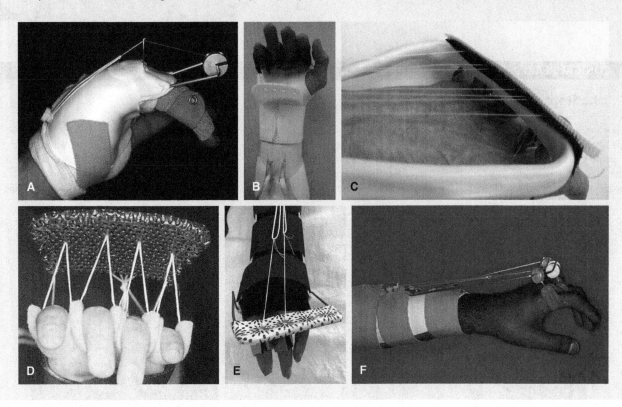

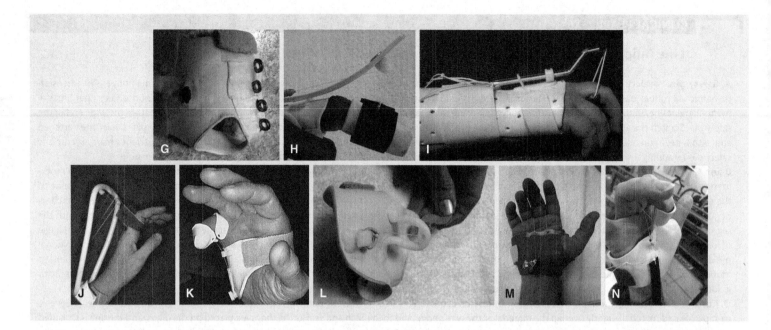

CLINICAL PEARL 2-X7

Adhering Components to Thermoplastic

A few key tips can make the process of component application success-ful. Firstly, prepare the thermoplastic by removing any protective coating with solvent, by scratching or scoring area thoroughly. Next, heat both the component by holding it over the heat gun using pliers for safety **(A)** and the targeted region on orthosis. Imbed this component into the prepared thermoplastic. To obtain optimal adherence, reinforce this area with a scrap piece of thermoplastic that has also been prepared by removing coating, heating, and adhering over the top of the component **(B)**. Obviously this process needs to be completed OFF the patient!

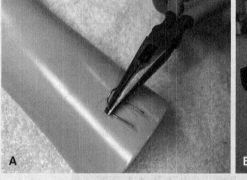

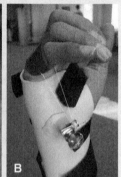

CLINICAL PEARL 2-X8

Line Stops

A–C, A line stop can be placed on the monofilament line to limit motion, as required with some extensor tendon and early mobilization protocols (Phoenix Outrigger System; Performance Health). This provides the therapist a way to restrict joint flexion to a specific degree. The patient is allowed to flex the joints actively within the range permitted by the stop bead; the dynamic component passively brings the digits back into extension. Commercial line stops (stop beads) are applied by placing the stop bead in the desired location and compressing it with pliers **(A and B)**. Stops can be repositioned to allow for a progres-sive increase in motion as healing allows, or the restrictive device can be simply fabricated by using tape **(C)** (although not as aesthetically pleasing).

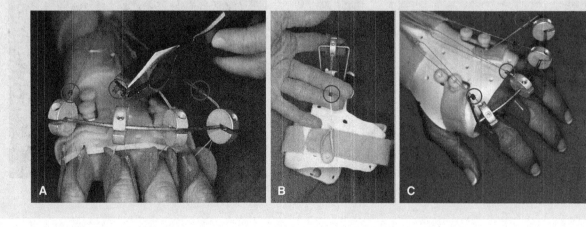

CHAPTER 2

CLINICAL PEARL 2–X9

Preparing Coated Materials for Bonding

When using thermoplastic material with a protective coating, the surfaces must be prepared if bonding of two pieces is necessary. To prepare the surfaces, use a commercially available solvent to eliminate the coating on the surface **(A)** or scratch and score the material's surface to disrupt the coating **(B)** either using an emery board or the ends of scissors. Use a heat gun to hyperheat the material, which helps make it tacky and more likely to adhere. To ensure a strong bond, press the materials firmly together. This is especially important if the bonded piece will be used as a line guide where forces will be placed upon or generated through this bonded piece **(C and D)**.

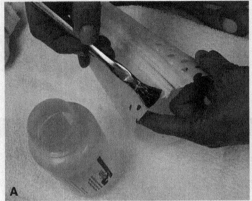
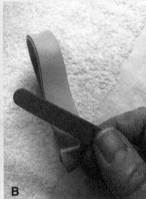
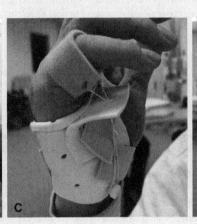
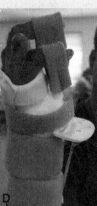

A   B   C   D

CLINICAL PEARL 2–X10

Forming Holes in Thermoplastic Material

A, Heated wire technique. To form holes in thermoplastic material in regions where a hole punch cannot reach, heat a 3/32″ piece of wire over a heat gun using flat-nose pliers. Pierce the hot end of the wire onto the premarked area. Move the heated wire around, forming a small hole, and immediately position the rubber band post or rivet in place. As an alternative, heat the end of an Allen wrench or awl instead of a wire. Note that this procedure should always be done with the orthosis off the patient.

B and C, Dremel. A small hand drill can be a useful tool to keep in a clinic; it provides a quick and easy way to make holes in difficult-to-reach areas. A Dremel can be used to form a hole or a slit in thermoplastic material. Making multiple holes can "perforate" a specific region of the orthosis to help improve air flow. Practicing these techniques on scrap pieces of material can help a therapist master this process. Caution should be taken to ensure the surface area that abuts the skin does not have residual sharp ridges/edges from the drilling process. Be mindful to immediately remove the shards of plastic while it is warm after making the hole, or try quickly heating the area with a heat gun and rubbing the underside of the holes; it can take away any debris from drilling.

D, Hole punch. The classic hole punch is the most accessible and convenient to use; however, it does not offer the depth necessary to make holes in the more central portions of an orthosis. Hole punches work well for holes on the border of an orthosis as shown on the radial border of this wrist immobilization orthosis.

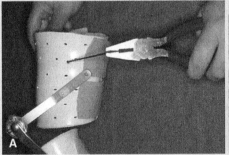
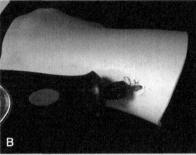

A   B

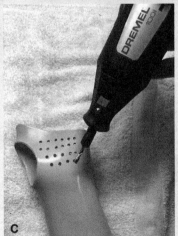
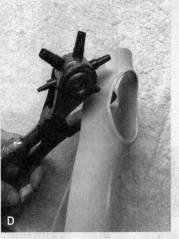

C   D

CLINICAL PEARL 2–X11

90° Line of Force Application

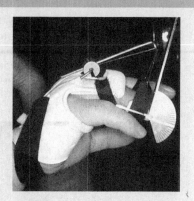

A goniometer ensures that a 90° line of application has been achieved (shown is Rolyan˚ Outrigger; Performance Health). This maximizes the effectiveness of the force application. Orthoses may need to be readjusted frequently, depending on the responsiveness of the tissue to the mobilization force. Another useful method includes holding an Allen wrench (perpendicular bend in metal) to the side of the segment mobilized to help visualize the 90° angle.

CLINICAL PEARL 2–X12

Mobilization Forces

A, Elastic cord. Wrapped elastic cord is a quick and commonly used method for providing a mobilization force for dynamic orthoses. The wrapped elastic can be directly fastened from the sling to the proximal attachment device. Be aware that if the cord traverses through line guides, the friction (or drag) may alter the force placed on the intended structures. Because the elastic cord is wrapped with cotton, it is less elastic and forgiving than rubber bands and should not be treated in the same way. Doubling the resting length of the cord will generate a much greater tension than doubling the length of a rubber band. There is a longer shelf life with this product versus traditional rubber bands that degrade over time. The dual-purpose orthosis shown is a combination of MCP flexion and PIP extension mobilization. MCP flexion is generated via elastic cord and a custom thermoplastic line guide, whereas the mobilization for PIP extension includes a Phoenix Outrigger (Performance Health).

B and C, Rubber bands. Rubber bands are the most commonly used component for generating tension in mobilization orthoses. They are readily available, inexpensive, and easy to apply and adjust and come in various lengths and widths. Be aware that the tension generated is directly related to the rubber band's length and width. Thinner rubber bands provide less tension and are more susceptible to fatigue and breaking; thus, they need to be replaced more often. It is recommended not to buy too many bands at one time since their shelf life is limited. The device shown is a forearm-based PIP extension mobilization orthosis (Phoenix Digit Outriggers [Performance Health]). Notice in **C** the use of a series of holes in the rubber band to allow for progressive change to dynamic force.

D, Spring coils. Graded spring coils offer a consistent way to control force accurately in a dynamic orthosis. Springs generate a given force based on their overall length and width, coil tightness, and the distance they have to travel from the proximal to distal attachment. Springs have been shown to be more durable and last longer than rubber bands. However, they are more expensive than rubber bands and wrapped elastic cord. A clinic should have various springs on hand to address a potential range of needs, although this may not always be feasible. The PIP dynamic traction orthosis shown includes a modified Digitec base outrigger (North Coast Medical).

E and F, TheraBand˚ or TheraTubing˚ (Performance Health). These work especially well with larger designs such as wrist, forearm, and elbow mobilization orthoses. The force delivered to the tissue depends on the tension property of the band. A custom wrist and digit extension mobilization orthosis is shown.

G, Tape. Microfoam™ tape (Performance Health) can be used to quickly fabricate a mobilization orthosis. The tape can be adjusted easily and be effectively reused several times. A custom small finger MCP flexion mobilization orthosis is shown.

H, Neoprene. Neoprene material, because of its elastic nature, can be used effectively in a cost-saving way to provide a mobilization force. Refer to Chapter 14 for further instruction. Shown here is a wrist, thumb, and digit extension mobilization orthosis applied to a radial nerve injured hand.

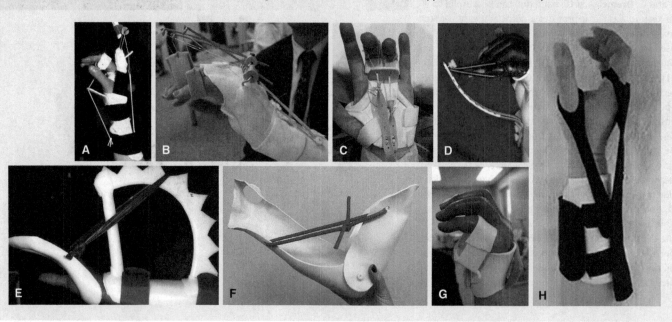

CLINICAL PEARL 2–X13

Proximal Attachment Devices

A, Aquatubes˚. An orthosis that is used as a mobilization device during the scar-remodeling phase of wound healing for a patient who sustained a severe crush injury. Rehabilitation focused on increasing digit ROM. Note the creative use of applying mobilization forces to the tissue. Static progressive stretch is applied to the MF via thin strapping material attached by hook on the nail and to the adhesive hook on the orthosis base proximally. The RF and SF are placed in PIP/DIP flexion mobilization straps. The SF has an additional sling that applies flexion force to the MP joint, creating a composite stretch to that digit. Note the Aquatubes˚ (Performance Health) used as the custom-made proximal attachment device; as an alternative, a scrap piece of thermoplastic can be fashioned into a hook as well. **B, Various.** Paper clips and dress hooks can be bent, heated, and applied to the thermoplastic material **(far right)**. Rubber band posts and thumb nuts are also easy devices to apply to an orthosis for attaching mobilization components **(middle)**. Another technique is to heat the small section where the proximal attachment device should be placed; then pierce through the material with scissors, lifting up from the orthosis base with a pencil (or similar object) to form an elongated hole that is approximately 4/5″. This forms a raised area where rubber bands can be attached **(far left)**.
C, Thermoplastic. Shown is a homemade line guide and proximal attachment device for a DIP mobilization orthosis.
D and E, Commercially available devices. These provide a quick and easy way to attach mobilization components. They can be easily reused and/or adjusted. The orthosis shown has several holes for the rubber band post to allow for quick adjustment as ROM improves **(D)** (Rolyan˚ Outrigger System; Performance Health). Note that more than one proximal attachment device may be needed, depending on the number of rubber bands to be attached. Wing nuts or similar devices can also be used as shown here **(E)**.
F and G, Loop and hook materials. F, Static progressive approach using a D-ring with simple loop and hook as the proximal attachment. **G,** Neoprene material attached directly to adhesive-backed hook in order to generate the elbow flexion mobilization force.
H and I, Orthosis base. Create a slit in the proximal end of an orthosis by either using a Dremel or making a series of holes with a hole punch. Feed the loop strapping through this slit and attach it back onto itself via double-sided adhesive hook. This technique allows the patient to adjust the tension distally similar to using a D-Ring—but no worries on that segment coming loose.

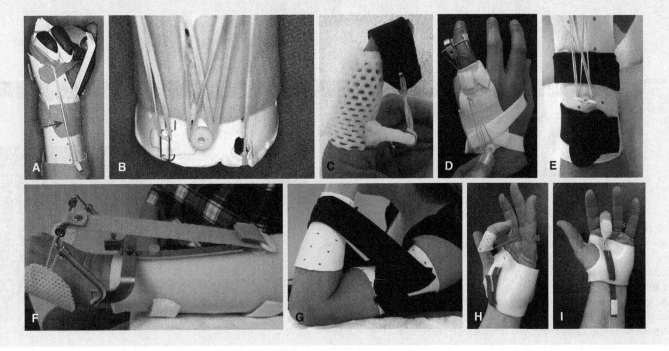

CLINICAL PEARL 2–X14

Homemade D-Ring

Homemade D-rings, often used as proximal attachment devices for mobilization orthoses, can easily be fabricated out of thermoplastic material to accommodate the standard 1″ and 2″ straps as well as wider strapping material. (Commercially available D-rings come in various sizes, commonly 1″, 1.5″, and 2″.) Use a scrap piece of thermoplastic material cut into a strip approximately ½″ wide. The length depends on how big the D-ring has to be. Heat the material, roll it onto itself for rigidity, overlap the ends, and pinch together firmly. Use your IFs to maintain the shape until the material is set. Be sure to prepare the surfaces of the material for bonding to ensure a strong attachment. Shown here is a homemade D-ring for the attachment of a static progressive strap for an elbow flexion mobilization orthosis.

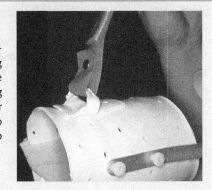

CLINICAL PEARL 2–X15

Preventing Orthosis Migration

There are a few products that can be helpful to have in the clinic to prevent orthosis migration which is a common consequence when a mobilization force is applied. **A,** Dycem can be adhered to the inside of the orthosis, and when this comes in contact with the skin, the orthosis will not move. **B,** Microfoam™ Tape is a low-tack foam tape that has a nonskid quality. Strips of this product can be added on the inside of both custom and prefabricated orthoses to prevent slippage with wear.

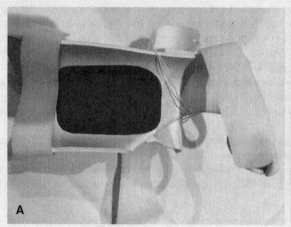

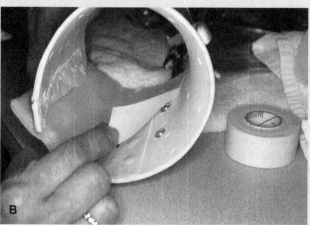

CLINICAL PEARL 2–X16

Elbow and Shoulder Harnesses

When designing a mobilization orthosis for the upper extremity, special consideration should be taken regarding potential migration. Some degree of migration will inevitably occur when the orthosis is worn secondary to the forces that are generated in order to mobilize tissue. A therapist can consider proximal stabilization that may assist in proper positioning and security of the orthosis onto the arm.

A, A shoulder harness can be fabricated from 2″ soft strapping material. The shoulder harness, which helps prevent distal migration of large arm orthoses, can be fabricated in various ways. The strapping is initiated on the posterior border of the orthosis and directed across the back and toward the opposite shoulder. It then passes across chest to attach to the anterior orthosis. An additional strap is initiated on the anterior aspect of the orthosis and traverses posteriorly to attach to the other strap. The straps can be riveted together.

B, For smaller orthoses that do not have a mobilization force yet need additional stabilization, consider a simple cross chest neoprene strap as seen in this nonarticular proximal humeral orthosis.

C, Forearm orthoses such as wrist flexion and/or extension mobilization orthoses can be anchored to the elbow to counteract the tendency for these devices to migrate distally on the forearm. When this occurs, there may be interruption of full mobility and irritation of bony prominences. There are numerous ways to secure orthoses to the proximal arm. Shown here is a simple foam strap that traverses about the posterior elbow and meets at the same proximal attachment device as the rubber bands. The elbow should be in flexion in order for this to be most effective.

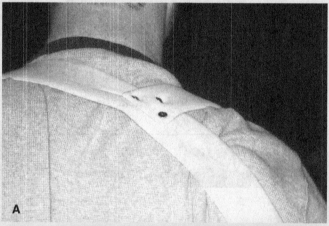

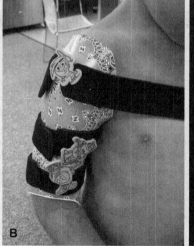

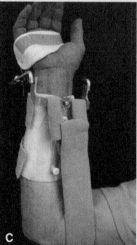

CLINICAL PEARL 2–X17

Orthoses and Modalities

A mobilization orthosis can be used to enhance the use of therapeutic modalities. For example, a static progressive IF MCP flexion mobilization orthosis (shown here) can be applied while ultrasound is being used on the adherent extensor tendons over the dorsum of the IF. Another example is stabilizing the wrist (blocking the wrist flexors and extensors) with a wrist immobilization orthosis while applying neuromuscular stimulation to the extrinsic digital flexors and/or extensors to facilitate tendon glide. Orthoses can be worn directly over electrodes as long as the patient is instructed in proper electrode application and maintenance.

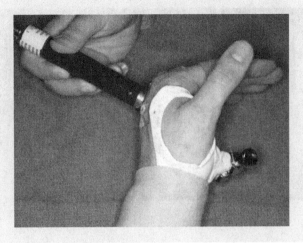

CLINICAL PEARL 2–X18

Measuring Tension

A, Tension can be measured using various tools; however, nothing can replace clinical judgment **(B)** and attention to the targeted tissue's response.

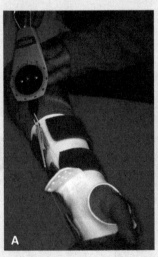

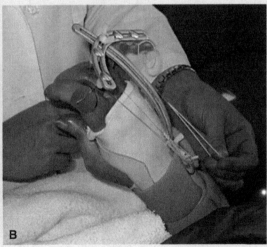

CLINICAL PEARL 2–X19

Sign of Too Much Tension!

A, Excessive tension is noted by the uniform blanching of the DIP joints. **B,** Note the blanching of the thumb dorsal IP joint and the volar MP joint and **(C)** dusky coloring distal to slings in this MCP mobilization orthosis. **D,** The dorsal sling shown here is applied directly over the middle phalanx (made from traditional loop material). A better choice would be to first fabricate a thermoplastic dorsal shell over the width and length of the middle phalanx and then apply the loop sling. The shear stress created by the loop sling alone can be dissipated over a larger surface area as shown in **(E)**, therefore making this a much more comfortable fit.

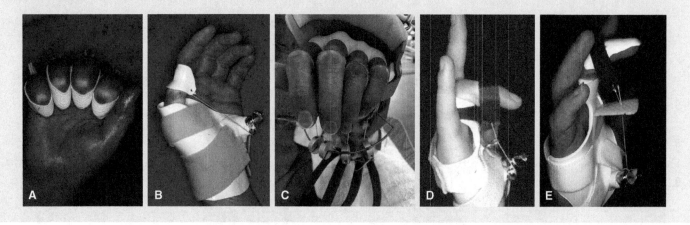

CLINICAL PEARL 2–X20

Combining Design Choices

Creating multipurpose orthoses that address more than one deficit can be helpful in situations when cost is an issue for one versus two orthoses. **A and B,** Shown here is a wrist extension mobilization/composite digit flexion orthosis. For the mobilization of the wrist, a dynamic design was used and for the digits a static progressive approach was chosen. Both choices depended on the severity and length of the stiffness and the ease of use for the patient. **C and D,** A dorsal wrist extension immobilization orthosis with an MCP extension assist (dynamic approach), combined with a static progressive IP flexion mobilization strap to address intrinsic tightness. **E and F,** Combined wrist extension and flexion mobilization orthosis using the Digitec system. **G,** Hand-based PIP extension and flexion mobilization orthosis using Phoenix outrigger for extension component.

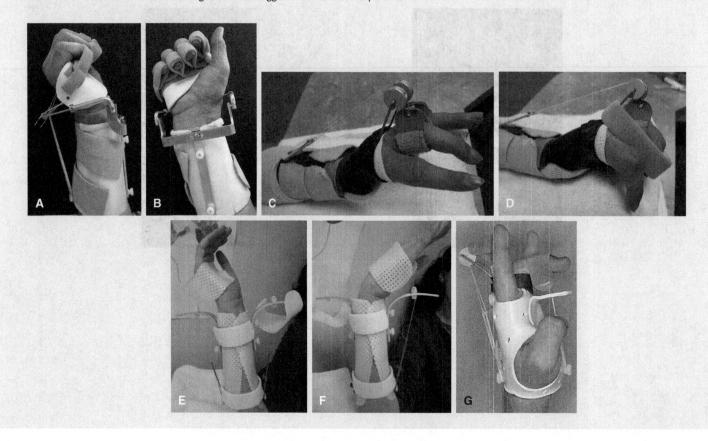

1 Digit- and Thumb-Based Orthoses

DISTAL INTERPHALANGEAL FLEXION MOBILIZATION ORTHOSIS (FO) (Fig. 2–1)

COMMON NAMES
- Dynamic DIP flexion orthosis

ALTERNATIVE ORTHOSIS OPTIONS
- Prefabricated orthosis
- Casting (serial static flexion)

PRIMARY FUNCTIONS
- Provide low-load, prolonged flexion mobilization force to DIP joint to facilitate lengthening of tissues.

Common Diagnoses	General Optimal Positions
DIP joint extension contracture	Proximal interphalangeal (PIP) 0°; DIP: terminal flexion

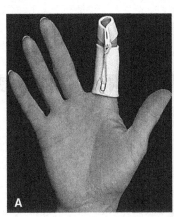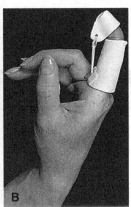

FIGURE 2–1

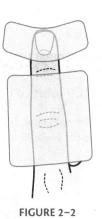

FIGURE 2–2

FABRICATION PROCESS

Pattern Creation (Fig. 2–2)

- For individuals with short digits, orthosis may need to include the metacarpophalangeal (MCP) joint to better stabilize PIP joint for optimal force application distally.
- For proximal attachment device, prepare one scrap (½″ by 1″) of thermoplastic material.

Refine Pattern

- Make sure that digital web spaces are cleared and that PIP joint is held in 0° extension.
- DIP flexion crease should be cleared proximally.

Options for Materials

- Use nonperforated 1/16″, 1/32″, or ⅛″ material.
- Plastic materials conform well to contours of digit.

Cut and Heat

- Position patient with hand supinated, digits slightly abducted, resting over platform.

- Warm material.
- Prepare mobilization components: sling, line, rubber band, and proximal attachment device.

Evaluate Fit While Molding

- Fabricate PIP orthosis.
- Clear distally to allow unimpeded DIP flexion.

Strapping and Components

- Circumferential design does not require straps.
- Sling must be wide enough to distribute pressure over dorsum of DIP joint and short enough to prevent interference with line guide if used.
- Secure proximal attachment device at most proximal border of orthosis along longitudinal axis of proximal phalanx.
- Connect rubber band to sling and loop at proximal device.

Survey Completed Orthosis

- Adjust tension per patient and/or tissue tolerance; goal is low-load stretch over prolonged period of time.

PATTERN PEARLS 2–1 AND 2–2

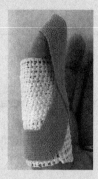

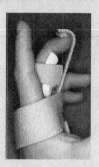

FIGURE PP2–1 Circumferential stabilization of PIP joint, with Kinesio° Tex Tape (Performance Health) strap applying gentle flexion force to DIP joint.

FIGURE PP2–2 Dynamic force via elastic strapping attached to adhesive hook on nail.

CLINICAL PEARL 2–1

Including MCP Joint to Increase Effectiveness of DIP Stretch

To better secure the PIP joint, consider including the MCP joint in the orthosis. The additional length allows for a longer line of application, which can increase the effectiveness of this type of device. This is especially helpful when fabricating an orthosis on a small hand.

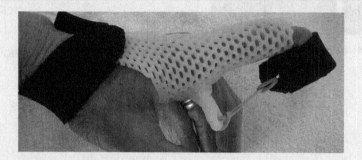

CLINICAL PEARL 2–2

Creating 90° Angle of Application on a Digit Orthosis

It is often challenging and cumbersome to add an outrigger to a digit orthosis. When compliance and functionality are not an issue, consider a simple "home-made" thermoplastic outrigger applied to the most proximal base of the digit orthosis; this can be easily modified to obtain the optimal angle by heating and reshaping.

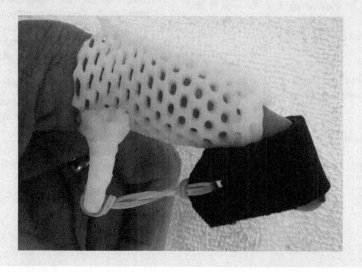

CLINICAL PEARL 2–3

Serial Static Approach to Mobilize a Stiff DIP Joint

Application of a circumferential orthosis such as QuickCast 2 **(A)** or Orficast™ or a plaster of paris (POP) digit cast **(B and C)** can be an effective way to provide a low-load, prolonged flexion force (serial static) to a DIP extension contracture. Including the PIP joint and the entire length of the proximal phalanx will increase the purchase of the orthosis/cast and its overall effectiveness.

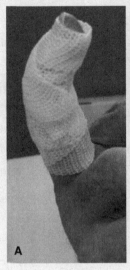
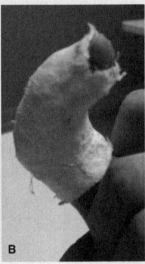
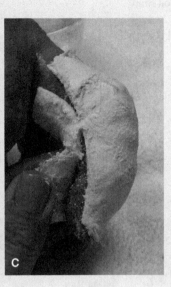

CLINICAL PEARL 2–4

Thermoplastic Distal Phalanx Caps

Slings used to mobilize DIP joint extension contractures frequently slip during use. One solution is to fabricate a circumferential cap from 1/16″ material to form a joined volar tab for the line attachment. Heat the material, and place it dorsally over the distal phalanx, quickly stretching to form a small volar tab. Pinch both ends to seal. Once set, punch a hole through the tab to serve as the attachment for the monofilament line. This can also be used when designing composite IP flexion mobilization orthoses as shown here.

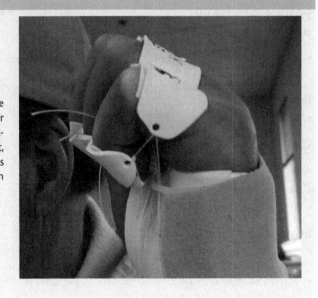

PIP/DIP MOBILIZATION ORTHOSIS (FO) (Fig. 2–3)

COMMON NAMES

- PIP/DIP strap
- Interphalangeal (IP) flexion strap

ALTERNATIVE ORTHOSIS OPTIONS

- Taping in flexion
- Elasticized wrap
- Neoprene orthosis
- Flexion glove
- Prefabricated straps

PRIMARY FUNCTIONS

- Provide low-load, prolonged flexion mobilization force to DIP and PIP joints to facilitate lengthening of tissues.

ADDITIONAL FUNCTIONS

- Facilitate extensor digitorum communis (EDC) function and glide during exercise.

Common Diagnoses	General Optimal Positions
Intrinsic tightness	PIP/DIP terminal flexion
PIP and DIP joint tightness	PIP/DIP terminal flexion
Extension contracture	PIP/DIP terminal flexion

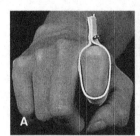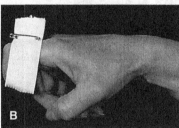

FIGURE 2–3

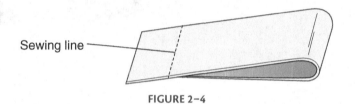

Sewing line

FIGURE 2–4

FABRICATION PROCESS

Pattern Creation (Fig. 2–4)

- Cut strip of 3/4″ elastic strapping (pajama elastic) to approximately 1½ times length of digit.

Refine Pattern

- Be sure width of elastic is adequate for size of digit.

Options for Materials

- 3/4″ elastic strap is generally appropriate for adult digits; ½″ for children.

Cut and Heat

- Be sure length is adequate to secure around digit.

Evaluate Fit While Molding

- While placing center of strip along dorsal distal phalanx, have the patient flex PIP and DIP joints of affected digit (claw position).
- Stretch strap ends to meet across dorsum of proximal phalanx, hold together, and adjust tension to tolerance.

- Apply strap at an oblique angle with light downward pressure to increase force in DIP flexion.
- Mark both pieces of elastic and remove slowly from digit.

Strapping and Components

- Sew straps together on sewing machine, if available.
- Use safety pin or staples for simple, quick closure technique.
- May add a piece of soft foam under portion of straps that comes in contact with nail to soften contour of elastic over this sometimes sensitive area.

Survey Completed Orthosis

- As range of motion (ROM) increases, tension in strap must be adjusted accordingly.
- Periodically check elasticity of strap; may need to be replaced with prolonged use.
- When fabricating straps for more than one digit, label them to ensure correct strap is placed on each digit.
- Adjust tension per patient and/or tissue tolerance; goal is low-load stretch over prolonged period of time.

PATTERN PEARLS 2-3 TO 2-5

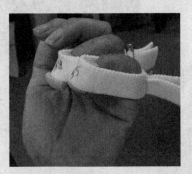

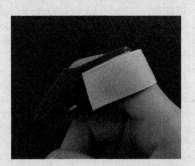

FIGURE PP2-3 Use of foam over distal phalanx to dissipate pressure and provide conforming fit.

FIGURE PP2-4 Rolyan® PIP/DIP finger flexion strap (Performance Health, Warrenville, IL).

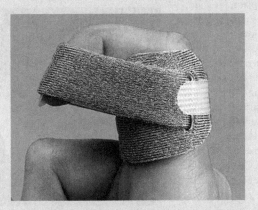

FIGURE PP2-5 Final flexion wrap. (Photo courtesy of 3-Point Products, Stevensville, MD.)

CLINICAL PEARL 2-5

Sewing Technique for Increasing Strap Effectiveness

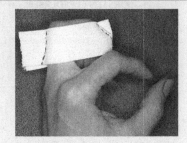

When DIP joint flexion is extremely limited, applying a PIP/DIP strap can be challenging. One way to help keep the strap in place and provide a more effective stretch at the DIP joint is to sew the distal end of the strap diagonally to form a "pocket" for the fingertip.

CLINICAL PEARL 2-6

PIP/DIP Strap for Increasing EDC Glide

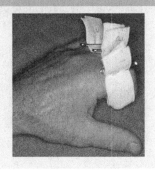

PIP/DIP straps can be used to position the joints in flexion during exercises to facilitate glide of the EDC tendons. Here, safety pins were used to secure the straps.

CLINICAL PEARL 2–7

PIP/DIP Mobilization Straps

Consider using a gentle dynamic or static progressive approach for mobilizing stiff IP joints. These techniques may be helpful for patients who have difficulty donning the traditional elastic PIP/DIP straps or for those who require frequent tension adjustments. Here are three ways to achieve this type of stretch.

A, Soft nonelastic strap method. This works best with less severe contractures because the foam strapping does not contour as well as an elastic-based strap and may cause tissue irritation. Use soft ½″ nonelastic foam strapping material. The severity of passive limitation determines the exact amount of strapping needed (i.e., the greater the contracture, the more material required). Use approximately two times the length of the digit. The fabrication method is the same as described for the PIP/DIP strap, except for the closure technique. A small strip of double-sided hook (adhesive hook folded onto itself) is placed on one end of the strap. Gentle tension is applied and then secured into place.

B, Neoprene (elastic type) strap. Neoprene strapping material contours well and typically has a layer of foam sandwiched between the outer layers. Because of this, patients find neoprene comfortable to wear for longer periods of time. The fabrication principles are the same as described previously. A simple safety pin can be used for closure or if the neoprene has loop material as one of the outer layers; double-sided hook can be considered for closure.

C, Thermoplastics and straps. For this method, fabricate a thermoplastic thimble over the distal phalanx and a thermoplastic sling on the proximal phalanx. Then apply a strip of adhesive hook on the lateral aspect of each thermoplastic piece. Connect the two segments with a ¼″ strip of nonelastic loop strapping material.

D, Cut the finger off an examination glove and stretch that around the digit to provide a dynamic stretch.

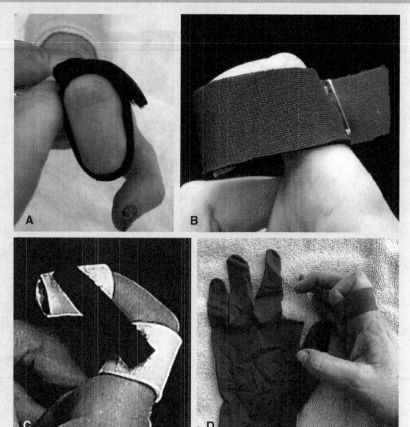

EXPERT PEARL 2–1

PIP/DIP Flexion Orthosis
KIRSTEN C. PEDERSEN, OT
Denmark

Use 1/16″ (1.6 mm) thermoplastic, elastic thread, and either a finger loop (prefabricated) cut to length or a piece of loop. A small piece of tube in thermoplastic (Orfitube shown), or a small residual thermoplastic that you form as a tube. Cut a piece of thermoplastic to the length of the proximal phalanx and wide enough so that a "bowl" can be formed. May apply padding under the thermoplastic segment for comfort. Attach a segment of tube across the thermoplastic that the elastic can run through. Tie the elastic to one side of the finger loop, pull the elastic through the tube, and tie on the opposite side of the finger loop after adjusting for the appropriate force.

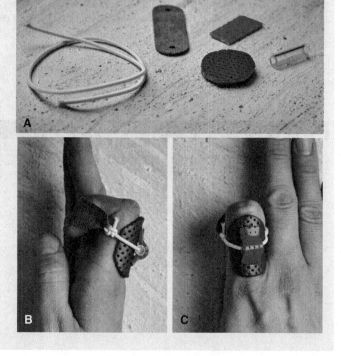

CHAPTER 2

PIP-DIP Strap
KIMBERLY GOLDIE STAINES, OTR, CHT
Texas

PIP-DIP static progressive flexion strap using scraps of loop and hoop strapping.

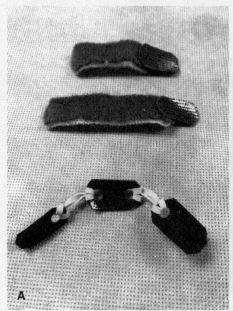
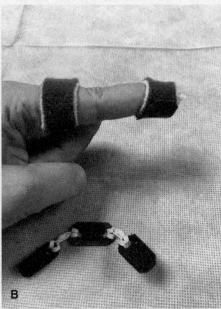
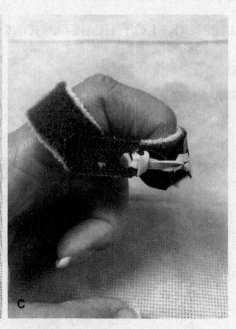

PIP Flexion Mobilization Orthosis
TRISH GRIFFITHS, OT, HAND THERAPIST
South Africa

Effective alternative when soft flexion straps slip off because available range is so limited. Dynamic component is elastic onto hook to allow the splint to be progressively changed. If the PIP joint is swollen, the "ring" portion can be opened volarly (not circumferential) for ease of donning/doffing.

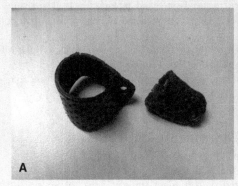
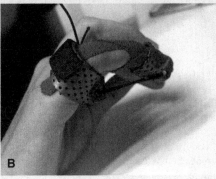
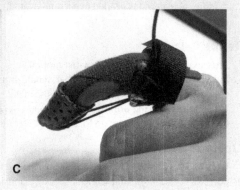

2 Hand-Based Orthoses

PIP EXTENSION MOBILIZATION ORTHOSIS (HFO) (Fig. 2–5)

COMMON NAMES

- Dynamic PIP extension orthosis

ALTERNATIVE ORTHOSIS OPTIONS

- Cast (serial static)
- Prefabricated orthosis

PRIMARY FUNCTIONS

- Provide low-load, prolonged extension mobilization force to PIP joint to facilitate lengthening of tissues.

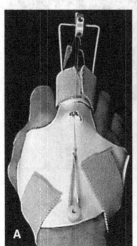
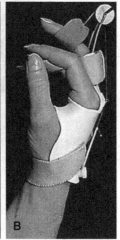

FIGURE 2–5

ADDITIONAL FUNCTIONS

- Facilitate extensor tendon function and glide during exercise.

Common Diagnoses	General Optimal Positions
PIP flexion contracture	MCP: 60°; PIP: terminal extension
Zone III or IV extension tendon repair	MCP: 0° extension; PIP: 0° extension (for complex injury)

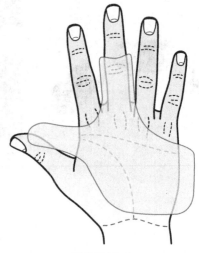

FIGURE 2–6

FABRICATION PROCESS (USING PHOENIX OUTRIGGER)

Pattern Creation (Fig. 2–6)

- Mark proximal border at wrist crease.
- If holding MCP joint at 0°, mark distal border only to mid-PIP crease. If holding MCP in flexion, mark distal border beyond PIP joint. Note: Additional material is needed to accommodate for flexion angle at MCP joint.

Refine Pattern

- Proximal border should allow wrist motion.
- Lateral borders of PIP extension bar should trough proximal phalanx, encompassing half to two-thirds of this segment.
- Ulnar aspect of hand orthosis should support hypothenar eminence.
- Make radial bar long enough to attach to volar ulnar border.

Options for Materials

- Use solid 3/32″ material, which is lightweight, yet strong enough to support MCP joint in flexion while accepting extension force.
- Plastic materials contour well, with minimal handling into arches and digital web spaces.
- If radial bar is intended to pop apart, coated material is necessary.
- If index finger (IF) and/or small finger (SF) MCPs are enlarged or if there is degree of thenar or hypothenar atrophy, the union must be popped open to ease donning and doffing.
- Use components of choice, following manufacturer's directions for correct application.

Cut and Heat

- Position patient with hand over platform, digits slightly abducted, and MCP joint positioned per diagnosis.
- Heat two additional pieces of material (1″ by 1″) for securing outrigger and safety pin.

Evaluate Fit While Molding

- Dry and apply warm material onto hand, making sure to clear all creases, trough around involved proximal phalanx, and encompass ulnar border of hand.
- Gently pull radial bar through thumb web space and across volar MCPs to meet with ulnar segment. Pinch and seal lightly.
- Make sure radial bar crosses proximal to MCP joints and incorporates arches to help maintain proper orthosis position.
- Maintain MCP joint position.

Strapping and Components

- Use ½″ to 1″ strap at proximal phalanx.
- Attach 1″ strap at ulnar-radial segment interface.
- Place an elasticized or soft foam strap at wrist to prevent orthosis migration.
- Mark desired outrigger attachment; position outrigger to extend distally over midportion of middle phalanx, extending it high enough so volar sling attached to line will clear pulley.
- Remove orthosis from patient and heat outrigger's proximal ends with heat gun. Press lightly to embed outrigger into marked area.
- Use extreme care when applying heated metal onto thermoplastic material. Metal may pierce through orthosis. Always perform this process off patient.

- Treat surfaces to be bonded with orthosis solvent. Place strip of heated thermoplastic material over outrigger and adhere to orthosis base.
- With flat-nose pliers, bend clasp part of safety pin at 90° angle. Heat same end over heat gun and embed into orthosis base over MCP joint.
- Position eye of safety pin along longitudinal axis of involved digit; secure with thermoplastic material scrap.
- Attach Phoenix wheel to outrigger using appropriately sized Allen wrench.
- Affix proximal attachment device for rubber band at most proximal border.
- Attach line on both sides of sling and apply sling to middle phalanx.
- Thread line through pulley and safety pin.
- Loop appropriate rubber band onto end of line and connect to proximal attachment device.

Survey Completed Orthosis

- Check for clearance of thumb, wrist, and uninvolved digits.
- Material should be flared about digital web spaces to avoid irritation.
- Check for equal traction on both sides of digit and for any possible rotational force.
- Adjust angles of pull to 90° by simply loosening pulley and rotating. Securely tighten in desired position with Allen wrench.
- Align pulley with longitudinal axis of proximal phalanx. Adjust by loosening pulley and sliding it transversely along width of outrigger. Securely tighten in desired position with Allen wrench.
- Adjust tension per patient and/or tissue tolerance; goal is low-load stretch over prolonged period of time.

PATTERN PEARLS 2–6 TO 2–10

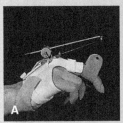 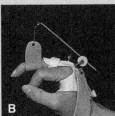 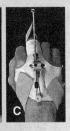

FIGURE PP2–6 A–C, Rolyan® Adjustable Outrigger (Performance Health) using same pattern.

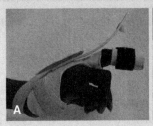 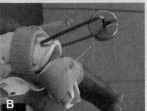

FIGURE PP2–7 To further isolate PIP joint, consider immobilization of DIP for increased purchase of sling: **(A)** circumferential and **(B)** volar.

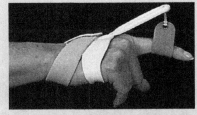

FIGURE PP2–8 Digit extension mobilization orthosis using Aquatubes® (Performance Health) or can use rolled thermoplastic.

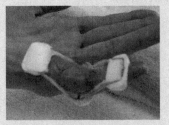

FIGURE PP2–9 LMB spring finger extension assist orthosis (North Coast Medical, Morgan Hill, CA).

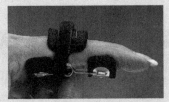

FIGURE PP2–10 Bunnell™ Mini modified safety pin splint. (Photo courtesy of North Coast Medical).

CLINICAL PEARL 2–8

PIP Extension Mobilization Used as Exercise Orthosis

A PIP extension mobilization orthosis can be used to facilitate PIP and DIP flexion by flexing against the resistance of the dynamic force. Sling can be applied at distal phalanx or at the middle phalanx to deliver resistance to DIP or PIP joint. Note use of Kinesio® Tex Tape beneath orthosis for edema management.

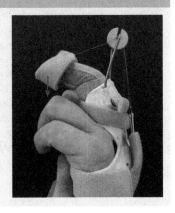

CLINICAL PEARL 2-9

Serial Static Casting to Mobilize Stiff PIP Joint

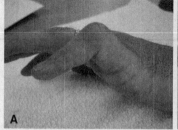

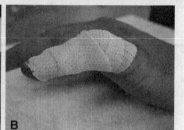

Casting tapes or plaster of paris can be used to apply a low-load, prolonged stress to PIP flexion contracture. In this case, QuickCast 2 (Performance Health) casting tape was applied; the DIP joint was included for better purchase on this small digit.

CLINICAL PEARL 2-10

Serial Static Extension Orthosis to Mobilize Stiff PIP Joint

A serial static orthosis can be utilized to stretch a PIP flexion contracture—commonly used at night for end range positioning to help maintain gains in motion made throughout the day with other stretching interventions. Create a volar recess overlying the PIP joint in the orthosis by using foam during the molding process. This forms the orthosis in greater PIP extension which then allows the dorsal strap to stretch the PIP joint to maximal extension.

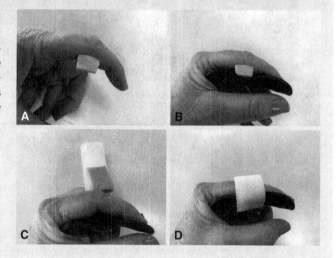

CLINICAL PEARL 2-11

Forearm-Based PIP Extension Mobilization Orthosis

When fabricating an orthosis on a patient with multiple PIP joint flexion contractures, or a PIP flexion contracture that is greater than approximately 60°, consider a forearm-based design **(A)**. The longer design may work well when addressing both MCP and PIP joint contractures within one orthosis. The pattern is similar to the hand-based PIP extension mobilization orthosis but includes the wrist. Shown is an RF-SF PIP extension mobilization orthosis. The patient had significant, long-standing PIP flexion contractures secondary to an ulnar nerve injury **(B)**. She presented with a 75° flexion contracture on the RF and a 45° flexion contracture on the SF. Note the length of the outrigger on the RF to achieve a 90° line of pull. The outrigger platform for the wheel had to be custom made to incorporate the height and achieve the optimal angle of force application. The detachable extension outrigger can be positioned higher or lower, moved proximally or distally, and (to a lesser degree) slide radially and ulnarly **(C)**. The more severe the contracture, the more distal and higher the rod will need to be. As the contracture resolves, the rod is retracted proximally and tightened back into place with the appropriate Allen wrench. The component shown here is the Rolyan® Adjustable Outrigger (Performance Health), which can be adjusted to hold single or multiple rod extenders.

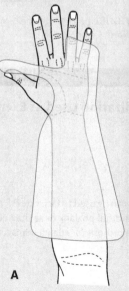

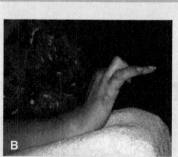

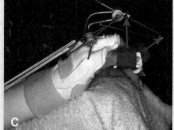

A

CLINICAL PEARL 2–12

Multipurpose Orthosis: Alternating PIP Flexion/Extension Mobilization

Creating an orthosis that incorporates two functions such as PIP flexion and PIP extension mobilization (**A**) can be a cost-saving measure and convenient for the patient. This hand-based orthosis addresses a stiff PIP joint with a custom outrigger for flexion mobilization and Phoenix Outrigger (Performance Health) for extension mobilization. The patient is effectively able to alternate between flexion and extension throughout the day using just one orthosis. **B,** A simple approach to combine both flexion and extension would be to add a static progressive approach via a composite IP flexion mobilization strap.

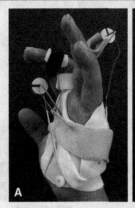
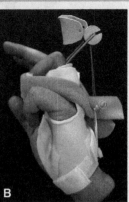

EXPERT PEARL 2–4

Dynamic Orthosis for PIP Extension
DEBBY SCHWARTZ, OTD, OTR/L, CHT
New Jersey

(Often referred to as the Capener orthosis)
The goal of this orthosis is to increase the extension of the PIP joint by exerting a sustained light traction on the tight ligamentous structures of the joint.
Materials needed:
- 1/16″ elastic-based thermoplastic material or Orficast (Orfit Industries, Belgium)

Prepare material as follows:
- Cut one strip of 2.5″-wide Orficast about 3″ long or similar in sheet material.
- Cut another strip of 2.5″-wide Orficast about 1″ long or similar in sheet material.
- Use two finger coil springs (Orfit Industries, Belgium). These can be custom made with spring wire or purchased from a supplier.
- The Orfit Industries finger coil springs have been calibrated and will allow a low-load traction. Each spring has a long leg and a short leg on either side of the coil.
- Bend the small leg of the spring upward in order to make a small hook which will allow you to anchor the coil spring into the material. Carefully cut away the excess length of the hook, preserving just a small hook. Repeat this on the other spring.
- Take the longer strip of Orficast material, activate it, pat dry, and fold it in half to create a piece of 2.5″ by 1.5″. Cut a small hole in the middle of the piece. Slip the intended finger through the material. Mold the upper part to the dorsum of the first phalanx, and twist the lateral edges of the material inward to avoid excess thickness of material between the fingers. Carefully mold the palmar piece under the metacarpal head while holding the finger in a 45° flexion.
- Take the smaller piece of the Orficast material, activate it, pat dry, and fold it in half as well and mold this underneath the DIP joint. Let these two pieces harden. Remove the two pieces.
- Trim the dorsal surface of the larger molded piece of Orficast and fully expose the PIP joint so that the finger coil springs can be correctly positioned in line at or slightly above the PIP joint axis of motion. Cut the palmar piece of the orthosis so that it does not interfere with the MCP flexion crease. Take the smaller piece and round all of the edges.
- Begin the assembly of the orthosis. Take one of the finger coil springs. Heat a small piece of Orficast with the heat gun and wrap this around the bent hook. Heat the base part of the orthosis. Attach the hook on the lateral side, at or slightly above the PIP joint axis of motion. Repeat with the second spring. Attach this spring exactly opposite to the first. Make sure to position the coils so that the thickest part of the coil is dorsal. Or in other words, place the coil so that the longer leg attaching to the distal cuff continues in the arc of the coil, and not upside down. The force applied distally follows the direction of the last coil.
- Place the orthosis on the finger. Measure the right length of the long leg of the finger coil spring. This should be the middle of the DIP joint. Bend the long leg downward to create a hook. Cut away the excess spring wire, leaving only the small hook. (When cutting the spring wire, hold onto the portion being cut away in order to avoid it flying.)
- Heat a small piece of Orficast with the heat gun and wrap this around both of the hooks. Heat both sides of the smaller part of the orthosis and secure the hooks to this portion.
- Check the fit of the orthosis on the client. Make sure the client can fully flex the PIP joint and that the orthosis assists with PIP extension. It is possible to adjust the coils slightly to increase or decrease the tension.
Note: Placing the coils slightly above the PIP joint axis of motion will influence more joint extension, but may make flexion more difficult.

(Continued)

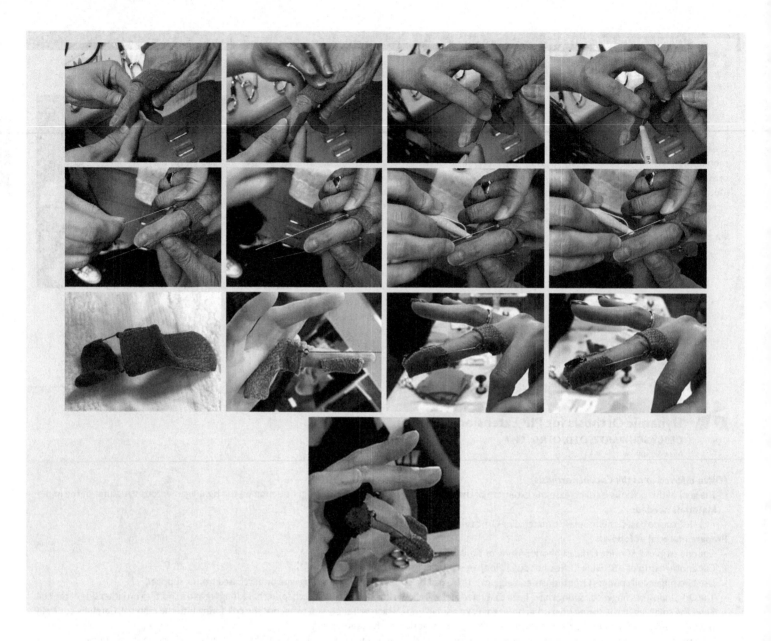

EXPERT PEARL 2-5

PIP Extension Mobilization Orthosis
TRISH GRIFFITHS, OT, HAND THERAPIST
South Africa

Shown fabricated from Woodcast (not currently available in the United States) but can be created with thermoplastics as well. The "bubble" below the PIP extends the lever and therefore increases the work of the strap to extend the PIP joint. Very important that the MCP and the DIP joints are supported in neutral. Consider using a thick, soft strap over the PIP joint to maximize surface area and reduce risk of pressure problems.

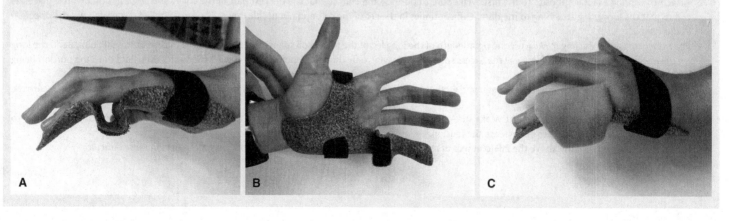

PIP FLEXION MOBILIZATION ORTHOSIS (HFO) (Fig. 2–7)

COMMON NAMES

- Dynamic PIP flexion orthosis

ALTERNATIVE ORTHOSIS OPTIONS

- Elastic wraps
- Flexion glove
- Prefabricated orthoses

PRIMARY FUNCTIONS

- Provide low-load, prolonged flexion mobilization force to PIP joint to facilitate lengthening of tissues.

Common Diagnoses	General Optimal Positions
PIP extension contracture	MCP: 0°; PIP: terminal flexion

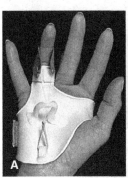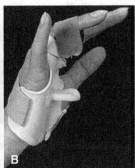

FIGURE 2–7

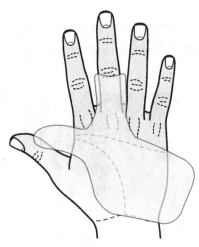

FIGURE 2–8

FABRICATION PROCESS

Pattern Creation (Fig. 2–8)

- Severity of contracture and number of joints involved determine whether orthosis is forearm or hand based.
- This hand-based pattern can easily be modified to include wrist.
- Mark proximal border at distal wrist crease.
- Mark distal border at proximal PIP crease.

Refine Pattern

- Lateral borders should encompass half to two-thirds of circumference of proximal phalanx (flush with dorsal surface).
- Borders should clear uninvolved MCP joint creases and encompass hypothenar eminence.
- When fabricating an orthosis for the IF and middle finger (MF), there should be enough material molded around thenar eminence to allow for line guide attachment.
- Radial bar should traverse through thumb web space, across dorsum of hand, and attach to ulnar border.

Options for Materials

- Use solid, coated 3/32″ material (elastic or plastic) for this orthosis; this makes for lightweight orthosis with adequate strength to support MCP joint in extension while accepting flexion force.
- Elastic materials allow excellent visualization of creases during molding.
- Plastic materials tend to contour well, with minimal handling, into arches and about digital web spaces.

- To seal off circumference of orthosis, choose an uncoated material; however, if dorsal segment is intended to pop apart, then coated material is recommended.
- Use components of choice (custom-fabricated line guide is shown).

Cut and Heat

- Position patient with hand supinated resting over platform, digits slightly abducted, and MCP joint extended.

Evaluate Fit While Molding

- Dry and apply warm material onto hand, making sure to clear all creases; trough about involved proximal phalanx; and encompass ulnar border.
- Gently pull radial bar through thumb web space and across dorsum to meet with ulnar segment. Pinch and seal lightly, and return focus to volar aspect.
- Make sure arches are incorporated into the orthosis to maintain orthosis position properly on hand.
- MCP joint should be positioned as close to 0° as possible.

Strapping and Components

- Use ½″ to 1″ across proximal phalanx.
- If necessary, attach 1″ strap dorsally at ulnar and radial segments. This area may be permanently sealed; however, if IF and SF MCPs are enlarged or if there is some degree of thenar or hypothenar atrophy, it will be difficult to doff orthosis without popping it open.
- Place elasticized or soft foam strap at wrist to prevent migration (if needed).

- Position sling over middle phalanx.
- Apply line guide at level of distal palmar crease, making sure it is extended far enough to create 90° angle of pull when force is applied to middle phalanx.
- Proximal attachment device should be attached at most proximal border of orthosis.
- Once force is applied, may need strap applied to proximal orthosis and about wrist to prevent tilt of the proximal edge of the device.

Survey Completed Orthosis

- Connect line to rubber band and loop about proximal device.
- Check for equal traction of both sides of digit and for any possible rotational force. Correct, if necessary, by adjusting monofilament line.
- Material should be flared, trimmed, and smoothed around digital web spaces to avoid irritation.
- Check that volar orthosis borders do not irritate uninvolved MCPs.
- Adjust tension per patient and/or tissue tolerance; goal is low-load stretch over prolonged period of time.

PATTERN PEARLS 2–11 TO 2–16

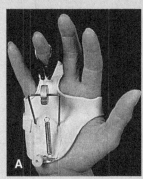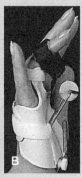

FIGURE PP2–11 A and B, Phoenix Outrigger System (Performance Health).

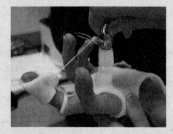

FIGURE PP2–12 Static progressive approach: note height of MERiT™ (Performance Health) component to achieve 90° angle of pull.

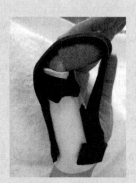

FIGURE PP2–13 Neoprene applied over DIP cast to isolate stretch to the PIP (Orficast™; North Coast Medical).

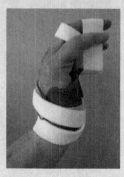

FIGURE PP2–14 Microfoam™ tape used to provide gentle flexion force (Performance Health).

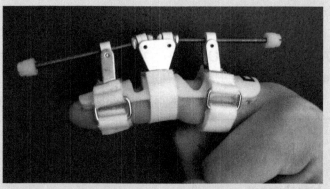

FIGURE PP2–15 Rolyan® Static progressive finger flexion orthosis (Performance Health).

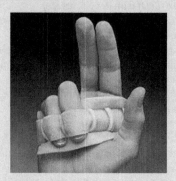

FIGURE PP2–16 Norco™ Cinch Strap. (Photo courtesy of North Coast Medical.)

CLINICAL PEARL 2–13

Convert Dynamic Orthosis to Static Progressive Using MERiT™ Component

These composite digit flexion orthoses have similar design characteristics as the hand-based mobilization orthoses previously described. The clinician can use creativity in "tweaking" the designs to meet particular patient needs. At times, a patient may have stiffness in all three joints (MCP, PIP, DIP), and the clinician is challenged to incorporate as many joints as possible to not burden the patient (and insurance carrier) with multiple orthoses. **(A)** SF composite flexion mobilization orthosis using a dynamic approach, which employs rubber band traction and homemade line guides (Aquatubes; Performance Health) to increase SF MCP, PIP, and DIP flexion. **(B)** MF composite flexion orthosis is using a static progressive approach, incorporating eyelets of safety pins as the line guides and a MERiT™ component to provide the static progressive force. The turn screw is gradually tightened to increase the tension applied to the MF.

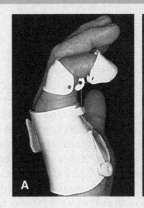
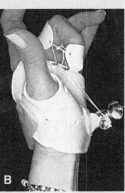

CLINICAL PEARL 2–14

Static Progressive Composite Digit Flexion Orthosis

Composite digit flexion orthoses can be used to address generalized stiffness in a digit involving MCP, PIP, and/or DIP joints. Fabrication involves two thermoplastic slings overlying the proximal and distal phalanx with monofilament weaved to attach proximally imparting the adjustable stretch. This can be converted to a dynamic approach if desired and can encompass more than one digit if required. Note the use of low-profile pulley incorporated into the orthotic base and the use of hook/loop proximally to provide the static progressive force.

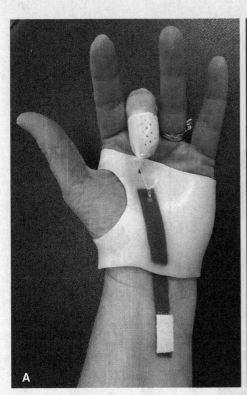
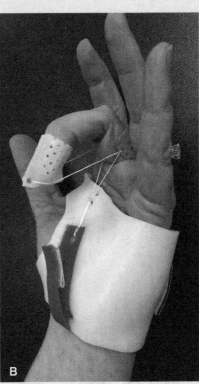
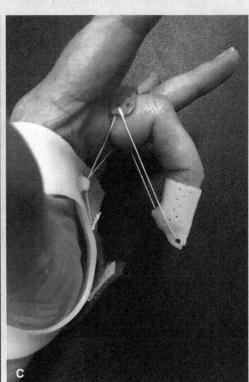

CLINICAL PEARL 2–15

Forearm-Based PIP Flexion Mobilization Orthosis

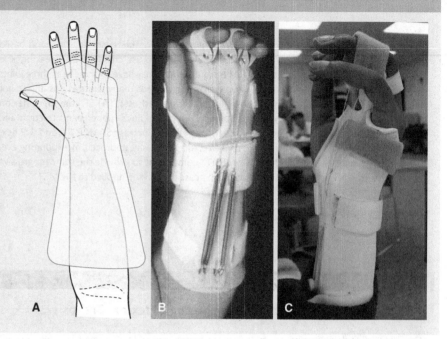

A, When fabricating an orthosis on a patient with multiple PIP joint extension contractures, consider a forearm-based design. The pattern is similar to the hand-based PIP flexion mobilization orthosis but includes the wrist; the additional material provides the surface for the proximal attachments. **B,** Shown is an IF-RF PIP flexion mobilization orthosis with a homemade outrigger and with dynamic force application via spring coils. **C,** A "dynamic" approach is used with this patient to isolate the very stiff PIP joint of the ring finger. The severity of this contracture would make it challenging to fit with a hand-based design.

CLINICAL PEARL 2–16

PIP Flexion Mobilization Straps

Elastic-, nonelastic-, or neoprene-type straps can be used to effectively mobilize a stiff PIP joint(s). **(A)** The strap is directed from the middle phalanx of the involved digit, through the thenar web space, and across the ulnar border of the hand to terminate on the dorsum of the hand as shown in this elastic-based strap. **(B)** The use of a thermoplastic cuff or foam over the middle phalanx will assist in comfort and optimal pressure distribution as noted in this foam (nonelastic strap). The tension should be gentle and adjusted appropriately to maintain the correct stretch on the joint. **C and D,** Pajama elastic or neoprene secured with safety pins dorsally; note isolated PIP flexion stretch on IF. **E–G,** Any of these mobilization straps can be used for simultaneous IP flexion.

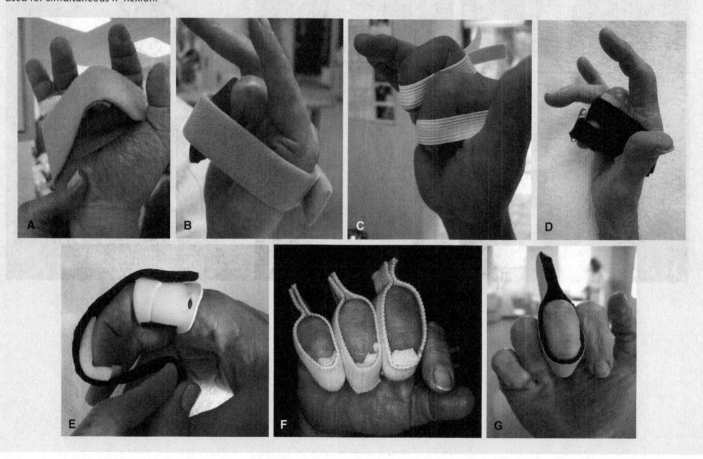

CHAPTER 2

Alternative Loop Option
THERESA BELL-NAGLE, OTR/L, CHT
Massachusetts

If slippage of loop is an issue, try using Dycem to create a custom loop by simply using hole punch.

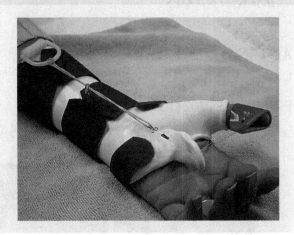

Line on Mobilization Orthosis
THERESA BELL-NAGLE, OTR/L, CHT
Massachusetts

Use safety pins to prevent the monofilament from sliding through the hole of the outrigger. Also it is easier for patients to don themselves because it gives them something to grab.

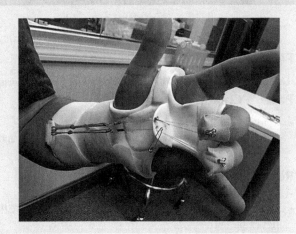

Composite Digit Mobilization
THERESA BELL-NAGLE, OTR/L, CHT
Massachusetts

Neoprene flexion loops attached proximally to hook on orthosis allow for adjustable dynamic end range stretch. Notice how cutting slit in neoprene and feeding material through form distal digit loop.

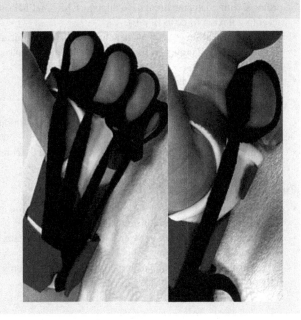

THUMB IP FLEXION MOBILIZATION ORTHOSIS (HFO) (Fig. 2–9)

COMMON NAMES

- IP flexion orthosis

ALTERNATIVE ORTHOSIS OPTIONS

- Elastic wraps

PRIMARY FUNCTIONS

- Provide low-load, prolonged flexion mobilization force to thumb IP joint to facilitate lengthening of tissues.

Common Diagnoses	General Optimal Positions
Thumb IP joint extension contracture	MCP: 0°; (carpometacarpal [CMC]): midpalmar-radial abduction; IP: terminal flexion

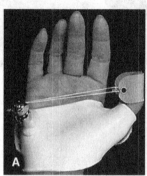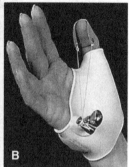

FIGURE 2–9

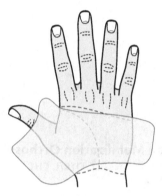

FIGURE 2–10

FABRICATION PROCESS

(Using Orthosis-Tuner™; North Coast Medical for Static Progressive Force)

Pattern Creation (Fig. 2–10)

- Mark proximal border at wrist crease.
- Mark distal border proximal to thumb IP flexion crease and distal palmar crease.

Refine Pattern

- Proximal border should allow full wrist motion.
- Distal border should allow unimpeded motion of digit MCP and thumb IP flexion.
- Provide appropriate amount of material within and dorsal to web space to support thumb CMC and MP position adequately and provide surface area for strap application dorsally.

Options for Materials

- Use solid, coated, 1/16″ or 3/32″ material; this makes for lightweight orthosis with adequate strength to support CMC and MP joints while accepting flexion force to IP joint.
- Elastic materials allow excellent visualization of creases during molding.
- Plastic material contours well, with minimal handling into arches and thumb web space.
- Use components of choice (Orthosis-Tuner™ is shown).

Cut and Heat

- Position hand supinated over an armrest, with thumb in midpalmar and radial abduction.
- Heat an additional piece of material (1″ by 1″) to secure Orthosis-Tuner™ component.

Evaluate Fit While Molding

- Lay warm material on towel, positioning thumb portion on correct side of material to place it on supinated hand.
- Place thumb section centrally over thumb proximal phalanx and guide rest of material evenly along palm.
- Take dorsal section of thumb material (between IF and thumb) and carefully contour through web space.

- Gently pull proximal volar thumb material and lightly overlap onto dorsal piece.
- While molding, avoid direct pressure over CMC joint and dorsal MP joint. Be sure to maintain thumb CMC and MP joints in appropriate positions.
- Carefully incorporate arches of hand by using smooth, even strokes and constantly redirecting material.
- Once material has cooled completely, pop apart overlapped pieces if necessary; otherwise, carefully remove orthosis.

Strapping and Components

- If necessary, attach ½″ strap dorsally at overlapped web space area.
- Attach 1″ strap dorsally at ulnar and radial segments.
- To attach Orthosis-Tuner™ component, first treat surfaces to be bonded with solvent (orthosis base and small thermoplastic piece).
- Heat small piece of material and wrap around component stem to form a cylinder.
- Reheat material over heat gun; then set at predetermined site on orthosis base.
- Firmly press component into orthosis base and gently rotate cylinder to achieve an intimate fit about grooves of stem onto orthosis base.
- Position Orthosis-Tuner™ component so axis of rotating cylinder is perpendicular to line.
- Apply sling to distal phalanx, and then attach static orthosis line, allowing enough so that orthosis can be easily donned and doffed but not so much that it is cumbersome to tighten up each time it is loosened.
- Make sure the Orthosis-Tuner™ component is completely cooled and set before applying line or it will pop off the orthosis base from the force/torque being applied.
- Thread line through hole in Orthosis-Tuner™ and tie line back onto itself.

Survey Completed Orthosis

- Check for clearance of wrist, especially around radial and ulnar styloids.
- Smooth and slightly flare all borders and around thumb IP opening.
- Pay careful attention to IF MCP, which frequently abuts radial portion of orthosis as it traverses through first web space.
- Make sure web tissue is not pinched under overlapped pieces.
- Adjust tension by rotating turn screw per patient and/or tissue tolerance; goal is low-load stretch over prolonged period of time.

PATTERN PEARLS 2–17 TO 2–19

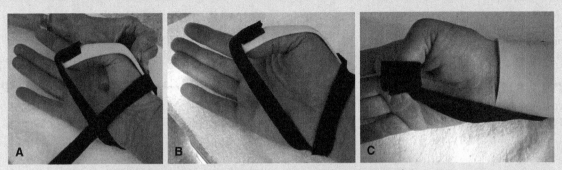

FIGURE PP2–17   A and B, Composite thumb MP/IP flexion using a dorsal approach with neoprene.
C, Simple IP neoprene loop directed to a wrist cuff.

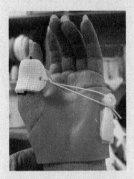

FIGURE PP2–18 Thumb MP flexion using elastic cord and neoprene/
QuickCast 2 sling (Performance Health).

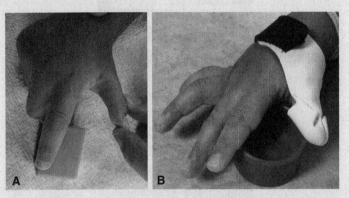

FIGURE PP2–19 Serial static design for congenital trigger thumb **(A)** IP
flexion contracture. **B,** Dorsal design promoting IP extension.

CLINICAL PEARL 2–17

Thumb MP/IP Flexion Mobilization

Often after injury to the thumb, both the MP and IP joints can be stiff, requiring mobilization. Stiffness may present after cast immobilization of the ulnar collateral ligament (UCL) or radial collateral ligament (RCL) sprain or repair, scaphoid or metacarpal fracture, scaphotrapeziotrapezoid (STT) fusion, CMC joint arthroplasty, or other thumb injury. To provide flexion forces to the MP and IP joints simultaneously, fabricate an orthosis similar to the thumb IP flexion mobilization orthosis, but the thumb portion should only extend as far as the MP joint flexion crease **(A)**. This allows adequate stabilization of the first metacarpal while forces are directed to the MP and IP joints. For a dynamic approach, use rubber band traction **(B)**. A small piece of hook is adhered to the nail to allow for loop attachment. For a static progressive approach, use adhesive hook-and-loop strapping for the proximal attachment device **(C)**. The adhesive hook is diagonally placed at the proximal border of the orthosis base, and the loop strapping is then directed to the hook and attached. This provides a gentle stretch that should be adjusted as the patient's tolerance permits.

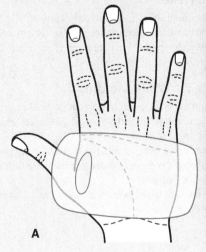
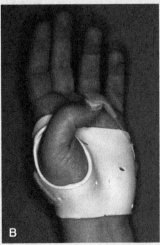
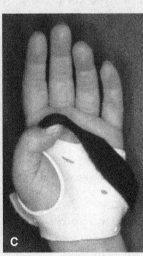

MCP EXTENSION MOBILIZATION ORTHOSIS (HFO) (Fig. 2–11)

COMMON NAMES

- Zero profile orthosis[a]
- Posterior interosseous nerve orthosis

ALTERNATIVE ORTHOSIS OPTIONS

- Dynamic MCP extension orthosis
- Prefabricated orthosis

PRIMARY FUNCTIONS

- Dynamically support MCP joints in extension while allowing active digit (and thumb) flexion.

Common Diagnoses	General Optimal Positions
Returning radial nerve function	MCP: 0°; PIP: free
Posterior interosseous nerve injury	MCP: 0°; PIP: free
Weak extrinsic extensor function	MCP: 0°; PIP: free

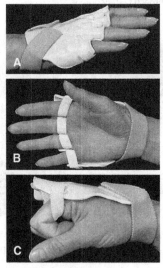

FIGURE 2–11

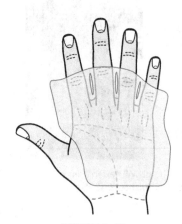

FIGURE 2–12

[a]Designed by Tina Steen, OTR/L, and Lois Carlson, OTR/L, CHT.

FABRICATION PROCESS

Pattern Creation (Fig. 2–12)

- Mark proximal border at wrist crease.
- Mark distal borders at middorsal PIP creases.
- Note small slits at digit web spaces for elastic to pass through.

Refine Pattern

- Radial aspect should extend enough to trough radial index and partially trough web space (just beyond proximal palmar crease); the trough should lie flush to volar surface and not interfere with digit flexion.
- Ulnar border should encompass hypothenar eminence but not interfere with MCP flexion.

Options for Materials

- Use solid 3/32″ plastic material; this makes for a lightweight orthosis with adequate strength to support MCP joints in extension while accepting flexion forces.
- Plastic material contours well, with minimal handling about metacarpal heads and between digital web spaces.

- Cut ¼″ to ½″ elastic strapping (pajama elastic), depending on size of hand, twice the width of hand (at MCP joint level); elastic should cover approximately two-thirds length of proximal phalanxes.
- Use three small pieces of scrap thermoplastic material (or Aquatubes®) to secure elastic loops dorsally.

Cut and Heat

- Heat thermoplastics, including small pieces.
- Position hand, pronated with digits slightly abducted; MCP joints should be positioned and held in extension. (Patient may need to support digits in extension with unaffected hand.)

Evaluate Fit While Molding

- Heat and apply material to dorsum of hand carefully, making sure that MCPs are extended and proximal phalanxes are precisely contoured, forming small troughs.
- Mold with care over metacarpal heads to avoid pressure areas.
- Wrap about hypothenar border volarly along fifth metacarpal to add stability to the orthosis.
- Radial border should be molded along radial aspect of IF and lie flush to its volar surface.

Strapping and Components

- Once set, use hole punch or hand drill to form slits that start approximately ½″ from distal orthosis border between the IF and MF, the MF and ring finger (RF), and the RF and SF.
- Weave elastic through slits to support each proximal phalanx.
- Tension of elastic strap should be just enough to hold proximal phalanx in extension; excessive tension can lead to neurovascular compromise.
- Prepare surface of dorsal loop areas with solvent for adhering rods.

- Place small pieces of warm thermoplastic material (rolled into rods) underneath each dorsal loop. Press rods into place, sealing elastic loop against orthosis base.
- Consider using rivets to secure radial and ulnar extensions of elastic.
- Use soft or elasticized 1″ strap through palm and at wrist crease to secure orthosis on hand.

Survey Completed Orthosis

- Check for pressure areas at dorsum of MCP joints during active flexion.
- Check tension on each proximal phalanx support, monitoring for signs of neurovascular compromise.

 PATTERN PEARLS 2-20 TO 2-26

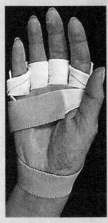

FIGURE PP2-20 Using wider elastic to better support larger digits.

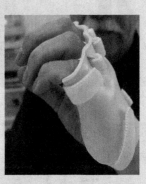

FIGURE PP2-21 Included hypothenar within the orthosis allows better purchase during digital flexion.

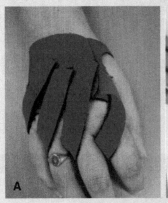
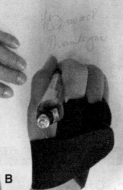
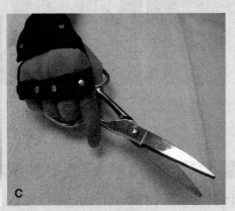

A   B   C

FIGURE PP2-22 A–C, Neoprene material can be used to provide gentle mobilization to MCP extension and radial deviation while allowing a degree of flexion for functional use. Many designs are possible.

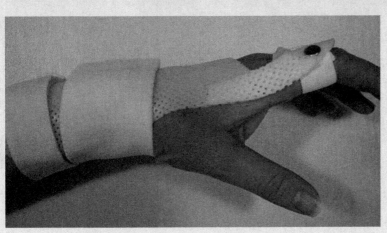

FIGURE PP2-23 Forearm-based MCP extension mobilization orthosis for proximal radial nerve injury—notice cut out to relieve pressure at MCP joints.

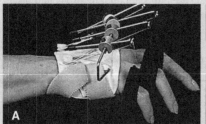
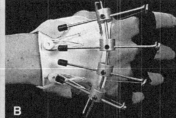

FIGURE PP2–24 A and B, Rolyan® Adjustable Outrigger System (Performance Health).

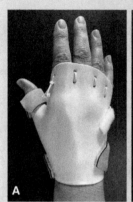
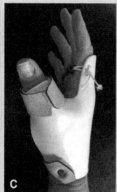
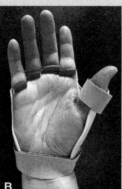
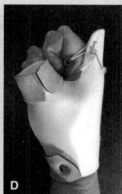

FIGURE PP2–25 A–D, Using wrapped elastic cord and pieces of Theratube to produce dynamic extension. Notice use of stretchy neoprene to assist thumb with extension.

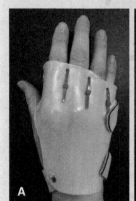
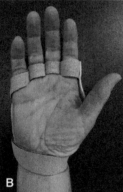
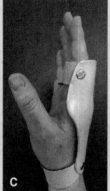
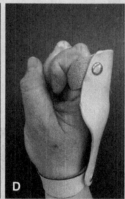

FIGURE PP2–26 A–D, Zip ties utilized to hold neoprene loops against orthosis. Notice ulnar side is adjustable via hook to allow patient to loosen allowing more flexion (grasping objects) or tighten to position the digits in more extension (typing).

 CLINICAL PEARL 2–18

Adding Thumb to Hand-Based MCP Extension Mobilization Orthosis

Loss of thumb extension is commonly seen after radial nerve injury and can impair functional use of the hand. To better position the thumb (out of a flexed and adducted posture) while awaiting reinnervation, consider adding a dynamic thumb MP extension assist to the MCP extension mobilization orthosis. The basic pattern does not change. A Phoenix Outrigger (Performance Health) shown here or similar system works well to support the thumb passively in extension while allowing active functional flexion.

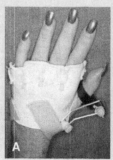
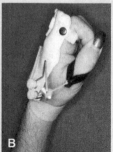

3 | Forearm-Based Orthoses

WRIST EXTENSION MOBILIZATION ORTHOSIS (WHO) (Fig. 2–13)

COMMON NAMES

- Dynamic wrist extension orthosis
- Wrist mobilization orthosis

ALTERNATIVE ORTHOSIS OPTIONS

- Casting (serial static)
- Adjustable wrist hinged orthosis
- Incremental wrist hinged orthosis
- Preformed dynamic wrist orthosis
- Static progressive wrist orthosis kit

PRIMARY FUNCTIONS

- Provide low-load, prolonged extension mobilization force to wrist joint to facilitate lengthening of tissue.

ADDITIONAL FUNCTIONS

- Restrict specific degree of motion by blocking movement through hinge device (restriction orthosis).

Common Diagnoses	General Optimal Positions
Wrist flexion contracture	Forearm: pronated; wrist: terminal extension

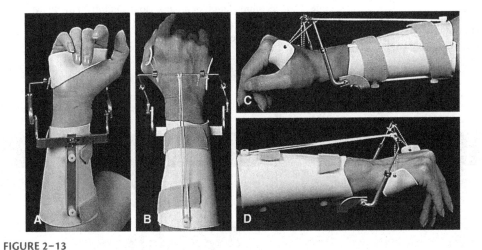

FIGURE 2–13

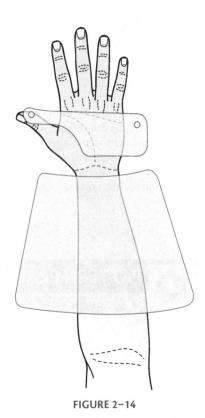

FIGURE 2–14

FABRICATION PROCESS (USING PHOENIX WRIST HINGE)

Pattern Creation (Fig. 2–14)

- Forearm orthosis
  - Length of orthosis should be at least 5″ to allow adequate attachment of outrigger.
- Hand orthosis
  - Width should be approximately 1.5 times width of hand (at distal palmar crease).
  - Length should extend ulnarly from distal palmar crease to hamate bone and radially allow enough material to contour through first web space.

Refine Pattern

- Allow adequate clearance for unimpeded wrist motion.

Options for Materials

- Use 1/16″ or 3/32″ material for both orthosis pieces; the thinness allows for easy removal and application.
- Use components of choice (Phoenix wrist hinge is shown).

Cut and Heat

- Heat and fabricate each piece separately.
- For forearm orthosis, position forearm in neutral rotation.
- For hand orthosis, position forearm supinated.

Evaluate Fit While Molding

- Forearm orthosis
  - Prepad ulnar styloid process.
  - After heating material, place material on volar surface of forearm and gently wrap around onto itself.

- Opening must be either on radial or ulnar aspect of forearm; volar or dorsal opening will impede outrigger placement.
- If using coated material, lightly overlap so it will adhere to itself; if using uncoated material, place wet paper towel between overlapped layers.
- Allow orthosis to set and then snap apart.
- Hand orthosis
  - Place material on volar hand and mold it around to dorsal surface.
  - Flare edges to clear thenar eminence and distal palmar crease.
  - Mark palmar orthosis for trimming just above ulnar and radial borders on dorsal surface.
  - Mark hole along ulnar and radial borders of hand orthosis for attaching nylon fasteners.
  - Remove orthosis, trim as needed, and smooth edges.

Strapping and Components

- Add straps once wrist hinge placement is determined.
- Forearm orthosis
  - With forearm orthosis on patient, position wrist hinge volarly.
  - Align long arm of wrist hinge with axis of motion.
  - Mark two holes on volar orthosis to match up with holes on long arm of wrist hinge.
  - Remove orthosis and punch out holes.
  - Attach hinge with rubber band posts (included with Phoenix wrist hinge).
  - Affix rubber band post to proximal dorsal border for attachment of mobilization component.
  - Apply forearm orthosis to hand.
  - Set screws on lateral bars allow proximal and distal height adjustment of 1½″. Loosen set screws with Allen wrench and adjust distal bar to accommodate appropriate position; tighten screws.

- Make necessary lateral adjustments for extreme radial or ulnar deviation by using screw on T-bar. Loosen with screwdriver and slide hinge radially or ulnarly to desired position.
- Hand orthosis
  - Punch holes on dorsal pieces.
  - Thread nylon fastener through dorsal holes on hand orthosis.
  - Apply hand orthosis.
  - Loop nylon fasteners around outrigger bar within movable collars of wrist hinge and adjoin fasteners.
  - Place wrist in maximum extension while adjusting fasteners to achieve 90° angle of pull with metacarpal bones.
  - Position two movable collars on distal bar of wrist hinge so they prevent nylon loops from slipping laterally.
  - Attach appropriate rubber band to distal bar, directing it to proximal attachment device.

Survey Completed Orthosis

- Add 1″ to 2″ strip of thin adhesive-backed padding (e.g., Moleskin) along length of inside border to prevent skin from being pinched when orthosis is overlapped and secured. Moleskin is doubled over (with thermoplastic edge in between adhesive sides of padding) and acts as flap.
- Line length of forearm orthosis and proximal and distal borders with nonskid material to decrease orthosis migration greatly. May use Microfoam™ tape, adhesive Dycem, or adhesive silicone gel sheets.
- Check for accommodation of ulnar styloid and full elbow ROM.
- Adjust tension per patient and/or tissue tolerance; goal is low-load stretch over prolonged period of time.

 PATTERN PEARLS 2–27 TO 2–30

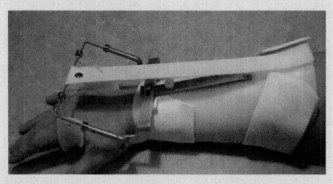

FIGURE PP2–27 Hook-and-loop strapping material used as static progressive force; loop riveted to bar and directed proximally onto strip of hook.

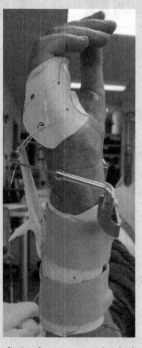

FIGURE PP2–28 Use of Microfoam™ tape at distal edge of forearm segment to prevent migration.

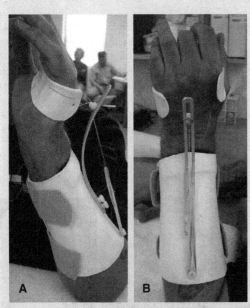

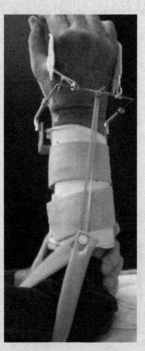

FIGURE PP2–29 A and B, Digitec Outrigger (Performance Health) with neoprene adhered to distal edge for padding.

FIGURE PP2–30 Use of elbow strap to prevent distal migration of forearm segment.

 CLINICAL PEARL 2–19

Rolyan® Incremental Wrist Hinge

As an alternative, the Rolyan® Incremental Wrist Hinge (Performance Health) can be used to fabricate a wrist mobilization orthosis. The pattern **(A)** differs from the Phoenix Wrist Hinge, as shown. The hinge can be locked in position for serial static positioning, and components can be added to provide the mobilization forces **(B–D)**. Follow the manufacturer's instructions for specific outrigger application.

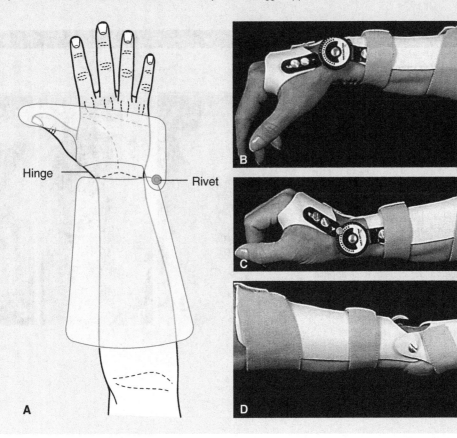

CLINICAL PEARL 2–20

Combined Wrist Flexion/Extension Mobilization Orthosis

Fabricating a wrist mobilization orthosis to address both extension and flexion limitations is a cost-effective way to address multidirectional wrist stiffness, which is common after cast immobilization. The hinge can be effective in both directions, as described for the wrist extension mobilization orthosis. When the patient has finished using the extension component, the hand is taken out of the palmar cuff, and the hinge is left to drop volarly. The dorsal cuff is then applied and directed to a volar proximal attachment device **(A)**. The patient can alternate use of wrist extension and flexion per therapist's recommendations **(B)**. Neoprene can be a choice in providing a mobilization force to solely wrist flexion or extension or can be used to deliver a combined wrist and hand extension **(C)** or flexion **(D)** stress as shown in the patient that had deficits in both directions of wrist mobility and extrinsic tightness. In image **E,** wrist flexion is delivered with elastic cord directly to a proximal rubber band post. Note the wrist extension palmar component. The arches of the hand are well defined creating a comfortable fit for the patient. This orthosis allows alternation of a wearing schedule between wrist extension and wrist flexion.

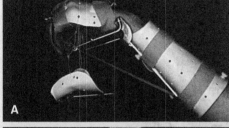
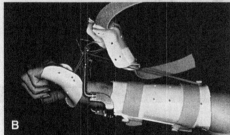
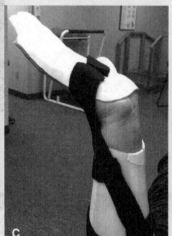
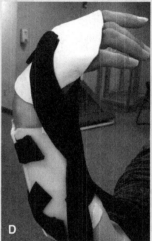
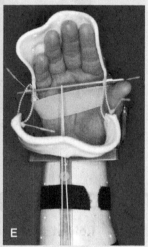

CLINICAL PEARL 2–21

Wrist Flexion Mobilization Orthosis

The pattern and instructions for the wrist extension mobilization orthosis (forearm orthosis and hinge) can be used to create a wrist flexion mobilization orthosis with minor changes. The material for the forearm orthosis is applied so that there is no overlapping material on the volar surface. Shown here, the forearm orthosis is not overlapping and nearly meets on the dorsum of the forearm. For the dorsal hand segment, place a rectangular piece of warm material on the dorsal surface of the hand and mold it well over the bony areas. Once set, line the inner surface of the orthosis to prevent migration and improve comfort (Microfoam™ tape works well). The Splint-Tuner™ (North Coast Medical) shown here is used to provide the wrist flexion mobilization force. Note **A** is fabricated without an outrigger and does not have an accurate 90° angle of force application. In **B and C**, a Digitec Outrigger (Performance Health) is used to achieve a better angle.

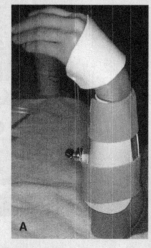
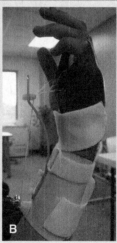
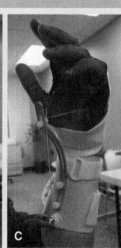

CLINICAL PEARL 2–22

Simultaneous Wrist/Thumb/MCP/IP Extension Mobilization Orthosis

Patients who have sustained severe wrist fractures or extrinsic flexor tendon repairs occasionally present with significant limitations in passive wrist extension and/or extrinsic flexor tendon adherence. A wrist extension mobilization orthosis can be converted to mobilize wrist extension and extrinsic flexor tendons simultaneously. The distal palmar bar of a wrist extension mobilization orthosis is replaced with a hand orthosis. To help achieve an intimate molding of the hand segment, make sure that the wrist is flexed to place the extrinsic flexors on slack and allow optimal positioning of the digits in maximal extension during molding. If the thumb is included, the first web space should be positioned in maximal palmar abduction and opposition. Once set, punch holes at the level of the SF and IF MCP joints. The nylon fasteners are attached at this level and directed to the distal bar of the hinge. The mobilization force is then connected and terminated on the proximal attachment device **(A)**.

Note that if the contracture is severe, the distal bar (the side arms) may be too short to create an accurate 90° line of pull. A custom-extended outrigger, fabricated from 3/32″ aluminum wire, can be fit in the side bar of the hinge. Several nylon fasteners may need to be linked together to accommodate the outrigger's extra length.

B, A serial static approach can address this same problem. Consider using QuickCast 2 (Performance Health) or Orficast™ (North Coast Medical) tapes for digit and thumb IP extension orthoses and a volar thermoplastic base (made of elastic or rubber material to allow for frequent remolding as mobility increases) to serially elongate the extrinsic flexor tendons and increase the passive wrist motion.

C, A static progressive approach (using the Using Splint-Tuner™; North Coast Medical) to gain simultaneous wrist and digit extension and thumb midpalmar abduction.

D, A similar orthosis design with forces being generated via rubber band traction from the Phoenix Wrist Hinge component.

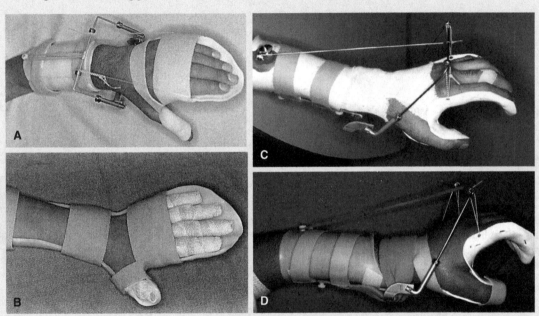

CLINICAL PEARL 2–23

Custom Hinges

A custom hinge can be fabricated as an alternative to a commercially available device. **A**, Scrap pieces of thermoplastic connected loosely via a rivet or carefully rolled thermoplastic can be used. **B**, Crimped Aquatubes® (Performance Health) were added to this mobilization orthosis to prevent migration of proximal segment.

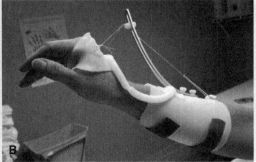

EXPERT PEARL 2–9

Homemade Hinge
DEBBIE FISHER, MS, OTR, CHT
Texas

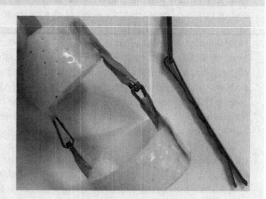

Use various size bobby pins to create a quick, inexpensive, durable hinge for a finger, wrist, or elbow orthosis. Use wire cutters to get the exact length for the appropriate size bobby pin, and close in the excess space with thermoplastic to prevent unnecessary migration with flexion and extension.

EXPERT PEARL 2–10

Dynamic Orthosis for Wrist Extension With Coils
(Adapted from "A Splinting Guide" by Paul Van Lede)
DEBBY SCHWARTZ, OTD, OTR/L, CHT
New Jersey

The goal of this orthosis is to assist with wrist extension through coils placed at the wrist joint axis.
Materials needed:

- 1/8″ elastic-based thermoplastic material: 6″ × 12″ to create a dorsal forearm piece and a palmar piece (Orfit Classic (Orfit Industries, Belgium) is shown here
- Orficast 1″(Orfit Industries, Belgium)
- Two wrist coils (Orfit Industries, Belgium)

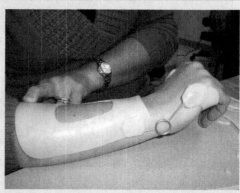

Prepare the thermoplastic material as follows:

- Make a palmar component for the orthosis. Use a strip of material 2″ wide and about 1″ wider than the client's palm. Mold so that it conforms to the palm and wraps around the second and fifth metacarpals laterally. Trim so that it allows full finger and thumb motion and does not block the wrist.
- Fabricate a dorsally placed forearm component, proximal to the wrist crease covering two/thirds of the forearm. Cut out the distal corners away so that the wrist joint axis of motion is cleared.
- The two wrist coil springs (Orfit Industries, Belgium) will be placed so that each coil aligns with the wrist joint axis of motion. These coils can be custom made with spring wire or purchased from a supplier.
- The Orfit Industries wrist coil springs have been calibrated and will allow a low-load traction toward wrist extension. Each spring has a long leg and a short leg with a hook.
- Start with placement of the coil on the ulnar side of the forearm. Wrap a small piece of Orficast that has been dry heated around the coil's hook. Using dry heat again, heat and press this into the thermoplastic material at the wrist level with the coil placed at the joint axis of motion. It is easier to see this on the ulnar side first. Make sure to place the coil so that the long arm coils away from the hand. Repeat this on the radial side, making sure each hook is firmly covered with Orficast and embedded into the dorsal forearm component.
- Place the orthosis on the client and check the alignment of the coils.
- Have the client hold the palmar component in a fist and rest the hand on the table. Take the longer leg of the coil, bend it down toward the table until it is parallel to the fifth metacarpal. Mark where this long leg meets the palmar component of the orthosis and mark the leg and the thermoplastic material. Bend the leg downward at the mark you just made, and create a hook using pliers. Carefully trim away the excess wire.
- Wrap a small piece of Orficast that has been dry heated around this newly created hook. Using dry heat again, press this into the palmar component of the orthosis and repeat on the radial side.
- Apply a proximal forearm strap and one at the wrist if needed.
- Apply padding to the dorsal wrist if needed.

Wrist Mobilization

KIMBERLY GOLDIE STAINES, OTR, CHT
Texas

An inexpensive option for a patient who required a static progressive wrist flexion orthosis but had no insurance coverage. This was fabricated simply using R-Securable strapping (Performance Health) and a firm foam ball. The force can be modified by adjusting tension on the strap.

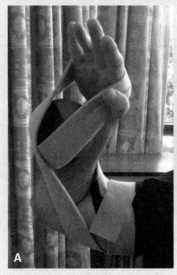

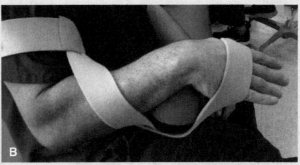

WRIST EXTENSION, MCP FLEXION/WRIST FLEXION, AND MCP EXTENSION MOBILIZATION ORTHOSIS (WHFO) (Fig. 2–15)[b]

COMMON NAMES

- Radial nerve palsy orthosis
- Tenodesis orthosis

ALTERNATIVE ORTHOSIS OPTIONS

- Phoenix Extended Outrigger Kit
- Rolyan® Static Radial Nerve Orthosis
- Wrist extension immobilization orthosis

PRIMARY FUNCTIONS

- Provide passive wrist and MCP extension, allowing finger flexion, active wrist flexion, and digit and thumb extension. (Grasp and release through natural tenodesis action.)

Common Diagnoses and General Optimal Positions

Radial nerve palsy

Posterior interosseous nerve palsy

The goal is to hold the wrist and MCPs in a comfortable degree of extension, allowing functional flexion

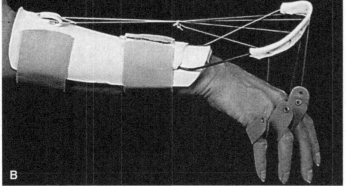
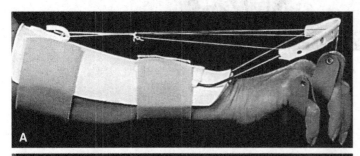

FIGURE 2–15

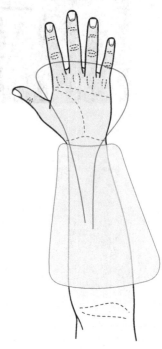

FIGURE 2–16

[b]Designed by Judy C. Colditz, OTR/CHT.

FABRICATION PROCESS

Pattern Creation (Fig. 2–16)

- Mark for dorsal forearm piece; proximal to wrist joint and 1″ to 1½″ distal to elbow crease.
- Consideration could be given to making the orthosis base a circumferential design (in this case, thinner material can be used as shown in wrist extension mobilization orthosis pattern).
- Circumference is half to two-thirds of forearm.

Refine Pattern

- Adjust length and width appropriately.

Options for Materials

- Use ⅛″ thermoplastic material for orthosis base (unless a circumferential design is chosen where a thinner material such as a 1/16″ material can be considered).
- Consider foam- or gel-lined materials to decrease distal orthosis migration.
- Cut three extra pieces of thermoplastic material (preferably noncoated) for
  - Adherence of outrigger onto orthosis base (2″ by 2″)
  - Formation of pulleys over distal outrigger wire (4″ by 3″) for individual proximal phalanx slings
  - Creation of the proximal attachment for the nylon line

Cut and Heat

- Heat forearm piece while arm is resting pronated on table.
- Heat additional two pieces (one piece approximately 6″ by 3″; the other 1″ by 3″).

Evaluate Fit While Molding

- Apply heated material to forearm.
- Mold radial and ulnar aspects of forearm piece so they cup slightly.

Strapping and Components

- Apply distal and proximal strap to secure forearm orthosis. Elastic-based or D-ring–type straps may help prevent distal orthosis migration.
- Per pattern, bend an outrigger of 3/32″ wire into desired shape.
- Bend outrigger at level of wrist joint at approximately 40° of wrist extension.
- Off patient, heat proximal end of outrigger and apply it to orthosis. When placed on patient's hand, outrigger should rest at middle of each proximal phalanx with fist position.
- Check location of outrigger; if correct, apply solvent to orthosis surface around outrigger.
- *Line guide*: Adhere warm piece of thermoplastic material intimately about outrigger (use solvent before heating) to form sturdy attachment, remembering that this area must accept weight of hand.
- Take warmed second strip of the orthosis material and apply to distal width of outrigger end, draping it over onto itself. Immediately trim to ½″ to 3/4″ width.
- When cool, mark and punch hole over middle of each proximal phalanx.
- *Proximal attachment*: Take third piece of warmed material; apply to center of most proximal end of orthosis (having applied solvent to this area prior); roll and press into the base, leaving half unattached and rolling back onto form a "C" (refer to picture). Hold this "C" or hook in order for it to cool. Do not allow the piece to touch the base. Make sure enough room is provided for the nylon line to "hook" onto this segment.
- Apply slings to cover two-thirds length of proximal phalanxes. Premade leather slings work well because they are soft, comfortable, and not bulky.
- Tie long piece of nylon line to each sling.
- Place sling under each proximal phalanx and direct cord through hole punched in the orthosis material on distal outrigger.
- Hold cords while patient lifts arm off of tabletop and passively opens and closes fist.
- Adjust tension on nylon lines so that MCP joints are in 0° extension with neutral wrist and wrist is in 20° to 30° extension with full finger flexion. Adjustment process may be easier with help of assistant.
- If dorsum of patient's hand touches outrigger during finger flexion, bend outrigger into greater extension.
- Once correct line tension has been determined, ask patient to again rest full fist on tabletop so weight of hand is not on lines.
- Tie cords with firm knot and apply glue to secure it.
- Another option is to have individual lines converge at the proximal attachment.

Survey Completed Orthosis

- Flare distal edge and make sure that there is no abutment or irritation at ulnar styloid.
- If unlined material was used, consider lining orthosis with adhesive Dycem, gel, or Microfoam™ tape.

 PATTERN PEARLS 2–31 TO 2–36

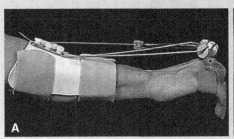
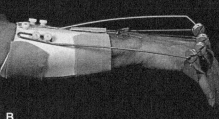

FIGURE PP2–31 **A and B,** Custom-bent wire secured with thermoplastic material, neoprene slings, and individual lines to proximal attachment device.

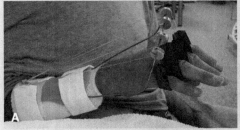
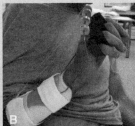
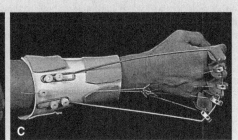

FIGURE PP2–32 **A–C,** Phoenix Extended Outrigger Kit (Performance Health) includes prebent wire.

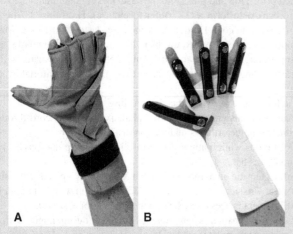

FIGURE PP2–33 A and B, Robinson Forearm-Based Radial Nerve Splint. (Photo courtesy of AliMed, Dedham, MA.)

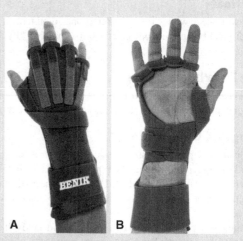

FIGURE PP2–34 A and B, Benik W711 Forearm-Based Radial Nerve Splint; this device is also offered in hand-based design. (Photo courtesy of Benik Corporation, Silverdale, WA.)

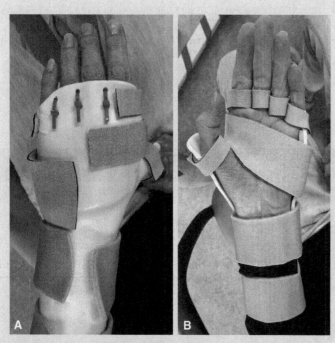

FIGURE PP2–35 A and B, Zip ties utilized to hold neoprene loops against orthosis. Notice ulnar side is adjustable via hook to allow patient to loosen allowing more flexion (grasping objects) or tighten to position the digits in more extension (typing). Optional palmar strap to support dorsal hand against inside of orthosis if needed.

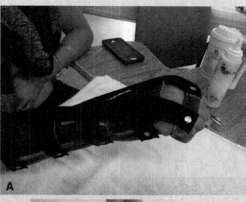

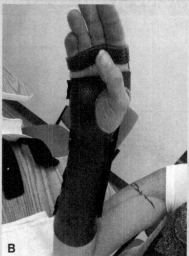

FIGURE PP2–36 A and B, Distal nonarticular proximal phalanx segment connected to proximal base using elasticized loop provides MCP extension—chosen to prevent excessive pressure over sensitive dorsal MCP joints. Utilized in this patient s/p humerus fracture ORIF with resulting radial nerve palsy.

THUMB CMC PALMAR/RADIAL ABDUCTION MOBAILIZATION ORTHOSIS (WHFO) (Fig. 2–17)

COMMON NAMES

- CMC abduction orthosis
- Palmar abduction orthosis
- Thumb abduction orthosis

ALTERNATIVE ORTHOSIS OPTIONS

- Hand-based CMC abduction orthosis (serial static)
- Hand cones
- Air orthoses

PRIMARY FUNCTIONS

- Provide low-load, prolonged abduction mobilization force to first CMC joint to facilitate lengthening of tissue.

Common Diagnoses	General Optimal Positions
Thumb CMC adduction contracture	Wrist: 10°–20° extension; CMC: terminal midpalmar and radial abduction

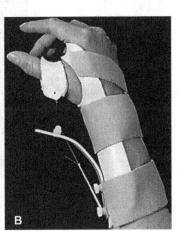

FIGURE 2–17

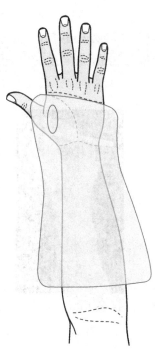

FIGURE 2–18

FABRICATION PROCESS (USING DIGITEC SYSTEM)

Pattern Creation (Fig. 2–18)

- Mark proximal border two-thirds length of forearm.
- Mark distal border at distal palmar crease.
- Mark for thumbhole in distal central portion of pattern, approximately 1″ down and in.
- Allow enough material to encompass half to two-thirds circumference of forearm, remembering that forearm tapers distally.

Refine Pattern

- Proximal border should allow full elbow motion.
- Distal border should allow unimpeded motion of IF to MF MCP joints and full thumb mobility.
- For average adult, thumbhole should be about the size of elongated half dollar.

Options for Materials

- Consider ⅛″ thermoplastic material to provide needed rigidity to withstand mobilization forces.
- Gel- or foam-lined materials may help decrease distal migration and increase comfort.
- Use components of choice (Digitec Outrigger System shown).

Cut and Heat

- Position patient with elbow resting on table and forearm supination for gravity-assisted molding; thumb should be held in gentle palmar abduction while molding.
- Cut out thumbhole in material either by making a series of holes with a hole punch before heating or by carefully piercing the slightly warm material with sharp scissors.

Evaluate Fit While Molding

- Lay warm material on towel, positioning thumbhole on correct side of material to be placed on forearm.
- Using IFs, gently open hole, making it slightly larger and more elongated (egg shaped).
- Place thumbhole over thumb and guide rest of material evenly along volar wrist and forearm.
- Carefully incorporate arches of hand by using smooth, even strokes and constantly redirecting material into arches.
- Allow for clearance at base of CMC joint; as thumb abducts in orthosis, base of thumbhole may need to be adjusted.
- Rotate forearm at end of molding to check for possible abutment of ulnar and radial styloid processes, and flare as necessary.

Strapping and Components

- Distal strap: 1″ strap directed from volar to dorsal border.
- Middle strap: 2″ strap applied proximal to dorsal wrist crease; use piece of adhesive foam to further stabilize wrist in orthosis and prevent migration. Foam should not overlap orthosis edges.
- Proximal strap: depending on size of forearm, 1″ or 2″ strap.
- Position Digitec Outrigger along radial volar aspect of orthosis base.
- Position soft sling (sling made of QuickCast 2 shown) in web space proximal to ulnar side of thumb MP (around metacarpal head). Positioning sling in this way directs forces to CMC joint, not MP joint ulnar collateral ligament.
- Check that sling and monofilament lines are directed at 90° angle from first metacarpal; attachment on outrigger may appear more proximal than anticipated.

- Next, thread monofilament line to line guide on outrigger, attach mobilization force, and secure to proximal attachment device.

Survey Completed Orthosis

- Make sure sling does not irritate web space. Fabricating wider sling may assist in distributing pressure and increasing comfort.
- Adhesive-backed Dycem or silicone gel sheet may help sling stay in place.
- Smooth and slightly flare distal and proximal borders.
- Gently flare around thenar hole, especially at base; avoid rolling, which can make future orthosis modifications difficult and can lead to an unnecessarily bulky orthosis.
- Check clearance of elbow, irritation at radial and ulnar styloid processes, and digital MCP motion.
- Adjust tension per patient and/or tissue tolerance; goal is low-load stretch over prolonged period of time.

PATTERN PEARLS 2–37 AND 2–38

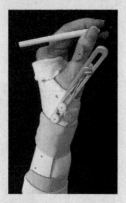

FIGURE PP2–37 Dorsal approach to obtain exact thumb placement for function.

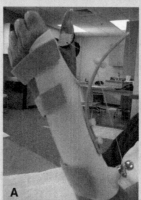
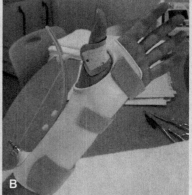

A   B

FIGURE PP2–38 **A and B,** Static progressive approach using a Splint-Tuner™ device (North Coast Medical) (note combination of neoprene/QuickCast 2 sling).

CLINICAL PEARL 2–24

Thumb CMC Abduction, MP/IP Extension, or Flexion Mobilization Orthosis

Thumb flexion and adduction contractures can sometimes develop after flexor pollicis longus (FPL) repair or thumb fracture immobilization. Fabricating a mobilization orthosis can be a way to stretch the volar and ulnar soft tissue structures of the thumb. **A,** The dorsal wrist immobilization pattern is used for the orthosis base. The outrigger is aligned with the dorsal longitudinal axis of the thumb column and secured to the orthosis (Digitec Outrigger; Performance Health). A thermoplastic sling is molded to the volar thumb surface, supporting the proximal phalanx. Monofilament line is attached, threaded through the line guide on the outrigger, and attached proximally via a rubber band. Tension is adjusted per patient's tolerance. **B,** Neoprene straps or similar can also be used directly over case immobilization to provide a gentle stress to a potential adherence of the FPL tendon. **C,** A similar approach can be used when trying to gain palmar abduction and MP flexion. Shown here is a static progressive approach with the dorsal thermoplastic sling placed over the dorsum of the thumb proximal phalanx with forces directed in MP flexion and midpalmar-radial abduction.

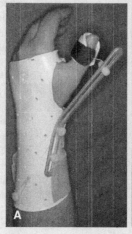
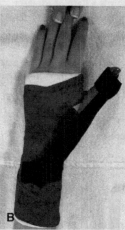
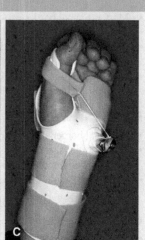

A   B   C

Adjustment of the Elastic Thread

KIRSTEN C. PEDERSEN, OT

Denmark

Adjusting the pull on elastic tread can be made easy by using a "lark head" knot. This knot can be loosened if the elastic is to be tensioned or released, and the knot acts as a stop block in the tube.

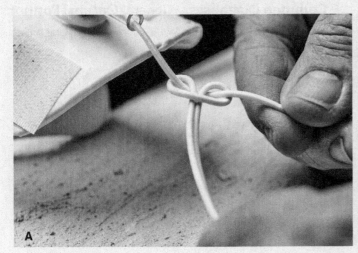

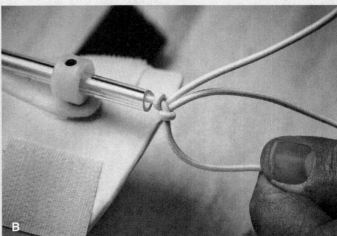

Thumb Strapping

SABRINA CASSELLA, MED, OTR/L, CHT

Massachusetts

Wide strap applied over prefabricated orthosis for thumb abduction stretch after cast removal.

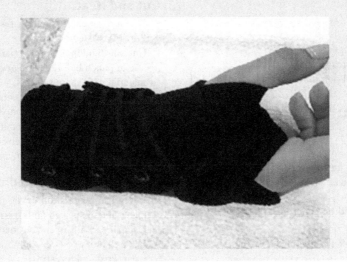

MCP FLEXION MOBILIZATION ORTHOSIS (Fig. 2–19)

COMMON NAMES

- Dynamic MCP flexion orthosis

ALTERNATIVE ORTHOSIS OPTIONS

- Prefabricated orthosis
- Flexion glove

PRIMARY FUNCTIONS

- Provide low-load, prolonged flexion mobilization force to MCP joint to facilitate lengthening of tissue.

Common Diagnoses	General Optimal Positions
MCP extension contracture	Wrist: 10°–20° extension; MCP: terminal flexion

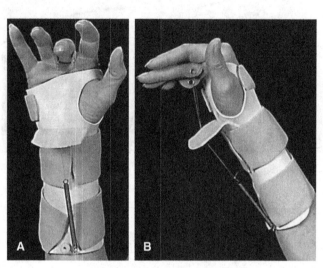

FIGURE 2–19

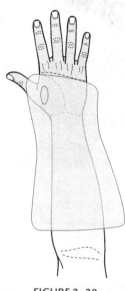

FIGURE 2–20

FABRICATION PROCESS

Pattern Creation (Fig. 2–20)

- Mark proximal border two-thirds length of forearm.
- Mark distal border at distal palmar crease.
- Mark for thumbhole in distal central portion of pattern, approximately 1″ down and in.
- Allow enough material to encompass half to two-thirds circumference of forearm.

Refine Pattern

- Proximal border should allow elbow motion.
- Distal border should allow unimpeded motion of IF to MF MCP joints and full thumb mobility.
- For average adult, thumbhole should be about size of elongated half dollar.
- Distal portion of orthosis should clear proximal palmar crease to allow MCP flexion.

Options for Materials

- Use ⅛″ material to provide needed rigidity to withstand mobilization forces.
- Gel- or foam-lined materials may help decrease distal migration and increase comfort.
- Custom-fabricated outrigger, made from ⅛″ perforated material, acts as line guide. The best material choice for the outrigger is a material that is not coated. Solid thermoplastics can be used; however, smooth holes can be made using quality hole punch.

Cut and Heat

- Position patient with elbow resting on table and forearm supination for gravity-assisted molding.
- Cut out thumbhole in material either by making a series of holes with a hole punch before heating or by carefully piercing the slightly warm material with sharp scissors.
- Determine where outrigger should be positioned to achieve 90° angle of pull. Ideal outrigger position should allow for line of pull to scaphoid. General placement at or about wrist crease should be long enough to address degree of MCP extension contracture.
- Prepare surface with solvent and heat thermoplastic outrigger.

Evaluate Fit While Molding

- Lay warm material on towel, positioning thumbhole on correct side of material to be placed on forearm.
- Using IFs, gently open hole, making it slightly larger and more elongated.
- Place thumbhole over thumb and guide rest of material evenly along volar wrist and forearm.
- Carefully incorporate arches of hand by using smooth, even strokes and constantly redirecting material into arches.
- Allow for clearance at base of CMC joint. As thumb abducts in orthosis, base of thumbhole may need to be adjusted.
- Rotate forearm to check for possible abutment of ulnar and radial styloid processes, and flare as necessary.

Strapping and Components

- Distal strap: 1″ strap directed from volar to dorsal border.

- Middle strap: 2″ strap applied proximal to dorsal wrist crease; use piece of adhesive foam to further stabilize wrist in orthosis and prevent migration. Foam should not overlap orthosis edges.
- Proximal strap: depending on size of forearm, 1″ or 2″ strap.
- Affix outrigger at correct angle on base.
- Mark holes on outrigger where monofilament will be threaded to apply correct angle of pull.
- Affix proximal attachment device; several are needed if multiple digits are involved.
- Affix individual slings to proximal phalanxes, thread monofilament through predetermined holes, attach mobilization force, and attach to proximal attachment devices.
- Line of pull should be directed toward scaphoid bone, which follows natural cascade of digits.

Survey Completed Orthosis

- Make sure that sling does not irritate web space.
- Adhesive-backed Dycem or silicone gel sheet may help sling stay in place.
- Smooth and slightly flare distal and proximal borders.
- Gently flare around thenar hole, especially at base; avoid rolling, which can make future orthosis modifications difficult and can lead to an unnecessarily bulky orthosis.
- Check clearance of elbow, irritation at radial and ulnar styloid processes, and digital MCP motion.
- As MCP flexion gains are made, line of pull (changing hole in outrigger) must be adjusted, and outrigger can be cut down.
- Adjust tension per patient and/or tissue tolerance; goal is low-load stretch over prolonged period of time.

 PATTERN PEARLS 2–39 TO 2–41

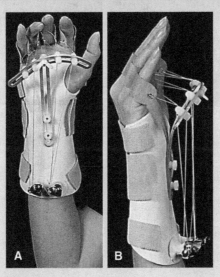

FIGURE PP2–39 A and B, Base 2™ Outrigger System; note the use of a Splint-Tuner™ (North Coast Medical).

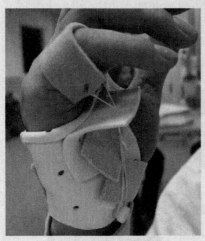

FIGURE PP2–40 Hand-based design using scrap thermoplastic piece as line guide.

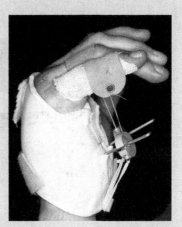

FIGURE PP2–41 Phoenix Outrigger (Performance Health) turned on side to achieve optimal angle of force application; note SF casting for improved leverage.

CLINICAL PEARL 2–25

Clearance of Distal Palmar Crease

Be mindful to check for full clearance of MCP flexion to allow unrestricted mobilization. The orthoses tend to migrate distally once the force is applied; achieving good contour can help combat this tendency. Also try applying the orthosis directly on the skin or place strips of nonskid material such as Microfoam™ tape to minimize slippage. In this orthosis, the SF MCP flexion crease is blocked **(A)**, limiting full flexion potential; this border needs to be cleared to the line shown. **B** shows the clearance of the distal border.

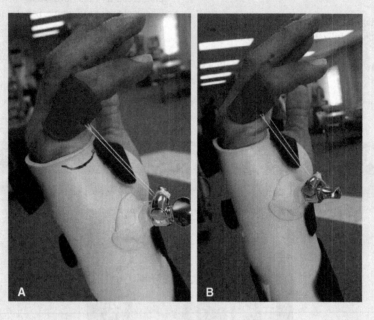

EXPERT PEARL 2–14

Rubber Band Application

KIMBERLY GOLDIE STAINES, OTR, CHT
Texas

Use a small (3 mm) crochet hook to ease the process of getting rubber bands through holes on straps or slings.

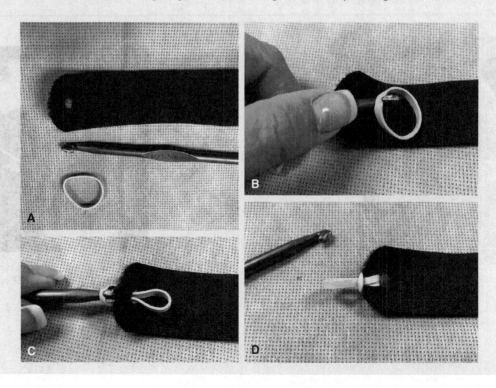

MCP/PIP/DIP FLEXION MOBILIZATION ORTHOSIS (WHFO) (Fig. 2–21)

COMMON NAMES

- Final finger flexion orthosis
- Composite flexion orthosis

ALTERNATIVE ORTHOSIS OPTIONS

- Finger flexion glove
- Phase II composite finger flexion loop attachments
- Prefabricated orthoses
- Splint-Tuner™ Final Finger Flexion Kit
- Rolyan® Biodynamic Flexion System

PRIMARY FUNCTIONS

- Provide low-load, prolonged flexion mobilization force to MCP, PIP, and DIP joints to facilitate lengthening of tissue.

Common Diagnoses	General Optimal Positions
Extrinsic extensor tightness	Wrist: 10°–20°; MCP/PIP/DIP: terminal flexion
MCP, PIP, or DIP extension contractures	Wrist: 10°–20° extension; MCP/PIP/DIP: terminal flexion

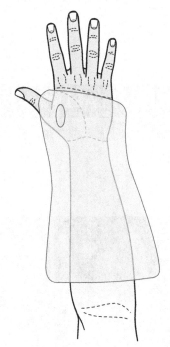

FIGURE 2–22

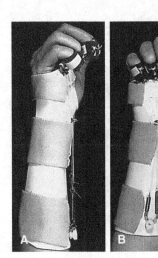

FIGURE 2–21

FABRICATION PROCESS

Pattern Creation (Fig. 2–22)

- Orthosis is most effective when MCP and IP joints have approximately 50% passive range of motion (PROM).
- Mark proximal border two-thirds length of forearm.
- Mark distal border at distal palmar crease.
- Mark for thumbhole in distal central portion of pattern, approximately 1″ down and in.
- Allow enough material to encompass half to two-thirds circumference of forearm, remembering that forearm tapers distally.

Refine Pattern

- Proximal border should allow full elbow motion.
- Distal border should allow unimpeded motion of IF to MF MCP joints and full thumb mobility.
- For average adult, thumbhole should be about size of elongated half dollar.
- Distal volar portion of orthosis should clear proximal palmar crease to allow unimpeded MCP flexion.

Options for Materials

- Consider $^1/_8$″ thermoplastic material to provide needed rigidity to withstand mobilization forces.
- Gel- or foam-lined materials may help decrease distal migration and increase comfort.

Cut and Heat

- Position patient with elbow resting on table and forearm supination for gravity-assisted molding. Thumb should be held in gentle palmar abduction while molding.
- Cut out thumbhole in material either by making series of holes with hole punch before heating or by carefully piercing the slightly warm material with sharp scissors.

Evaluate Fit While Molding

- Lay warm material on towel, positioning thumbhole on correct side of material to be placed on forearm.
- Using IFs, gently open hole, making it slightly larger and more elongated (egg shaped).
- Place thumbhole over thumb and guide rest of material evenly along volar wrist and forearm.

- Carefully incorporate arches of hand by using smooth, even strokes and constantly redirecting material into arches.
- Allow for clearance at base of first CMC joint. As thumb abducts in orthosis, base of thumbhole may need to be adjusted.
- Rotate forearm to check for possible abutment of ulnar and radial styloid processes, and flare as necessary.

Strapping and Components

- Distal strap: 1″ strap directed from volar to dorsal border.
- Middle strap: 2″ strap applied proximal to dorsal wrist crease; use piece of adhesive foam to further stabilize wrist in orthosis and prevent migration. Foam should not overlap orthosis edges.
- Proximal strap: depending on size of forearm, 1″ or 2″ strap.
- Apply line guides as close to the distal palmar crease as possible (approximately where digits would rest if composite fist were possible).
- Rolyan® Wrap-On Finger Hooks, used as distal attachment device, are shown.

- One or two lines guides per digit can be used. If using one line guide per digit, place in alignment with longitudinal axis of involved digit(s). If using two line guides, place in alignment with web spaces of involved digit(s).
- Line of pull should be directed to the line guide.
- Static line should be approximately triple length of hand; fold in half and guide from sling through line guides.
- Proximally, line is attached to rubber band post via springs.

Survey Completed Orthosis

- Smooth and slightly flare distal and proximal borders.
- Gently flare around thenar hole, especially at base; avoid rolling, which can make future orthosis modifications difficult and can lead to an unnecessarily bulky orthosis.
- Check clearance of elbow, irritation at radial and ulnar styloid processes, and digital MCP motion.
- Adjust tension per patient and/or tissue tolerance; goal is low-load stretch over prolonged period of time.

 PATTERN PEARLS 2–42 TO 2–47

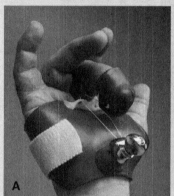 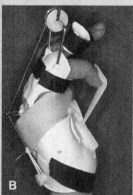

FIGURE PP2–43 A, Hand-based design using static progressive approach via the Splint-Tuner™ and thermoplastic line guides (North Coast Medical). A static progressive approach via simple hook and loop can be used to gain composite flexion. **B,** Shown here is a combination orthosis which gives the patient the ability to work on dynamic PIP extension via the rubber band traction using the Phoenix Outrigger System; Performance Health.

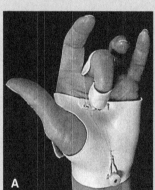 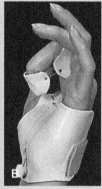

FIGURE PP2–42 A and B, Hand-based design using rubber band "dynamic" approach, embedded safety pins as line guides, and 1/16″ thermoplastic slings.

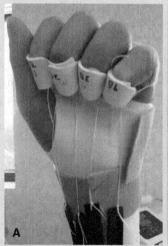 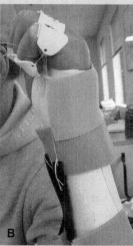

FIGURE PP2–44 A and B, Hook and loop being used for a static progressive approach with each digit numbered and adjusted individually.

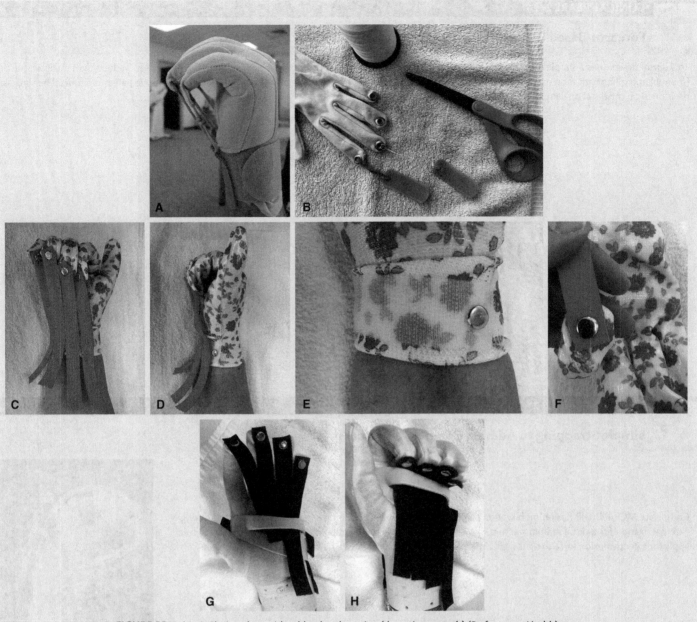

FIGURE PP2–45 A, Flexion glove with rubber band traction (dynamic approach) (Performance Health). **B,** Flexion glove being modified to provide a static progressive approach—elastics replaced with static line. **C and D,** Custom-made flexion glove using a garden glove with "homemade" digit mobilization using a static progressive approach via hook/loop strapping. **E,** Strip of hook riveted on proximal cuff of glove. **F,** Scrap 1/16″ thermoplastic "washer" to prevent rivet from pulling off at fingertip. **G and H,** Flexion glove modification—utilization of transverse palmar bar to feed loop beneath providing DIP flexion. Also note use of thermoplastic wrist cuff for proximal attachment of flexion force.

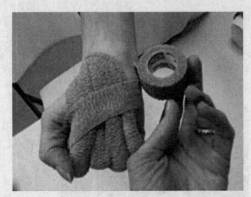

FIGURE PP2–46 Coban™ wrap for composite MCP and PIP flexion stretching (Performance Health).

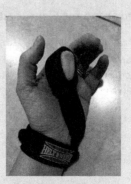

FIGURE PP2–47 Frap Strap® (Performance Health) multiuse device can be used to provide composite stretch.

CLINICAL PEARL 2–26

Forearm-Based Dorsal Design PIP/DIP Flexion Mobilization Orthosis

This dorsal design uses a simple and cost-effective static progressive approach to composite mobilization of the IP joints to address tight intrinsic muscles (monofilament line with loop material attaching proximally to adhesive hook). Note the foam-lined slings, which improve patient comfort. The slings are positioned on the distal phalanx, and the forces are dorsally directed.

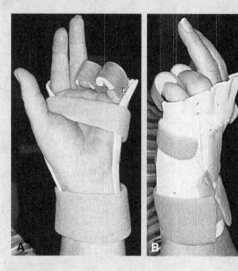

CLINICAL PEARL 2–27

Simple Strapping to Address Composite Stiffness

Composite MCP/PIP/DIP flexion mobilization can be initiated following an initial observation of stiffness during external fixation for a distal radium fracture. Shown here is a simple foam strapping system that the patient can apply for a gentle flexion force to tight digits. This patient is not yet a candidate for thermoplastic application.

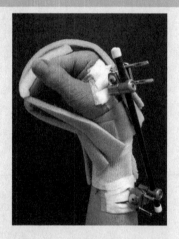

CLINICAL PEARL 2–28

Use of Neoprene for Composite Flexion Stretch

Neoprene can be used effectively to provide a gentle composite force as shown here, status post extensor tenolysis (**A and B**). Neoprene can also be added to an orthosis base to provide a similar composite flexion stretch while the wrist is stabilized. This orthosis places the wrist in neutral and the MCP joints in maximum passive flexion. Conforming neoprene is used to encompass the distal joints and provide a gentle stretch (**C**) (see Chapter 14 for more instructive detail on the use of neoprene).

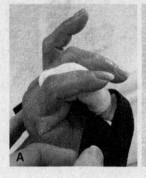
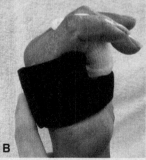
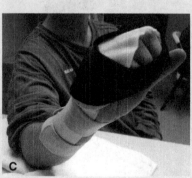

EXPERT PEARL 2–15

MCP Flexion Restriction Orthosis
JULIANNE LESSARD OTR/L, CHT
Massachusetts

Can be worn with or without a flexion glove to encourage passive or active PIP/DIP flexion.

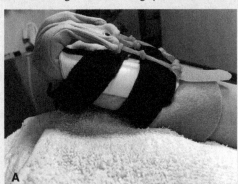 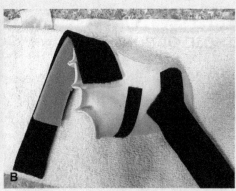

 EXPERT PEARL 2–16

Homemade Flexion Glove: Steps of Fabrication
DEBBY SCHWARTZ, OTD, OTR/L, CHT
New Jersey

Garden Glove orthosis for dynamic or static progressive composite finger flexion.

1. Fabricate a circumferential wrist orthosis from a square of coated 1/12″ thermoplastic material. Apply straps and also adhesive-backed hook to the volar orthosis.
2. Place a 3″ piece of Orfitube at the distal palmar edge close to the distal palmar crease. Attach by wrapping the ends with heated scraps of Orfit material and bond to the orthosis.
3. Punch holes in the fingers of an inexpensive garden glove.
4. Slip an elastic pony tail holder through one of the finger holes and secure with a knot. Add another elastic pony tail holder for length as needed (dynamic). Slip a doubled piece of upholstery thread through a finger hole and secure with a knot (static progressive). Attach a small square of adhesive-backed loop strap through the elastic pony tail holder and/or the thread.
5. The client slips on the glove and then puts on the wrist orthosis. The loop strap of each finger is pulled underneath the Orfitube pulley and attached to adhesive-backed hook on the volar orthosis. The tension on each finger can be adjusted individually so that a tolerable end range position is maintained.
6. Begin with a low load of tension and gradually increase, but never to the point of pain. Suggested evidence-based wearing schedules: 3 to 4 times/day × 30 minutes for static progressive orthoses versus 6 to 12 hours/day for dynamic orthoses.
7. Another option is to work on passive PIP and DIP flexion while blocking MCP flexion in a hand-based orthosis.

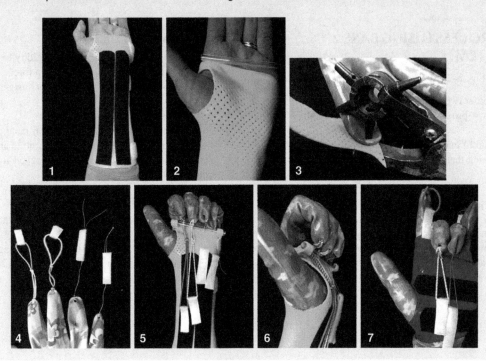

THUMB MP AND IP EXTENSION MOBILIZATION ORTHOSIS (WHFO) (Fig. 2–23)

COMMON NAMES

- Dynamic thumb extension orthosis
- Extensor pollicis longus (EPL) orthosis

ALTERNATIVE ORTHOSIS OPTIONS

- Casting (serial static)

PRIMARY FUNCTIONS

- Provide low-load, prolonged extension mobilization force to thumb MP and IP joints to facilitate lengthening of tissue.

ADDITIONAL FUNCTIONS

- Maintain thumb MP and IP joints in extension, allowing restricted flexion within predetermined range, to facilitate tendon healing, tendon glide, and prevent tendon adherence (restriction orthosis).

Common Diagnoses	General Optimal Positions
IP and MP flexion contracture	Wrist: 20°–30° extension; CMC: mid rad/palmar abduction; MP/IP: terminal extension

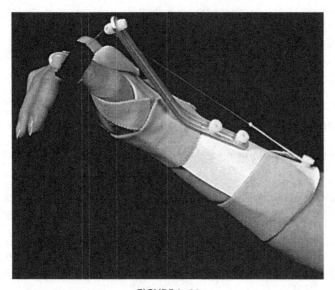

FIGURE 2–23

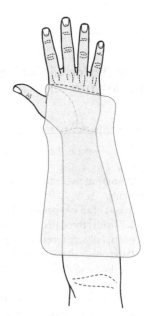

FIGURE 2–24

FABRICATION PROCESS (USING BASE 2™ OUTRIGGER SYSTEM)

Pattern Creation (Fig. 2–24)

- Mark for proximal border two-thirds length of forearm.
- Mark distal border, just proximal to dorsal digit and thumb MP joint skinfolds.
- Allow enough material to encompass half to two-thirds circumference of forearm, remembering that forearm tapers distally.

Refine Pattern

- Proximal border should allow full elbow motion.
- Distal border should allow unimpeded motion of digital MCP and thumb MP and IP joints.
- Allow appropriate amount of material radially to provide surface area for component application.

Options for Materials

- Use ⅛″ material to provide needed rigidity to maintain wrist joint position and accept extension mobilization force.
- Use components of choice (Base 2™ Outrigger System shown).

Cut and Heat

- Position patient with elbow resting on table and forearm pronated for gravity-assisted molding. Position thumb in abduction and opposition.
- Prepad ulnar styloid with adhesive-backed foam, putty, cotton ball, or silicone gel.

Evaluate Fit While Molding

- Position material on dorsum of involved hand and wrist just proximal to MP joints.
- Make sure desired wrist position is maintained. Some patients tend to flex and deviate wrist while orthosis is being formed.

Strapping and Components

- Thumb strap: apply volarly, allowing MP motion.
- Distal strap: 1″ strap connecting distal radial and distal ulnar borders.
- Middle strap: 2″ strap just proximal to dorsal wrist crease; use piece of adhesive foam to further stabilize wrist in orthosis and prevent migration. Foam should not overlap orthosis edges.
- Proximal strap: 2″ soft or elasticized strap is good choice.
- Attach Base 2™ Outrigger to orthosis base using rubber band posts. Be sure outrigger aligns with thumb column and extends distally in entire length of thumb.
- Apply sling to distal phalanx. Next, thread the monofilament line through line guide on outrigger and secure the mobilization component to proximal attachment device.

Survey Completed Orthosis

- Smooth and slightly flare distal and proximal borders.
- Gently flare around dorsal thumb region; avoid rolling, which can make future orthosis modifications difficult and can lead to an unnecessarily bulky orthosis.
- Check clearance of elbow, radial and ulnar styloid processes, and MCP joints.
- Adjust tension per patient and/or tissue tolerance; goal is low-load stretch over prolonged period of time.

CLINICAL PEARL 2–29

Serial Static Approach for MP and IP Extension

A and B, Oftentimes, MCP and IP stiffness is in combination with other injuries. The therapist should consider a serial static approach when faced with multiple injuries. When thumb extension is restricted because of extrinsic flexor shortening, the wrist must be included. **C and D,** Shown is maximizing wrist extension while simultaneously positioning the thumb into extension and radial abduction. Note the spiral design that wraps around the thumb from volar radial to ulnar dorsal. This helps keep the thumb from positioning into adduction and IP flexion.

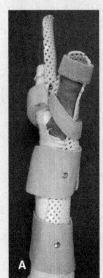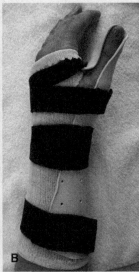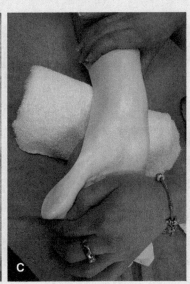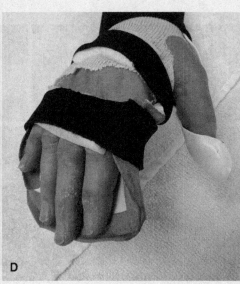

MCP EXTENSION MOBILIZATION ORTHOSIS (WHFO) (Fig. 2–25)

COMMON NAMES
- Dynamic MCP extension orthosis

ALTERNATIVE ORTHOSIS OPTIONS
- Preformed adjustable outrigger kits
- Prefabricated orthosis

PRIMARY FUNCTIONS
- Provide low-load, prolonged extension mobilization force to MCP joints to facilitate lengthening of tissue.
- Passively support MCP joints in extension while allowing active digital flexion.

Common Diagnoses	General Optimal Positions
MCP joint arthroplasty	Wrist: 30°–45° extension; MCP: 0°–10° flexion and slight RD
Extensor tendon repair (zones V to VII)	Wrist: 30°–45° extension; MCP: 0°–10° flexion (thumb zones IV to V) (if thumb involved: CMC extension and 45° radial abduction)
Radial or posterior interosseous	Wrist: 30°–45° extension, MCP: 0° nerve injury
Extrinsic flexor tightness	Wrist: 451°, IP: 0°, MCP: terminal extension

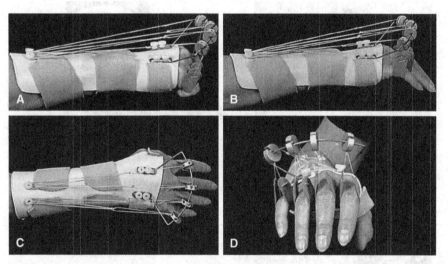

FIGURE 2–25

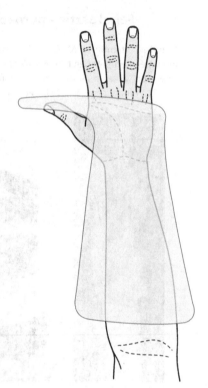

FIGURE 2–26

FABRICATION PROCESS (USING PHOENIX OUTRIGGER SYSTEM)

Pattern Creation (Fig. 2–26)

- Mark for proximal border two-thirds length of forearm.
- Mark distal border just distal to dorsal digit MCP joint skinfolds.
- Make radial tab (palmar bar) long enough (approximately 30) to traverse through palm and secure on distal ulnar border.
- Allow enough material to encompass half to two-thirds circumference of forearm, remembering that forearm tapers distally.

Refine Pattern

- Proximal border should allow full elbow motion.
- Extend distal portion of orthosis to MCP head level.

Options for Materials

- Consider ⅛″ thermoplastic material to provide needed rigidity to maintain wrist joint position and accept extension mobilization force.
- Use components of choice (Phoenix Outrigger System shown).

Cut and Heat

- Position patient with elbow resting on table and forearm pronated for gravity-assisted molding.
- Prepad ulnar styloid using adhesive-backed foam, putty, cotton ball, or silicone gel.

Evaluate Fit While Molding

- Position material on dorsum of involved hand and wrist just distal to MCP joints.
- Gently pull radial bar through thumb web space and across volar MCPs to meet ulnar segment. Pinch and seal lightly, and return focus to molding dorsum.
- Make sure desired wrist position is maintained. Some patients tend to flex and deviate wrist while orthosis is being formed.

Strapping and Components

- Distal strap: 1″ strap connecting distal radial and distal ulnar borders (if needed).
- Middle strap: 2″ strap just proximal to wrist crease; use piece of adhesive foam to further stabilize wrist in orthosis and prevent migration. Foam should not overlap orthosis edges.
- Proximal strap: 2″ soft or elasticized strap.
- Mark desired outrigger attachment, positioning to extend distally over middle portion of proximal phalanx and extending high enough that when volar sling is attached to monofilament line, it clears pulley.

- Use rubber band posts to secure outrigger on orthosis.
- Attach Phoenix wheels to outrigger using Allen wrench.
- Attach line on both sides of sling, apply sling to middle phalanx, and thread line through Phoenix wheels.
- Loop appropriate rubber band onto end of monofilament line, and connect to proximal attachment device.

Survey Completed Orthosis

- Material should be flared distally to prevent irritation of MCP heads during flexion exercises; if necessary, use layer of thin padding to increase patient comfort.
- Check that mobilization force is strong enough to support and return MCP joints to desired position after active digital flexion.
- Check that mobilization force is not too strong, impeding patient's ability to flex digits in the desired amount.
- Instruct patient to monitor for signs of increased pressure over ulnar styloid and radial and ulnar sensory nerve branches.
- Consider padding of the radial styloid and Lister tubercle, especially for patients with frail skin such as those with rheumatoid arthritis.

PATTERN PEARLS 2–48 TO 2–53

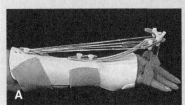
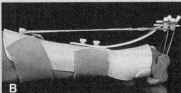
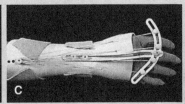
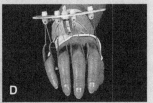

FIGURE PP2–48 **A–D,** Digitec Outrigger System (Performance Health).

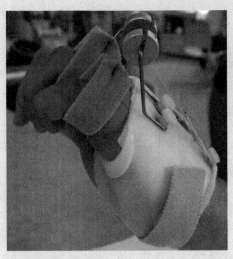

FIGURE PP2–49 Hand-based design: Phoenix Outrigger System (Performance Health) for RF and SF.

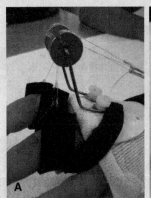
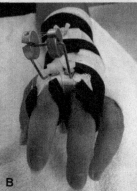

FIGURE PP2–50 **A and B,** Hand-based design: Phoenix Outrigger System (Performance Health) for IF and MF only. Notice slight radial deviation pull used post-MCP arthroplasty.

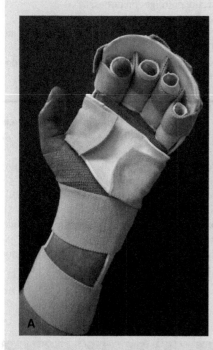

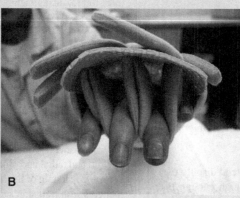

FIGURE PP2–51 **A and B,** Static progressive approach for simultaneous MCP/PIP/DIP extension.

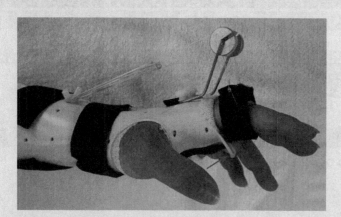

FIGURE PP2–52 Volar MCP flexion block can be incorporated into the base design.

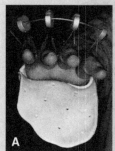
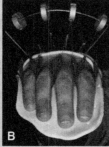
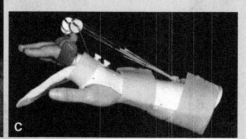

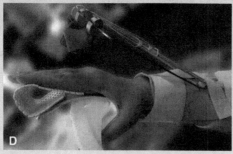

FIGURE PP2–53 **A–D,** MCP flexion block secured as separate removable segment.

CLINICAL PEARL 2–30

PIP/DIP Extension Orthoses to Assist With a Mobilization Orthosis

A, A PIP/DIP extension mobilization orthosis or cast can be slipped under the slings of an MCP extension mobilization orthosis to prevent or address concurrent PIP flexion contractures. These orthoses can be worn periodically throughout the day as an exercise tool to stretch tight IP joints or to isolate/facilitate MCP flexion with exercise. Commonly, the SF can have difficulty with isolating MCP flexion; this technique of using a cast can be especially helpful with addressing this often problematic digit. Shown is QuickCast 2 (Performance Health).

B and C, An IP extension mobilization orthosis (Orficast™; North Coast Medical) is used to simultaneously treat an SF PIP flexion contracture and to more effectively direct gentle tension to extrinsic tightness of the SF flexor tendons. A simple neoprene strap is shown providing a dynamic approach. This same patient had MCP capsular tightness especially in flexion; therefore, the same neoprene strap was used, intermittently, to provide MCP flexion. Note how well the IP extension orthosis aids in directing all the forces of flexion to the MCP joint.

D, A hand-based version of an IP extension orthosis (QuickCast 2, Performance Health) is used to dynamically mobilize the SF MCP into flexion. The orthosis allows isolation of flexion forces to the MCP joint. Shown is the Phoenix Outrigger System; Performance Health.

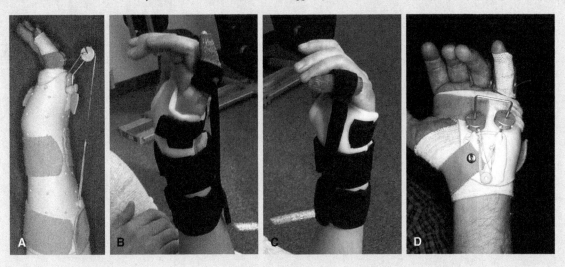

CLINICAL PEARL 2–31

Modification of Small Finger Sling

Oftentimes, the SF sling needs to be customized for the short proximal phalanx; notice sling shown is too wide, limiting PIP flexion **(A)**. Trim the width of the sling to the appropriate length, allowing for unrestricted MCP and PIP motion **(B)**. The length may also need to be modified accordingly. Also, commonly when using this orthosis for exercise following an MCP joint arthroplasty, using a separate elastic of very light tension or releasing the tension completely for exercise is necessary to allow for the desired amount of MCP flexion. When the digit is at rest, the elastic must not be so tight that the MCP is held in hyperextension. **C,** Take caution to avoid this by having the patient bring the orthosis into the clinic for therapy sessions to check these joint angles.

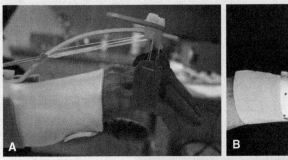

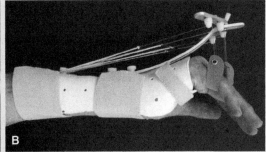

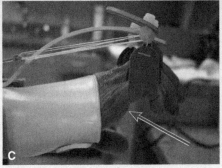

CLINICAL PEARL 2–32

IF Radial Outrigger to Prevent Pronation and Ulnar Deviation

An IF outrigger attachment is most often found in combination with an MCP extension mobilization orthosis for patients who have undergone MCP joint arthroplasty involving reconstruction of the IF radial collateral ligament. Consider applying an ulnarly positioned dress hook (with gel-based glue) or a piece of hook material to the fingernail. If using the dress hook, attach a thin strip of loop material (via a hole) directed ulnarly, crossing the volar aspect of the fingertip. Fasten a thin rubber band to the other end and attach it to the radial outrigger. If using adhesive hook material glued to the nail, place a thin strip of loop directed as described for the dress hook. This should provide a gentle radial deviation and supination force to the IF. Note: If pronation is not an issue, a sling can be applied to the digit directed radially.

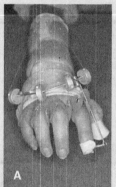
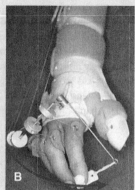

PIP INTRA-ARTICULAR MOBILIZATION ORTHOSIS (WHFO) (Fig. 2–27)[c]

COMMON NAMES

- Dynamic traction orthosis
- Schenck orthosis
- Hoop orthosis

ALTERNATIVE ORTHOSIS OPTIONS

- Swing design dynamic traction[d]

PRIMARY FUNCTIONS

- Provide gentle, controlled distal distraction to involved PIP joint to reduce articular fragments and realign joint surfaces.

Common Diagnoses and General Optimal Positions

- Note: Direction of distal traction, tension on rubber band, and passive arc of flexion and extension are set by the surgeon in the operating room. Any alteration to these placements should be discussed with the surgeon. This orthosis can be modified to accommodate intra-articular MCP and thumb MP/IP joint injuries (Kearney & Brown, 1994; Schenck, 1986, 1994)
- Pilon fracture of PIP
- Fracture dislocation of PIP
- Severe fracture of grade 3 or 4; grade 2 if combined with subluxation or dislocation
- Condylar fracture
- Oblique or spiral phalangeal shaft fracture

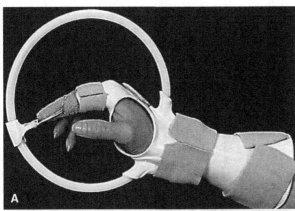

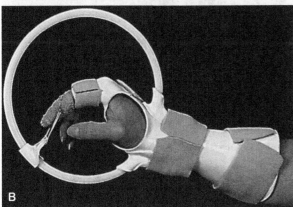

FIGURE 2–27

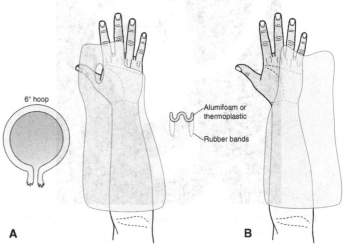

FIGURE 2–28

---

[c]Developed by Robert Schenck, MD; Laura Kearney, OTR/L, CHT; and Krista Brown, OTR/L, CHT. Schenck, R. R. (1986). Dynamic traction and early passive movement for fractures of the proximal interphalangeal joint. *Journal of Hand Surgery (American)*, *11*(6), 850–858.

[d]Designed by Griet Van Veldhoven, modified by Kadelbach, D. (2006). Swing design dynamic traction splinting for the treatment of intra-articular fractures of the digits. *Journal of Hand Therapy*, *19*(1), 39–42.

FABRICATION PROCESS

Pattern Creation (Fig. 2–28)

- Orthosis should be fabricated preoperatively or in operating room as physician places wire.
- Choose appropriate base pattern for digit.
  - IF or MF (**A**): radial wrist extension and MCP flexion immobilization orthosis
  - RF or SF (**B**): ulnar wrist extension and MCP flexion immobilization orthosis
  - Thumb: wrist and thumb MP immobilization orthosis or wrist immobilization orthosis
  - Fabricate 6″ hoop or partial hoop.

Refine Pattern

- Make sure wrist is extended approximately 30°, and MCP joints are flexed to approximately 60°.
- Orthosis can encompass bordering digit for maximal orthosis stabilization if necessary. Do not interfere with motion of uninvolved digits.
- Clear PIP flexion crease proximally.

Options for Materials

- Use 3/32″ or ⅛″ material.
- Hoop can be made from rolled thermoplastic material or wide Aquatubes®.

Cut and Heat

- Prepare hoop by warming material around 6″ cylindrical form (e.g., 5-lb therapy putty container), leaving about 1″ extension on each end for attachment onto orthosis base.
- Position patient with forearm in neutral and digits slightly abducted.

Evaluate Fit While Molding

- Fabricate appropriate ulnar or radial wrist extension and MCP flexion immobilization orthosis.
- Clear distally to allow unimpeded PIP flexion.

Strapping and Components

- Attach hoop to orthosis so involved joint is equidistant from hoop; align longitudinally with involved digit.
- Fabricate movable component with either thermoplastic material or AlumaFoam® (see pattern).
- Apply rubber band traction (no. 19) or spring coils to interosseous wire and measure tension so it applies approximately 300 g of force.

- Mark flexion and extension limits (as set by physician) on hoop with tape or marker.
- Strap orthosis base at orthosis's distal border, wrist crease, and proximal orthosis border.
- Apply ½″ strap about proximal phalanx.

Survey Completed Orthosis

- Carefully instruct patient on use of orthosis. Generally, patients should alternate between positions of flexion and extension. Beginning on first day of orthosis application, patient should change positions every 10 minutes while awake. When sleeping, rubber bands should be placed midway between flexion and extension. Orthosis should be worn for 6 to 8 weeks (Schenck, 1994).

 PATTERN PEARL 2–54 TO 2–56

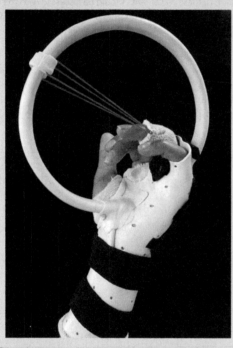

FIGURE PP2–54 Hoop, in this case, was positioned on dorsum of the hand and volar hand/wrist.

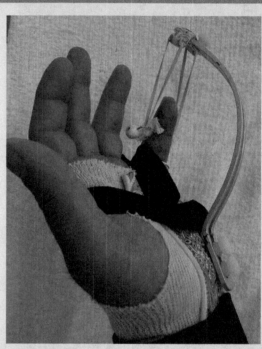

FIGURE PP2–55 Creative use of Digitec Outrigger (Performance Health) as a lower profile option for dynamic traction.

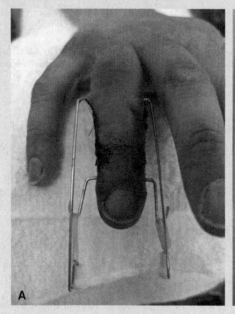 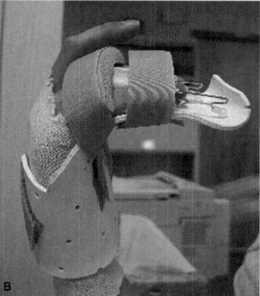

FIGURE PP2–56 A and B, Alternative dynamic traction treatment of an intra-articular PIP joint fracture.

CLINICAL PEARL 2–33

Adjusting Tension of Intra-articular Dynamic Traction Orthosis

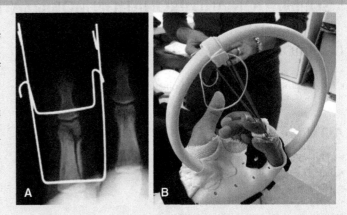

Rubber bands play a significant role in this orthosis design for the treatment of intra-articular fractures of the digit(s). Over time, rubber bands will lose some of their elasticity when under tension. A selection of rubber bands, each of which generates slightly different degrees of tension, should be sent with the patient to each medical doctor (MD) visit **(A)**. Most often, the digit is x-rayed weekly with the rubber bands in place to confirm proper tension **(B)**. Having rubber bands accessible of varying tensions can give the MD options to correct forces, ensuring proper fracture alignment with the goal of preserving articular symmetry and space. If too much tension is generated through the fracture, the space will fill in with scar. Too little tension will be ineffective in maintaining fracture alignment.

CLINICAL PEARL 2–34

Measuring Tension of Intra-articular Dynamic Traction Orthosis

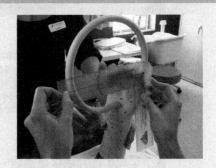

Use a goniometer or ruler to ensure equidistance from the horizontal wire on the middle phalanx to the hoop. This needs to be measured throughout the requested ROM to ensure that the traction force is applied at a constant level to the healing fracture.

4 Arm-Based Orthoses

SUPINATION AND PRONATION MOBILIZATION ORTHOSIS (EWHO) (Fig. 2–29)[e]

COMMON NAMES

- Forearm rotation orthosis
- Static progressive or dynamic supination/pronation orthosis

ALTERNATIVE ORTHOSIS OPTIONS

- Dynamic supination-pronation orthosis[f]
- Cast (serial static)
- Tone and positioning (TAP) orthosis
- MERiT™ SPS forearm rotation kit
- Dynamic/static progressive orthosis
- Neoprene and thermoplastic combination orthosis (Chapter 14)

PRIMARY FUNCTIONS

- Provide low-load, prolonged rotation mobilization force to proximal and distal radioulnar joints to facilitate lengthening of tissue.

Common Diagnoses	Optimal Positions
Supination or pronation contracture	Elbow: 90°; wrist: 0°–10° extension (comfortable wrist position)

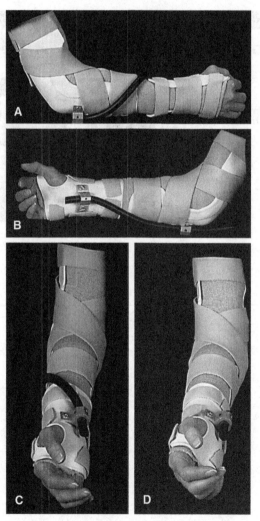

FIGURE 2–29

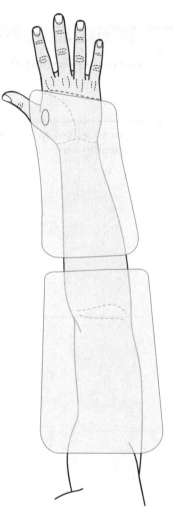

FIGURE 2–30

[f]Designed by Kay Collelo-Abraham.

[e]Designed by Kay Collelo-Abraham.

FABRICATION PROCESS (USING ROLYAN® PRONATION/SUPINATION KIT)

Pattern Creation (Fig. 2–30)

- Proximal orthosis
  - Fabricate orthosis per posterior elbow immobilization orthosis design.
  - Orthosis should extend distally approximately 5″ along ulnar border.
- Distal orthosis
  - Fabricate orthosis per volar wrist immobilization orthosis design.
  - Orthosis should extend proximally, leaving approximately 1″ of space between proximal and distal orthosis, which should not overlap.

Refine Pattern

- Be sure to allow for clearance of MCPs and thumb.
- Proximal orthosis border should allow full shoulder movement.

Options for Materials

- Use either perforated or nonperforated ⅛″ materials.
- Lightweight materials may not provide rigid support necessary for length and width of this orthosis.

Cut and Heat

- Position each orthosis as described for the individual orthosis.
- Heat and cut materials accordingly.

Evaluate Fit While Molding

- Mold dorsal elbow orthosis in 90° of elbow flexion and as close to neutral forearm rotation as possible.
- Check for clearance of medial and lateral epicondyles.

- Fabricate volar wrist immobilization orthosis, making sure to clear ulnar and radial styloids.

Strapping and Components

- Mark for housing units as described here; then apply straps so they do not interfere with cable.
- Using screws, apply two metal housing components, oriented transversely, on midportion of posterior elbow orthosis (just below olecranon) and on midportion of wrist orthosis.
- Large cable is set into proximal and distal housing units; distal end of tube is set in with Allen wrench and secured.
- For supination, cable is run from volar aspect of wrist around radial border to lateral elbow area and terminates in proximal housing unit on elbow orthosis (Fig. 2–29**A** and **B**).
- For pronation, cable is run from volar wrist around ulnar aspect of forearm to medial aspect of elbow and terminates on proximal housing unit of elbow orthosis (Fig. 2–29**C** and **D**).
- Twisting cable in opposite direction of desired motion controls force.
- Cut excess cable.
- Instruct patient in wearing schedule, donning and doffing techniques, and self-adjustments.
- Adjust tension as tissue accommodates.

Survey Completed Orthosis

- Line length of proximal and distal orthosis as well as proximal and distal borders with nonskid material; this greatly decreases orthosis migration. Consider Microfoam™ tape, adhesive Dycem, or adhesive silicone gel sheets.
- Check for clearance of ulnar styloid and epicondyles.
- Check for pressure on radial sensory nerve with supination design; cable may apply pressure directly over this area.

 PATTERN PEARLS 2–57 TO 2–59

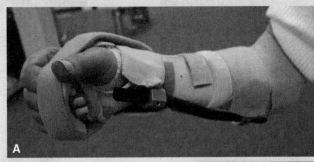

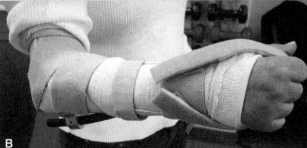

FIGURE PP2–57 **A and B,** Additional soft strap applied for gentle digital composite flexion stretch.

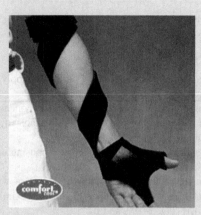

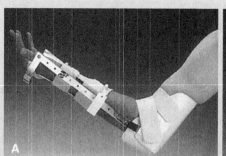

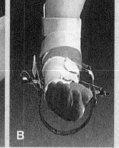

FIGURE PP2–58 Comfort Cool® Spiral Arm Splint. (Photo courtesy of North Coast Medical.)

FIGURE PP2–59 **A and B,** MERiT™ Static Progressive Forearm Rotation Orthosis Kit (Performance Health).

 CLINICAL PEARL 2–35

Combination Neoprene and Thermoplastic Forearm Rotation Orthosis

Distal wrist stabilization with addition of a neoprene wrap can provide a "dynamic" rotation mobilization force. **A,** Wrist immobilization with neoprene strapping wrapped in the direction of pronation. **B,** Wrist and thumb immobilization with a supination mobilizing force. **C and D,** Proximal thermoplastic cuff to anchor strap may help with proper donning of orthosis. Also notice how rivets assist with obtaining correct angle of pull to maximize supination end range positioning.

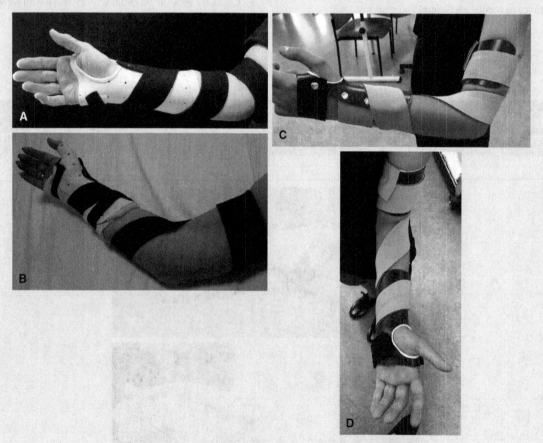

Colello Orthosis

LAURA CARTER, OT, HAND THERAPIST
Australia

The Colello design is used to encourage supination or pronation. Fabrication can be tricky, and having two pairs of hands can be invaluable. Here is a 10-step guide to making this two-part dynamic orthosis:

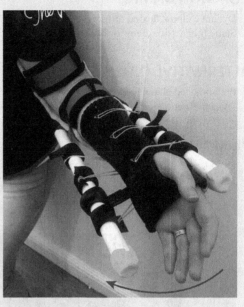

1. Gather all necessary material prior to fabrication.
   a. thermoplastic of choice
   b. hook and loop
   c. adequate padding
   d. anchor loops—can use paper clips, dress hooks, hook/loop
   e. rubber bands for dynamic force
   f. outrigger of choice—aluminum rods, PVC pipe
   g. splinting pan and heat gun
   h. wax pencil
2. Fabricate a circumferential wrist immobilization orthosis with the seam at the dorsum of the forearm. Fabricate with the forearm in neutral/midrotation and be sure to pad over bony prominences or potential pressure areas (ulnar head).
3. Fabricate a short dorsal elbow immobilization orthosis with the elbow positioned at ~90° flexion. Needs to be long enough to adequately stabilize elbow in this position but allow for rotation at the forearm. Approximately one-third of the way down the forearm and one-half the length of the upper arm is a good estimate; however, length depends on the patient's anatomy.
4. Cut the outrigger material to length if not already presized. In these images, we use PVC piping. The length was determined by measuring the length of the forearm and hand, taking into consideration that the outrigger piping needs to be fixated at the posterior elbow.
5. This is where two sets of hands are helpful—position each outrigger rod so that they align with the longitudinal axis of the forearm when the forearm is in neutral rotation. It is easiest to mark this position with a wax pencil to ensure you secure it in the right location. You will then need to fixate the outriggers onto the dorsal elbow segment in their correct positions. Wrapping thermoplastic around the end of the outrigger and then dry heating it to adhere to elbow orthosis is effective, reinforcing this seal with additional thermoplastic is helpful.
6. Once the outriggers are in place longitudinally, use a piece of thermoplastic (or bendable aluminum) to create the "cradle" of the orthosis. This will help keep the outriggers in place laterally and maintain the correct axis of movement. Hold the thermoplastic in the "cradle" position as it cools to ensure it clears the forearm during rotation.
7. Apply anchor loops along the length of the forearm on both the ulnar and radial sides. May use bent paper clips that are dry heated and inserted into forearm segment and then reinforce with dry heated thermoplastic.
8. Positioning of these anchors depends on degree of rotation the patient has and whether the orthosis is being designed to gain supination or pronation. In this supination orthosis, the radial anchors were applied more volarly, while the ulnar anchors were more dorsally located.
9. Be sure to know what way you are wanting to rotate the forearm before you apply the anchors! This will ensure you orientate the anchors correctly so the rubber bands pull into the anchor (and do not slide off).
10. Apply adhesive hook onto each outrigger in line with each anchor—this will provide the attachment point for the dynamic component.
11. Select appropriate size/strength rubber bands to use—you will need a minimum of six in total. Attach one end of each rubber band to a length of loop material that can be secured around the hook on the outrigger. Cut a small hole in the top of the loop and thread the rubber band through this and then through itself to secure.
12. Attach the rubber bands to each of the anchors on the orthosis. Apply each dynamic force couple (the pair of bands opposing each other along the length of the orthosis) in opposite directions to create the rotational force in your desired direction. Adjust tension as deemed appropriate.

ELBOW FLEXION MOBILIZATION ORTHOSIS (EO) (Fig. 2–31)

COMMON NAMES

- Dynamic elbow flexion orthosis
- Static progressive elbow orthosis

ALTERNATIVE ORTHOSIS OPTIONS

- Prefabricated elbow flexion/extension kits
- Dynamic/static progressive orthoses

PRIMARY FUNCTIONS

- Provide low-load, prolonged flexion mobilization force to elbow joint to facilitate lengthening of tissue.

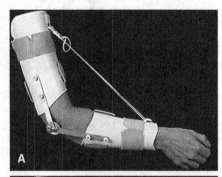
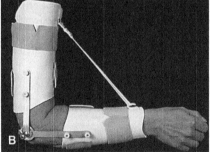

FIGURE 2–31

ADDITIONAL FUNCTIONS

- Restrict full elbow extension or flexion.
- Restrict or prevent forearm rotation.
- Minimize medial or lateral stress at elbow.

Common Diagnoses	General Optimal Positions
Elbow extension contracture	Terminal elbow flexion

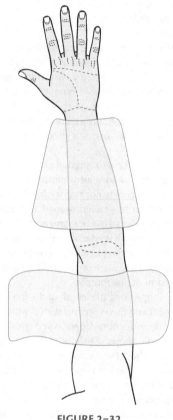

FIGURE 2–32

FABRICATION PROCESS (USING PHOENIX ELBOW HINGE)

Pattern Creation (Fig. 2–32)

- Proximal orthosis
  - Fabricate nonarticular humerus orthosis.
- Distal orthosis
  - Fabricate nonarticular forearm orthosis.
  - If hand is extremely edematous, painful, arthritic, or weak, consider incorporating wrist in forearm orthosis.
  - If forearm rotation needs to be controlled, include wrist in forearm design.

Refine Pattern

- Proximal orthosis borders should allow full shoulder motion and unimpeded elbow motion.
- Distal orthosis borders should allow unimpeded elbow and wrist motion.
- Check for irritation at epicondyles, olecranon, axilla, ulnar nerve (cubital tunnel), median nerve (wrist), ulnar styloid, and radial sensory nerve.

Options for Materials

- Use coated material so circumferential overlapped section can be popped open without permanent sealing.
- Remember that elastic materials tend to shrink around orthosis part; do not remove until orthosis is completely set.
- Use material that has some degree of flexibility when set (slightly perforated 1/8″ and 3/32″ materials); important because orthoses need to give slightly when removed for hygiene and guarded exercise (if appropriate).

Cut and Heat

- When molding distal orthosis, make certain that forearm is in desired amount of forearm rotation.

Evaluate Fit While Molding

- Once both orthoses are formed, mark for hinge placement; align center (axis) of hinge with axis of rotation at elbow joint.
- Line inside of orthosis opening with Moleskin as described in orthosis pattern; consider using lining over border of axilla region for comfort.

Strapping and Components

- Plan and attach hinge before securing straps.
- D-ring straps work well because of ease of application.
- Direct straps so they secure on medial aspect of arm; may be applied over hinge arms.
- With both orthoses on and forearm in desired amount of rotation and elbow in flexion, line up axis of hinge with elbow joint and mark specific placement of hinge arms.
- Remove orthoses and attach hinge to proximal and distal orthoses using rubber band posts.
- Form hook with scrap material and attach to distal third of distal orthosis.
- Attach D-ring to proximal third of proximal orthosis.
- Apply elastic cord to attachment devices.

Survey Completed Orthosis

- Consider a trial use in clinic because adjustments are frequently necessary.
- Make certain that lines of pull are appropriate for diagnosis (e.g., supination and flexion common for biceps repair, not pronation and flexion).
- Check for unwanted stress on collateral ligaments of elbow.
- Make sure orthosis allows clearance at elbow; there may be potential for abutment of distal and proximal orthosis segments as flexion increases, causing compression of skin in flexion crease and possible pressure areas. May need to trim distal border of proximal orthosis as flexion increases.
- Proximal portion of orthosis may migrate distally as tension is applied. Consider lining orthosis with adhesive Dycem, adhesive silicone gel, Microfoam™ tape, or foam. If this does not help, application of shoulder harness may be necessary.
- Adjust tension per patient and/or tissue tolerance; goal is low-load stretch over prolonged period of time.

 PATTERN PEARLS 2–60 AND 2–61

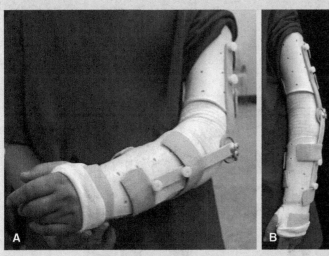
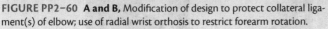

FIGURE PP2–60 A and B, Modification of design to protect collateral ligament(s) of elbow; use of radial wrist orthosis to restrict forearm rotation.

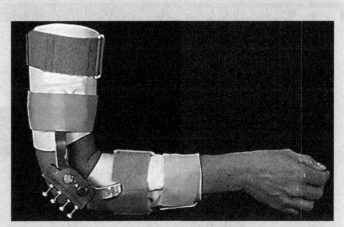

FIGURE PP2–61 Rolyan® Adjustable Hinge (Performance Health).

 CLINICAL PEARL 2–36

Clearance of Elbow Flexion Crease

During the fitting process, be sure to clear for unrestricted elbow flexion; note the pinching of soft tissue when flexion is attempted here. Simply trimming the volar edges of the two segments can fix this issue. Also, be sure to minimize orthosis migration by taking advantage of friction force: placing proximal cuff directly against the skin or apply strips of Microfoam™ tape within this segment.

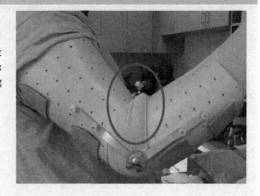

CLINICAL PEARL 2–37

Neoprene for Creative Wrist and Elbow Mobilization

Neoprene was used in this orthosis as a creative alternative for combined elbow and wrist stiffness. The soft contouring nature of the neoprene material joined with the gentle "dynamic" force it generates when stretched offers the therapist a versatile option. See Chapter 14 for additional information on using neoprene.

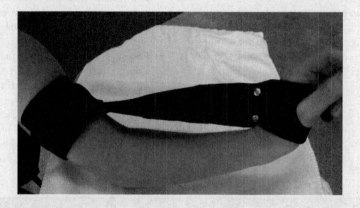

CLINICAL PEARL 2–38

Proper Hinge Placement

Center of elbow hinge must be placed at elbow's axis of rotation **(A)**. Improper placement of hinge can lead to abnormal forces on the joint and shifting of the thermoplastic material on the body segment as noted here **(B)**.

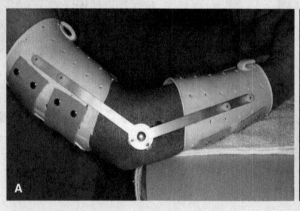

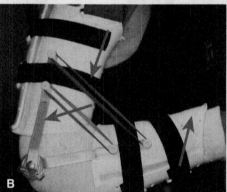

CHAPTER 2: MOBILIZATION ORTHOSES DISCUSSION POINTS

1. What are the three types of approaches for a mobilization orthosis?
2. Give an example of each type of mobilization orthosis including the rationale for use.
3. Explain what the appropriate angle of application should be and why this is important. Include the harmful effects if application is not correct.
4. Given the diagnosis of a PIP flexion contracture, what are the choices for mobilization? Why would you choose one over the other?
5. Name a minimum of three types of:
   • proximal attachments devices
   • elastic force applications
   • slings
   • line guides

REFERENCES

Kearney L. M., & Brown K. K. (1994). The therapist's management of intra-articular fractures. *Hand Clinics*, 10, 199–209.

Schenck R. R. (1986). Dynamic traction and early passive movement for fractures of the proximal interphalangeal joint. *Journal of Hand Surgery (American)*, 11, 850–858.

Schenck R. R. (1994). The dynamic traction method. Combining movement and traction for intra-articular fractures of the phalanges. *Hand Clinics*, 10, 187–197.

3 Restriction Orthoses

MaryLynn Jacobs, MBA, MS, OTR/L, CHT
Noelle M. Austin, MS, PT, CHT

1 Digit- and Thumb-Based Orthoses

PROXIMAL INTERPHALANGEAL EXTENSION RESTRICTION ORTHOSIS (FO) (Fig. 3–1)

COMMON NAMES

- Anti–swan-neck splint
- Antideformity splint
- Figure-8 splint
- Proximal interphalangeal (PIP) hyperextension block splint

ALTERNATIVE ORTHOSIS OPTIONS

- Buttonhole orthosis
- Ring-designed orthoses
- Taping

PRIMARY FUNCTION

- Maximize functional use of digit by preventing PIP joint hyperextension while allowing PIP flexion.

Common Diagnoses	General Optimal Positions
Swan-neck deformity	PIP: slight flexion
PIP volar plate injury	PIP: 10°–30° flexion
PIP dorsal dislocation	PIP: 15°–30° flexion (depends on severity)

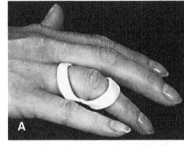
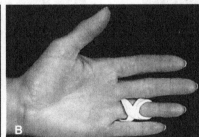
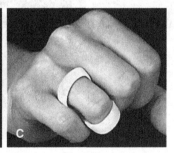

FIGURE 3–1

FABRICATION PROCESS

Pattern Creation (Fig. 3–2)

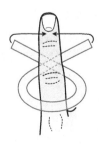

4"–6" long

¹/₄"–¹/₂" wide

FIGURE 3–2

- Thermoplastic material for this orthosis should be approximately 4" long and ¼" to ½" wide when folded.

Refine Pattern

- The width of the material should be judged by the size of the digit; the larger the digit, the wider the strip of material.

Options for Materials

- Use thin (3/32" or 1/16") elastic-based material; the memory characteristic allows for excellent contouring and intimate fit.
- Plan to overlap and/or roll material to increase strength.
- Medium to thin Aquatubes® (Patterson Medical) (flattened out) provide another option; size depends on strength required and the size of the digit.
- The wider the dorsal segment, the more evenly distributed the pressure and the more comfortable the fit.

Cut and Heat

- Consider placing a light layer of lotion on the digit before molding to ease removal of the orthosis.

Evaluate Fit While Molding

- Center strip on middle of proximal phalanx dorsally.
- Wrap both ends volarly around to PIP joint crease (clearing the flexion crease), returning dorsally onto the middle phalanx, ending dorsally.
- Cut and pinch ends so they overlap; smooth.
- While material is setting, position PIP joint in desired amount of flexion by gently providing pressure over volar crossed segment; make sure two dorsal ring pieces are contoured well around phalanges.
- Position dorsal segments close to metacarpophalangeal (MP) and distal interphalangeal (DIP) joints to maximize leverage and improve orthosis effectiveness.

Strapping and Components

- No strapping required.

Survey Completed Orthosis

- Remove orthosis from patient and prepare overlapped pieces with solvent, spot heat, and bend.
- Carefully spot heat volar crossed segment with heat gun to secure adherence and smooth edges.
- If DIP or PIP joints are enlarged owing to trauma or arthritis, gently flare rings laterally to allow extra space for removal.

PATTERN PEARLS 3–1 TO 3–5

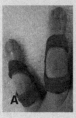
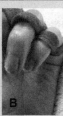
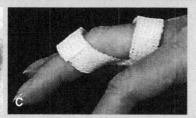

FIGURE PP3–1   Casting tapes: **A and B,** Orficast™ (North Coast Medical, Morgan Hill, CA) or **(C)** QuickCast (Performance Health, Warrenville, IL).

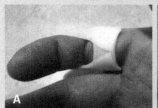
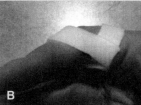
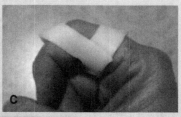

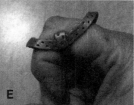
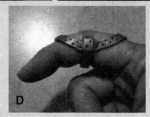

FIGURE PP3–2   A–C, Ring around proximal phalanx with dorsal block. **D and E,** Lateral ring with volar strip support.

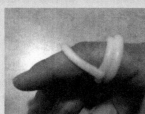

FIGURE PP3–3   Rolyan® Aquatubes® (Performance Health).

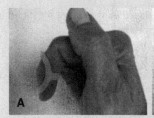
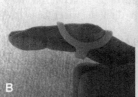
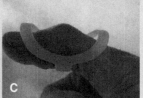

FIGURE PP3–4   A–C, Oval-8® finger splints (3-Point Products, Stevensville, MD).

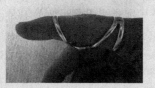

FIGURE PP3–5   Silver Ring™ splints (Silver Ring Splint Company, Charlottesville, VA).

CLINICAL PEARL 3–1

Buttonhole PIP Extension Restriction Orthosis

The buttonhole design is another option for the PIP extension restriction orthosis. This design can be more challenging to fabricate than the figure-8 design. Remember that the degree of restriction for PIP extension depends on the diagnosis as well as the specific digit you are treating.

Use thin (3/32" or 1/16") elastic material because its memory characteristic allows for a contoured intimate fit. Cut out the pattern on a scrap piece of thermoplastic material (approximately 2" by 1" piece). Prior to heating, make the slits with the widest setting on a hole punch. Once material is heated, be careful not to overstretch; gently feed the material onto finger through both holes, orienting the proximal orthosis border on the dorsum of the proximal phalanx, the middle section volar, and the distal orthosis border on the dorsal surface of the middle phalanx.

Position the PIP joint in the desired amount of flexion and fold the lateral orthosis pieces onto themselves to minimize bulk in this area. Overlap any excess volar material onto the volar PIP piece to allow PIP joint flexion. Once set, remove the orthosis from the finger and smooth the edges, especially at the volar portion of the orthosis.

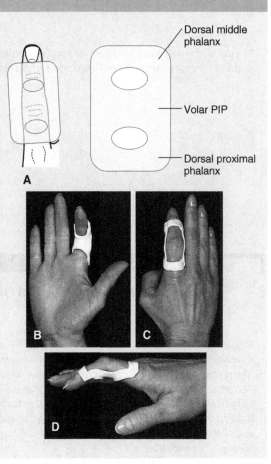

CLINICAL PEARL 3–2

Thumb MP Extension Restriction Orthosis

This orthosis is extremely effective for managing instability of the thumb MP joint and a tendency to posture in MP hyperextension while writing or engaging in activities requiring opposition. If left untreated, over time, the CMC joint may become unstable, resulting in pain and metacarpal subluxation. To fabricate this orthosis, use a 1/16" material, measuring the length from the crease of the dorsal thumb interphalangeal (IP) to just distal to the radial wrist crease. Allow the width to be approximately ¼" wider on each side of the thumb metacarpal and phalanx (see pattern). Create two slits horizontally in the center of the material approximately ¼" to ½" apart, leaving the ¼" on each side. The material between the slits will form a "sling" that will rest across the volar thumb MP crease, supporting the first metacarpal into gentle extension.

Heat material, and then, working quickly, begin to feed the widest piece onto the dorsum of the metacarpal followed by gently pulling down on the material between the two slits that have formed the sling and feeding it directly under the most distal portion of the metacarpal head (volar MP crease). The distal portion will rest on the dorsum of the proximal phalanx. Once the material is fully set, position the MP joint in the desired amount of flexion, making sure that there is adequate counterpressure on the first metacarpal (dorsal-oriented pressure from the volar sling and volar-directed pressure from both the proximal and distal dorsal segments).

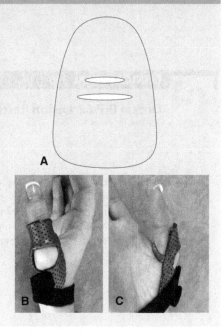

CLINICAL PEARL 3-3

Thumb MP and IP Extension Restriction Orthosis

The pattern for the thumb MP extension restriction orthosis can be modified slightly to include flexion of the IP joint for added stability. The pattern just needs to be lengthened approximately 1" distally.

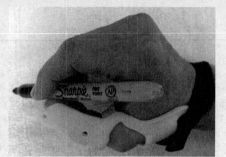

CLINICAL PEARL 3-4

Thumb MP Flexion Restriction Orthosis

Chronic thumb MP flexion can lead to a boutonniere-type deformity with progressing pain along the thumb column. This is often seen in massage therapists and in individuals who use their thumbs in daily work or recreational tasks. This small design can be used during the activity to restrict MP flexion yet allow thumb MP/IP extension to neutral.

To fabricate this orthosis, use a 1/16" material measuring the length from the crease of the dorsal thumb IP to just distal to the radial wrist crease. Allow the width to be approximately ¼" wider on each side of the thumb metacarpal and phalanx (see pattern). Create one slit horizontally approximately 1" to ½" from the distal border of the material, leaving ¼" on each side.

Heat material, and then working quickly, feed the widest piece onto the dorsum of the metacarpal followed by gently pulling down on the slit to form a volar "pan" for the proximal phalanx to rest in. Once the material is set in place, place the MP joint in the desired amount of extension, making sure there is adequate counterpressure on the proximal phalanx (dorsal-oriented pressure) and the first metacarpal (volar-oriented pressure).

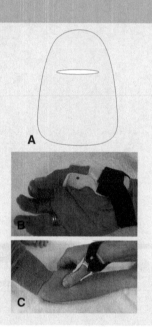

CLINICAL PEARL 3-5

Dorsal PIP Extension Restriction Orthosis

Restriction of full PIP joint extension may be required to allow adequate healing of structures such as the volar plate. The dorsal orthosis is fabricated in much the same way as the dorsal PIP immobilization orthosis (see Chapter 1), except for positioning the PIP joint in the desired amount of flexion. Once the proximal strap is secured, the distal strap can be periodically removed to allow active-restricted (to the limit of the dorsal block) flexion and extension exercises of the PIP joint if appropriate. Early motion can help prevent capsular tightness and allow tendon gliding.

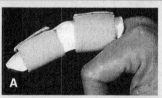

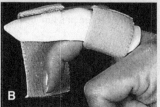

CLINICAL PEARL 3–6

Volar PIP Flexion Restriction Orthosis

The volar orthosis can be used as part of a specific extensor tendon protocol to limit a particular range of PIP joint flexion when treating zone III and IV injuries. The orthosis allows early-protected motion to promote gliding of the injured or repaired extensor mechanism. The volar orthosis is fabricated in the same way as a volar PIP immobilization orthosis, except for positioning the PIP joint in the desired amount of maximum flexion (see Chapter 1). The orthosis is secured with a single proximal strap because it is generally used only for exercise sessions. The patient may flex the PIP joint to the limits of the volar block and actively extend to neutral. The orthosis can be modified weekly as the healing progresses. The patient is immobilized in PIP extension between exercise sessions. Note: This protocol requires specific patient selection and physician's approval; the therapist must have a full understanding of the theoretical basis behind any particular protocol before implementing it.

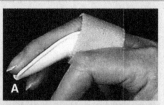
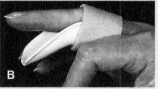

CLINICAL PEARL 3–7

Spiral Design for Digit Extension/Flexion Restriction Orthosis

This spiral design is fabricated with a strip of 1/16″ material. In this case, the design is used intermittently for lateral stabilization and guarded motion post–PIP joint arthroplasty (6 weeks). Note the use of plastic wrap for edema control and as an orthosis liner.

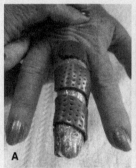
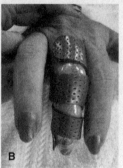

EXPERT PEARL 3–1

Swan-Neck Orthosis Using Orficast: "X" Design
KIRSTEN C. PEDERSEN, OT
Denmark

A piece of 3-cm-wide Orficast is cut to a length corresponding to MCP to DIP joint. Cut up the middle from both ends. Heat the material and place the cross so that it lies at the PIP joint or slightly proximal. Take the two proximal ends up dorsally and press them together. Repeat with the two distal ends. Cut away the excess material. As the material hardens, keep the joint slightly flexed so that hyperextension is not possible.

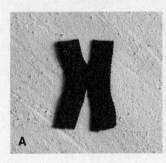
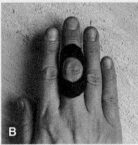
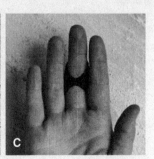

Figure-8 Design Used to Address "Locking Finger"

SABA KAMAL, OTR, CHT
California

Due to attenuation of lateral bands, this finger is stuck in extension; but when kept in 30° of flexion, the finger does not lock. This position advances the lateral bands below the PIP joint axis, to make them flexors. In order to keep the "loops" as far apart as possible to prevent full extension, use an extra strip of thermoplastic and wrap around the intersection of the figure-8 volarly. Notice use of nail polish used to identify the proximal and distal ends.

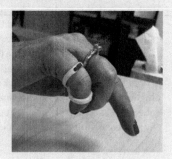

2 | Hand-Based Orthoses

MCP EXTENSION RESTRICTION ORTHOSIS (HFO) (Fig. 3–3)

COMMON NAMES

- Lumbrical blocking splint
- Anticlaw splint
- Ulnar nerve splint
- MCP blocking splint
- Figure-8 MCP blocking splint

ALTERNATIVE ORTHOSIS OPTIONS

- Prefabricated orthoses: (spring coil, figure-8 designs)
- Dynamic MCP flexion orthosis
- Immobilization orthosis

PRIMARY FUNCTION

- Maximize functional use of hand by preventing MCP joint hyperextension while allowing MCP flexion for grasp.

ADDITIONAL FUNCTIONS

- Prevent MCP collateral ligament tightness.
- Facilitate PIP extension.

Common Diagnoses	General Optimal Positions
Low-lesion ulnar nerve injury	Ring finger (RF) and small finger (SF) MCPs: 45°–75° flexion
Combined ulnar and median	Index finger (IF) to SF MCPs: nerve lesion 45°–75° flexion

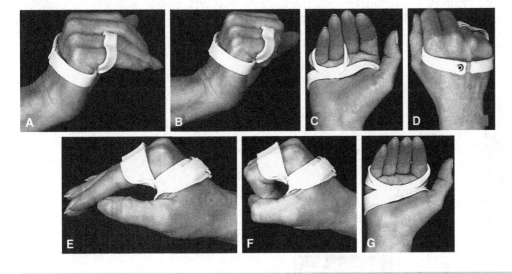

FIGURE 3–3

FABRICATION PROCESS

Pattern Creation (Fig. 3–4)

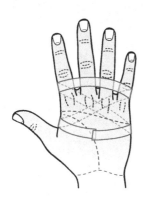

8"–12" long

1"–1½" wide

FIGURE 3–4

- Depending on combination of nerve injury, fabricate orthosis to include two to four MCP joints (ulnar nerve: RF and SF; median and ulnar nerves: IF to SF).
- Thermoplastic material should be 8″ to 12″ long and 1″ to 1½″ wide.

Refine Pattern

- Width of material depends on the size of the hand.

Options for Materials

- Use thin (3/32″ or 1/16″) elastic materials; memory characteristic allows for excellent contouring and intimate fit.
- When using elastic materials (recommended for the novice fabricator), constantly mold and redirect material over dorsum of metacarpal heads and proximal phalanges until material sets.
- If the clinician is experienced with the use of thermoplastic materials, consider the use of plastic-based materials; they tend to allow for the effective use of gravity to contour between digits, forming comfortable troughs over proximal phalanges.
- Rolled thermoplastic or Aquatubes® are not recommended; surface area in contact with skin is not wide enough to provide well-molded orthosis with adequate pressure distribution in most cases.
- Allow enough material to encompass minimum of one-third length of proximal phalanxes; the wider the dorsal segments, the more evenly distributed the pressure and the more comfortable the fit.

Cut and Heat

- Position patient with elbow resting on table, wrist extended, in an intrinsic plus position: MCPs flexed and IPs extended (patient may need to help position using the unaffected hand).
- Warm material thoroughly.

Evaluate Fit While Molding

- Be sure to accommodate for natural descent of MCPs; in fist, SF MCP is lower than RF MCP, which is lower than middle finger (MF) MCP.
- Drape material centrally over middle of proximal phalanges, gently contouring material between digits; there should be an equal length of material draped on each side.
- Cross two draping pieces over each other on volar surface at distal palmar crease level.
- Press and flatten out intersection of two crossed pieces, forming less bulky bar. Constantly work material in palm to provide needed volar support for arches.
- Position remainder of pieces: one through radial web space and other over mid-ulnar border; pinch together dorsally.

- While material is still warm, pull down and overlap excess material on ulnar SF MCP and radial RF (or IF MCP) areas to allow unimpeded MCP flexion.

Strapping and Components

- None, unless there is significant atrophy.
- Many patients with long-standing ulnar nerve injury have significant atrophy of first web space and hypothenar eminence, which may make it difficult to remove the orthosis. Pop open orthosis dorsally and apply straps to ease donning and doffing. (Orthosis shown has riveted strap.)

Survey Completed Orthosis

- Cut pinched dorsal piece, prepare surfaces with orthosis solvent, and spot heat to form permanent seal.
- If necessary, prepare surfaces and spot heat volar overlapped portion to adhere pieces together securely.
- May line dorsal bars with very thin adhesive silicone gel or wrap with Coban™ to help prevent orthosis migration during functional use and improve comfort.

 PATTERN PEARLS 3-6 TO 3-11

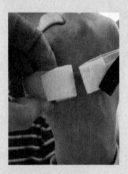

FIGURE PP3-6 To accommodate hand atrophy, create dorsal opening with flap from lining material on each end to avoid "pinching" skin during closure.

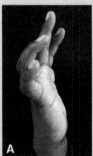 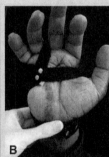 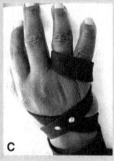 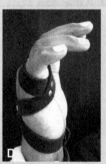

FIGURE PP3-7 A–D, Neoprene design for subtle clawing allows light restriction of MCP extension with full flexion.

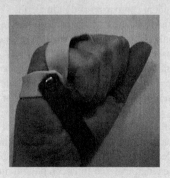

FIGURE PP3-8 Anchoring orthosis around wrist assists in preventing migration during active use.

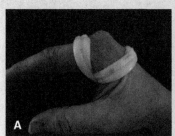 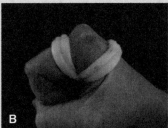 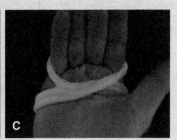

FIGURE PP3–9 A–C, Rolyan® Aquatubes® (Performance Health).

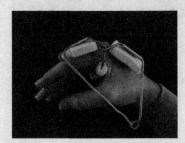

FIGURE PP3–10 Knuckle Bender Splint (Performance Health).

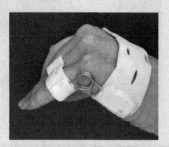

FIGURE PP3–11 Spring coil design (Orfit Industries, Norfolk, VA).

 CLINICAL PEARL 3–8

MCP Extension Restriction Orthosis With Thumb Included

With combined median and ulnar nerve injuries, the thumb is unable to abduct out of the palm because of the loss of thenar muscles, causing interference with functional use. A simple thumb abduction component can be incorporated into the MCP extension restriction orthosis to position the thumb in a functional position midway between palmar and radial abduction. The pattern is basically the same as described for the MCP extension restriction orthosis.

Heat a 12″ by 1″ piece of thermoplastic material. (Width depends on the size of the hand.) Place the thumb in the desired position (patient needs to position using the unaffected hand). Drape the material over the proximal phalanges as described, except provide the ulnar portion with 3″ to 4″ of additional material.

Working quickly, cross the ulnar strip radially across the palm; then guide it dorsally around the thumb MP joint, traversing back through the first web space onto the dorsum of the hand. Next, pull the radial strip ulnarward across the palm to join the strip on the ulnar dorsum of the hand. Finish as described for the MCP extension restriction orthosis. Hook and loop can be used to secure the closure and allow for easy donning and doffing. Note that the overlapped areas may need to be warmed with a heat gun to maximize adherence and minimize orthosis bulk within the first web space. This orthosis is stabilized onto the hand using a figure-8 strap closure. **(A)** Digit extension. **(B)** Digit flexion. **(C)** Volar view, note clearance of thumb MP crease.

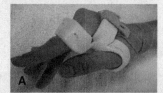
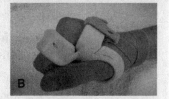
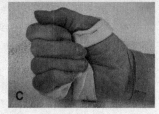

CLINICAL PEARL 3–9

Dorsal MCP Extension Restriction Orthosis

This dorsal design provides coverage of a wider surface area maximizing pressure distribution. For some patients who have increased digital extensor tone or severe MCP extension deformity, this may be the orthosis of choice. The additional material provides greater pressure distribution, and the open volar aspect allows digital flexion. The thumb can easily be incorporated, if desired **(A and B)**. Stable proximal phalanx fractures can sometimes be managed with fabrication of a restriction orthosis as shown here **(C and D)**. Note: See Chapter 1 for Additional Pattern Options.

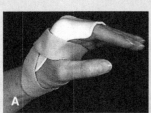
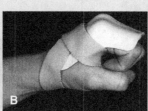
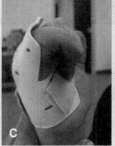
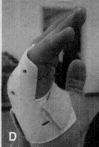

CLINICAL PEARL 3–10

Hand-Based Digit Extension Restriction Orthosis

Restriction of full MCP, PIP, and DIP joint extension may be required to allow adequate healing of structures such as repaired digital nerves. This hand-based orthosis is fabricated in much the same way as the dorsal hand immobilization orthosis, except for positioning the MCP, PIP, and DIP joints in the desired amount of flexion (refer to Chapter 1). Once the proximal strap is secured, the distal straps can be periodically removed to allow active-restricted (to the limit of the dorsal block) flexion and extension exercises of the MCP, PIP, and DIP joints if appropriate. Early motion can help prevent capsular tightness and allow tendon and/or nerve gliding. Note: See Chapter 1 for Additional Pattern Options.

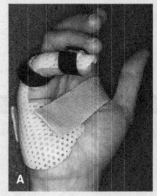
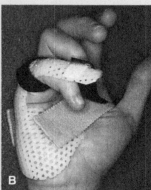

EXPERT PEARL 3–3

MCP/PIP Extension Restriction Orthosis
JULIANNE LESSARD OTR/L, CHT
Massachusetts

Patient presents post surgical manipulation to correct swan-neck deformities of digits 2 to 5. MD ordered an orthosis to restrict extension of the MCP and PIP joints. This design has a volar P1 strap to give the weakened volar plates support during active flexion. Notice rivet on radial side to reinforce and prevent breakage of thermoplastic bond in that vulnerable region of orthosis.

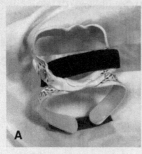
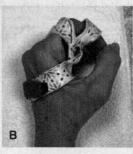
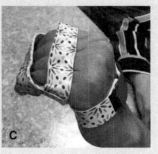

MCP DEVIATION RESTRICTION ORTHOSIS (HFO) (Fig. 3–5)

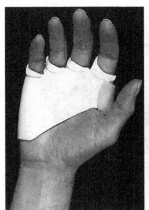 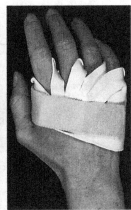

FIGURE 3–5

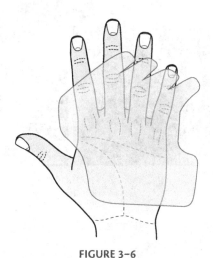

FIGURE 3–6

COMMON NAMES

- Ulnar deviation splint
- Ulnar drift orthosis
- Protective MCP splint
- Palmar MCP stabilization splint

ALTERNATIVE ORTHOSIS OPTIONS

- Prefabricated orthoses
- Custom neoprene orthoses

PRIMARY FUNCTION

- Maintain MCP joints in close to neutral alignment to protect from ulnar deviating or volar subluxation forces.

Common Diagnoses	General Optimal Positions
Arthritis of MCP joints	MCP: 0°–25° flexion with slight radial deviation

FABRICATION PROCESS

Pattern Creation (Fig. 3–6)

- Mark just distal to each PIP joint, appreciating the difference in their heights.
- Allow approximately 1″ additional material on ulnar border.
- Allow enough material radially to traverse through thumb web, contouring pattern to allow thumb mobility.
- Mark just distal to wrist crease, allowing unimpeded wrist mobility.

Refine Pattern

- Mark pattern from distal border to each digital web space, between IF and MF, MF and RF, and RF and SF.

Options for Materials

- Use thin (3/32″ or 1/16″) elastic material; memory characteristic allows for excellent contouring and intimate fit.
- Consider ⅛″ plastic material; thinner plastics may become weak as material is gently stretched about proximal phalanxes.

Cut and Heat

- Position patient with forearm supinated on table and digits slightly abducted. Digits may need to be supported in position by assistant, especially if joints are significantly deviated and/or subluxed.

- Warm material thoroughly.

Evaluate Fit While Molding

- Dry material quickly, and cut slits marked between digits; separate into four tabs. Each tab should be wide enough (approximately ½″) to encompass proximal phalanx comfortably. Do not make this wrapped portion too narrow.
- Place material on volar aspect of hand. While working quickly, pull each tab around ulnar aspect of each proximal phalanx (onto dorsum).
- Overlap tabs onto themselves (for quick closure) or trim to form separate small cuffs.
- Constantly work material in palm to provide needed volar support for arches.
- MCPs should be supported volarly and should rest in near neutral alignment.
- Check that material traversing between digits is not thick and is free of sharp edges.

Strapping and Components

- One strap to join radial and ulnar border.
- Consider riveted strap to allow for easy donning and doffing.

Survey Completed Orthosis

- Smooth edges and between digits.
- Be sure MCP joints are supported in optimal alignment.

PATTERN PEARLS 3-12 TO 3-15

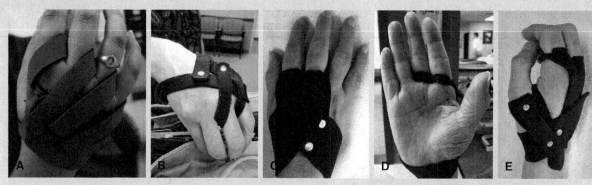

FIGURE PP3-12 **A-E,** Various neoprene orthoses providing MCP extension restriction. Refer to Chapter 14 for further instruction.

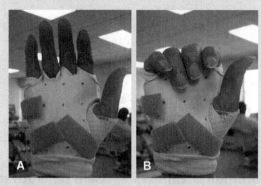

FIGURE PP3-13 **A and B,** Wrist strap assists to secure orthosis.

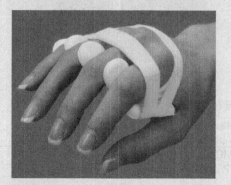

FIGURE PP3-14 LMB Soft Core Ulnar Deviation Splint (Photo courtesy of DeRoyal, Powell, TN).

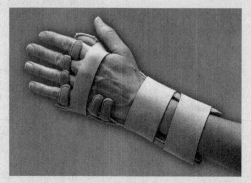

FIGURE PP3-15 Comforter™ Splint (Photo courtesy of 3-Point Products).

3 | Forearm-Based Orthoses

CIRCUMFERENTIAL WRIST FLEXION RESTRICTION ORTHOSIS (WHO) (Fig. 3–7)

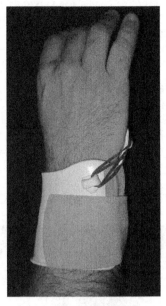

FIGURE 3–7

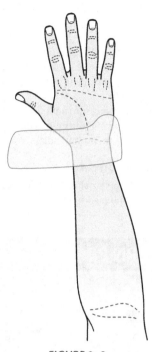

FIGURE 3–8

COMMON NAMES

- Midcarpal instability orthosis/splint (O'Brien, 2013; Skirven & DeTullio, 2006)
- Ulnar boost orthosis/splint (Chinchalkar & Yong, 2004)
- Pisiform boost orthosis/splint (Garcias-Elias, 2008)
- Palmar midcarpal instability orthosis/splint

PRIMARY FUNCTIONS

- Reduction of pain and wrist "clunking."
- To provide dorsally oriented pressure on the pisiform bone with simultaneous counterpressure over the head of the distal ulna to reduce volar sag of the carpus. This counterpressure corrects the volar flexed position of the proximal row.
- To achieve a more neutral carpal alignment by supporting the pisotriquetrial area (Chinchalkar & Yong, 2004; Garcias-Elias, 2008; Lichtman, Gaenslen, & Pollock, 1997; Skirven, 2011; Skirven & DeTullio, 2006; O'Brien, 2013).

ADDITIONAL FUNCTIONS

- Allows near full wrist extension, radial deviation, and ulnar deviation and *restricts* wrist flexion.

Common Diagnoses and General Optimal Positions

*This orthosis aims to give dorsally directed pressure on the pisiform bone with simultaneous counterpressure over the head of the distal ulna to restore a neutral alignment of the ulnar wrist.

Palmar midcarpal instability/ VISI (volar intercalated segment instability) deformity (hyper volar flexion of the lunate)	Position of wrist = neutral

* The orthosis assists to eliminate the "clunk," which occurs during ulnar deviation.

* Note: This orthosis is used in most cases in combination with midcarpal stabilization exercises and with activity modifications.

FABRICATION PROCESS

Pattern Creation (Fig. 3–8)

- Measure circumference of the wrist less than ½″.
- Mark for proximal border approximately 3″ proximal to the dorsal and volar wrist creases.
- The orthosis pattern is basically a rectangular piece of material with a rounded extension for application over the pisiform.
- The rounded extension measures approximately 1″ wide and 3/4″ high. This extension varies in size depending on the individual.
- The pattern opening is on the ulnar border.

Refine Pattern

- Distal borders should allow near full wrist extension, radial deviation, and ulnar deviation but restrict flexion.

- The rounded extension should not extend beyond the pisiform either distally or laterally (which would cause interference with deviation motions and fully impede wrist flexion).

Options for Materials

- Use nonperforated 3/32″ or ⅛″ material to achieve max stabilization. Material too thin or highly perforated may fold with attempted flexion.
- Noncoated material may be an option if homemade outrigger attachment posts are being used in the design. This would improve the adherence of the attachment device/homemade hook.

Cut and Heat

- Position patient's forearm in elbow flexion (resting on a table) and wrist in neutral.
- If using a stockinet under the orthosis, apply before heating material.

Evaluate Fit While Molding

- Starting on the ulnar volar aspect of the hand, place the extended piece over the pisiform.
- Wrap material around the radial aspect of the wrist/forearm just proximal to the wrist crease.
- Continue to guide the material over the dorsal aspect of the distal forearm ending along the ulnar lateral aspect covering the prominence of the ulnar head.
- When forming the orthosis, dorsally directed pressure is applied over the pisiform with counterpressure on the distal ulna.
- The opening is on the distal ulnar aspect of the wrist. This opening should be no wider than ½″.
- Continue with this counterpressure until the orthosis has hardened.
- Avoid inadvertently applying direct pressure over the dorsal radial aspect of the distal radius to prevent radial sensory nerve irritation.

Strapping and Components

- Once material has set, apply gel or foam discs properly sized over the head of the distal ulna and pisiform bones.

- Apply low-profile outrigger attachments over the pisiform rounded extension piece and directly over the distal ulna.
- Adhere securely to the thermoplastic material.
- Place a thin padding (such as Moleskin, Kinesio® Tex Tape) along the length of both lateral borders and allow for overlap. This will prevent any "pinching" that may occur upon orthosis closure.
- Apply one 2″ wide or two smaller 1″ straps to secure onto the wrist.
- Using an elastic band, starting on the pisiform outrigger attachment, pull from the pisiform to the ulna and back again. This angle of application is what will reduce the ulnar volar sag.
- Consider using rubber band posts as outrigger attachments.

Survey Completed Orthosis

- Smooth material borders.
- Consider rolling or flaring the distal borders along the dorsal/volar wrist creases to avoid potential irritation from edges during attempted motion.
- Check to confirm freedom of movement in wrist extension, radial deviation, and ulnar deviation.

 PATTERN PEARLS 3–16 TO 3–20

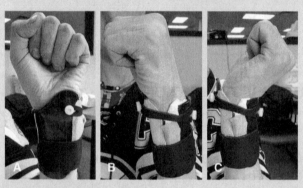

FIGURE PP3–16 A–C, Neoprene material used to create the dynamic force and rubber band posts for the attachment.

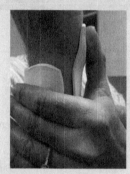

FIGURE PP3–17 Counterpressure applied as orthosis is being molded.

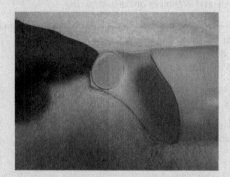

FIGURE PP3–18 Gel discs (or use foam) applied to the hardened material directly over pisiform and head of ulna.

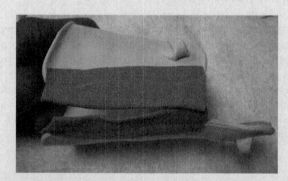

FIGURE PP3–19 Overlapped 2″ by 3″ piece of Kinesio® Tex Tape is used to prevent pinching of skin when the orthosis is closed.

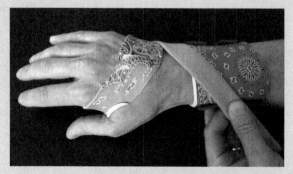

FIGURE PP3–20 Original design of ulnar boost orthosis for midcarpal instability (Chinchalkar & Yong, 2004).

WRIST AND IF/MF EXTENSION RESTRICTION ORTHOSIS (WHFO) (Fig. 3–9)[a]

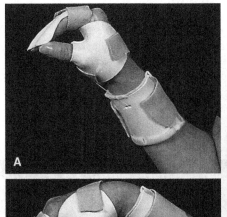

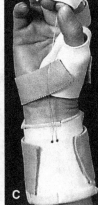

FIGURE 3–9

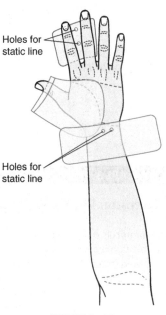

Holes for
static line

Holes for
static line

FIGURE 3–10

COMMON NAMES

- Tenodesis splint
- Rehabilitation Institute of Chicago (RIC) splint

PRIMARY FUNCTION

- Maximize available grasp and release action of digits by redirecting portion of power generated during wrist extension into functional flexion arc of IF and MF against thumb (tenodesis).

[a]Designed at the Rehabilitation Institute of Chicago.

Common Diagnoses and General Optimal Positions

Must have radial nerve function intact; loss of median and ulnar nerve function.

FABRICATION PROCESS

Pattern Creation (Fig. 3–10)

- There are three separate sections of this orthosis.
- Dorsal cap for IF/MF: Orthosis should encompass both proximal phalanges and terminate at tip.
- Thumb MP orthosis: Orthosis should stabilize thumb in mid-palmar abduction and opposition; thumb MP joint should be held in slight flexion.
- Thermoplastic wristband: Orthosis is fabricated to surround two-thirds circumference of wrist and is approximately 3½″ wide.

Refine Pattern

- Check that lateral borders of IF and MF dorsal orthosis do not irritate radial border of RF.

Options for Materials

- Use 3/32″ or 1/16″ material.

Cut and Heat

- Position patient with elbow resting on table, wrist extended, and MCPs flexed (tenodesis position).
- Warm material one section at a time.

Evaluate Fit While Molding

- Dorsal cap for IF/MF
  - Rest warm material over dorsum of IF and MF, making sure that PIPs are flexed to approximately 20°. There should be contouring between digits, distinguishing each one.
  - Proximal border of orthosis should extend just distal to MCPs.
- Thumb MP orthosis
  - This orthosis is fabricated per instructions for thumb carpometacarpal (CMC) immobilization orthosis.
  - Position thumb in mid-palmar/radial abduction and opposition; opposition should be to middle of IF and MF. MP joint should be slightly flexed.
- Thermoplastic wristband
  - This orthosis is fabricated proximal to wrist, allowing full passive wrist flexion and active extension.
  - Place material centrally over volar wrist and wrap about radial and ulnar wrist borders. Material should terminate flush with dorsal skin.

Strapping and Components

- Thin strap of loop material secures dorsal orthosis onto digits and should be placed at proximal phalanx level.
- If needed, place optional strap distal at middle phalanx level.

- Strap thumb orthosis from volar to dorsal.
- Wrist requires 2″ strap across dorsum of wrist, connecting radial and ulnar borders.
- To connect dorsal IF/MF orthosis and wristband, punch two holes along indentation of IF/MF proximal phalanx crease; punch two more holes at middle of wristband at distal border.
- Place double length of static line through holes onto dorsum of orthosis, tie securely, and feed between phalanges. Place wrist in extension and feed line through wristband holes.

- Line should have enough tension to pull MCP joints (along with dorsal orthosis) into flexion just to allow IF/MF tips to oppose thumb tip. Once proper tension is achieved, tie line through wristband holes.

Survey Completed Orthosis

- To obtain maximum benefits from this orthosis, it is crucial to achieve appropriate amount of tension.
- Line dorsal orthosis and wristband with very thin adhesive silicone gel or wrap digits and wrist with thin layer of Coban™ (or similar material) to help prevent orthosis migration during functional use and improve comfort.

CLINICAL PEARL 3-11

Digit Extension Restriction Strap

Some flexor tendon protocols call for the use of a restriction strap to protect the healing repairs once the dorsal orthosis has been discontinued (at 4–5 weeks). This strap protects the repaired structures from simultaneous wrist and digit extension. It also prevents excessive and forceful wrist extension (see Chapter 23 for details). **(A)** For the wrist strap component, use an 8″ by 2″ length of soft strap material (Rolyan˙ SoftStrap˙; Performance Health). Secure it about the wrist with a 3″ piece of adhesive hook (folded onto itself), placing the strap so that the closure is on the dorsum of the hand. Then punch a hole on the volar surface of the 2″ strap. Remember that the line of pull converges toward the scaphoid bone. Make a sling from 1″ by 4″ length of soft strapping and punch a hole on both ends of the sling. The overall length of the sling should be 1½″ to 2″. Finally, thread rubber band or elastic cord through the MCP sling and wrist strap holes. Adjust the tension so that as the wrist extends, the digit flexes; and as the wrist flexes, the digits extend. Watch for neurovascular compromise. **B and C,** This orthosis was designed with neoprene for both the wrist strap and proximal phalanx sling with wrapped elastic cord as the flexion force.

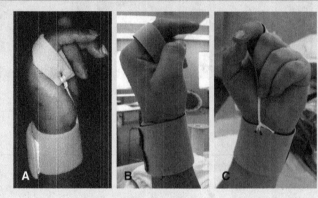

4 Arm-Based Orthoses

ANTERIOR/POSTERIOR ELBOW EXTENSION OR FLEXION RESTRICTION ORTHOSIS (EO)
(Fig. 3–11)

COMMON NAMES
- Anterior/posterior elbow splint
- Bi-surfaced static elbow splint
- Elbow extension-blocking splint
- Elbow flexion-blocking splint

ALTERNATIVE ORTHOSIS OPTIONS
- Prefabricated orthosis
- Hinged elbow orthosis

PRIMARY FUNCTION
- Restrict specific degree of elbow extension or flexion while allowing motion in opposite direction.

ADDITIONAL FUNCTIONS
- Limit or prevent forearm rotation.
- Statically position elbow flexion or extension contracture at maximum length to facilitate lengthening of tissue (serial static orthosis).

Common Diagnoses	General Optimal Positions
Rheumatoid arthritis	Position of comfort and support
Ulnar nerve compression	Elbow: 30°–45° flex; forearm neutral at cubital tunnel
Posterior/anterior dislocation	Elbow: 90°; forearm: neutral
Dislocation proximal radius	Elbow: 90°; forearm: supinated
Medial epicondyle fracture	Elbow: 90°–110°; forearm: pronated
Lateral epicondyle fracture	Elbow: 90°–110°; forearm: supinated
Olecranon fracture	Elbow: 20°–35° flex; forearm: neutral
Acute lateral epicondylitis	Elbow: 90°; forearm: neutral; wrist: 30°–45° extension
Acute medial epicondylitis	Elbow: 90°; forearm: neutral; wrist: 0°
Elbow extension contracture	Terminal flexion
Elbow flexion contracture	Terminal extension

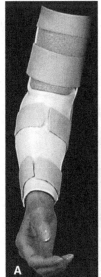
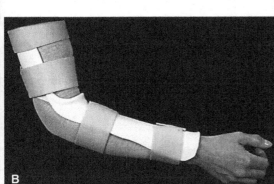
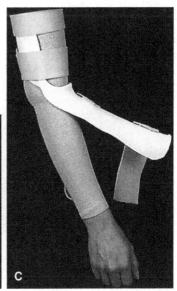

FIGURE 3–11

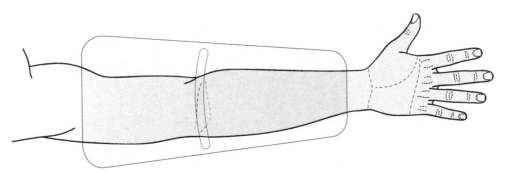

FIGURE 3–12

FABRICATION PROCESS

Pattern Creation (Fig. 3–12)

- This pattern may be alternative to anterior or posterior elbow immobilization orthosis design; consider when specific amount of flexion or extension must be restricted or when there are skin integrity issues (e.g., healing wounds or grafts).
- To restrict elbow extension: apply orthosis posteriorly on upper arm and anteriorly on forearm.
- To restrict elbow flexion: apply orthosis anteriorly on upper arm and posteriorly on forearm.
- Mark for proximal border two-thirds length of the humerus.
- Mark for distal border just proximal to ulnar styloid.
- Allow enough material to encompass half to two-thirds circumference of upper arm and lower forearm, remembering that forearm tapers distally.
- Mark slit for elbow at elbow flexion crease.

Refine Pattern

- Proximal border should allow unimpeded shoulder motion and not irritate axilla region when arm is positioned at side.
- Distal border should allow full wrist motion.
- Note that pattern is wider proximally because circumference of upper arm is greater than that of forearm.
- Make sure that opening for elbow is wide enough to allow forearm and hand to pass through.

Options for Materials

- Use ⅛″ material because strength is an important characteristic for this orthosis.
- Materials with high resistance to stretch (rubber) may offer more control for therapist.
- Consider material that has some degree of memory; material may stretch out as wrist and forearm pass through slotted piece.
- If patient has significant pain and swelling, consider uncoated materials or those that are slightly tacky to help prevent material from slipping, making it easier to position patient and mold orthosis.

Cut and Heat

- Position patient seated to allow for gravity-assisted molding.
- Gravity can assist with molding only one portion of orthosis; the rest of orthosis must be attended to by therapist.
- Have an assistant help to support proper elbow and forearm positions if possible.

Evaluate Fit While Molding

- Before molding orthosis, decide on which surface to apply material.
- Drape proximal piece either anterior or posterior on upper arm, simultaneously sliding elbow carefully through slot; then place forearm portion either anterior or posterior.
- As one hand supports non–gravity-assisted piece, fold elbow flaps onto themselves to reinforce this potentially weak section.
- Do not grab proximal or distal orthosis segments or try to secure with tight circumferential bandage. This may cause borders of orthosis to dig in. Instead, allow gravity to assist in forming one trough while gently supporting the other segment.
- Check for clearance of wrist distally.

Strapping and Components

- Stockinette or elasticized sleeve (if edema is present) is recommended before orthosis application to help eliminate pinching of skin once straps are applied.
- 2″ soft straps are recommended at most proximal and distal portions of orthosis.
- When used to restrict only one direction of elbow motion, forearm strap may be eliminated or released periodically to allow for exercise.

Survey Completed Orthosis

- Smooth and slightly flare all borders.
- Check for clearance and/or irritation of axilla, ulnar styloid, and epicondyles.
- Check for compression of ulnar nerve at cubital tunnel area as well as sensory branch of radial nerve.

PATTERN PEARLS 3–21 TO 3–22

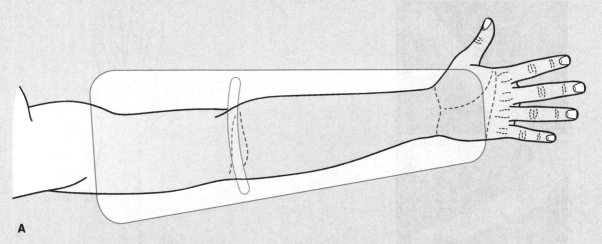

A

FIGURE PP3–21 A–C, Anterior/posterior design with supinated forearm and wrist included. Design allows near full elbow flexion.

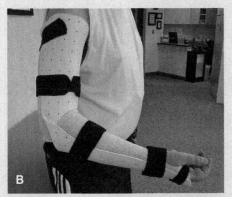

B

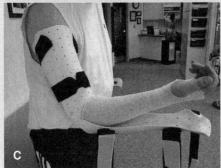

C

FIGURE PP3–21 Cont'd

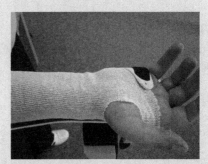

FIGURE PP3–22 Incorporating wrist will prevent distal migration and control forearm position.

FOREARM ROTATION/ELBOW EXTENSION RESTRICTION ORTHOSIS (EO) (Fig. 3–13)

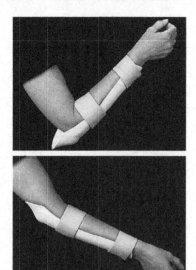

FIGURE 3–13

COMMON NAMES

- Muenster splint
- Sarmiento elbow brace

ALTERNATIVE ORTHOSIS OPTIONS

- Sugar tong orthosis
- Cast

PRIMARY FUNCTIONS

- Restrict elbow extension and provide full flexion to allow healing of involved structure(s).

ADDITIONAL FUNCTIONS

- Restrict some degree of forearm rotation.
- With wrist included, restrict forearm rotation and elbow extension.

Common Diagnoses	General Optimal Positions
Proximal or distal rotation radioulnar joint injury	Forearm: neutral
Interosseous membrane injury	Forearm: neutral rotation

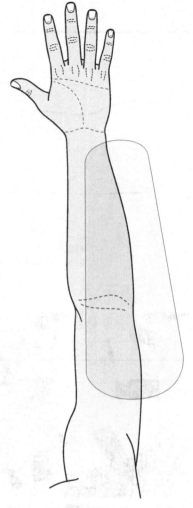

FIGURE 3–14

Common Diagnoses	General Optimal Positions
Proximal radius and ulna fracture	Forearm: neutral rotation; elbow: restricted in extension (per physician's orders)
Elbow dislocation	Depends on structures involved

FABRICATION PROCESS

Pattern Creation (Fig. 3–14)

- Mark for proximal border approximately 2″ above olecranon process.
- Mark for distal borders just proximal to wrist.
- Allow enough material to encompass half to two-thirds circumference of forearm, remembering that forearm tapers distally.

Refine Pattern

- Proximal border should allow limited elbow extension and unimpeded elbow flexion without irritating epicondyles or ulnar nerve.
- Distal border should allow full wrist and hand motion.

Options for Materials

- Use rubber materials (perforated or nonperforated).
- Consider elastic materials that are slightly tacky to help prevent material from slipping, making it easier to position patient and mold orthosis.

Cut and Heat

- Have patient lying supine with shoulder flexed or prone with shoulder extended to achieve gravity-assisted position. Place forearm in neutral and elbow in desired position.
- Have patient (or assistant) maintain this position during fabrication.
- While material is heating, pre-pad olecranon process and epicondyles with self-adhesive padding or silicone gel if desired.

Evaluate Fit While Molding

- While supporting entire piece of warm material, place centrally along ulnar border of forearm and distal humerus.
- Proximally, bring ends together and either cut warm material to form seam or overlap material ends. This seam can be reinforced with an additional piece of material later, if necessary.
- Make sure desired elbow and forearm positions are maintained. Some patients may tend to flex their elbows excessively while orthosis is being formed.
- When almost set, check for clearance of ulnar styloid and epicondyles. If patient complains of abutment, simply push material out.

Strapping and Components

- Distal strap: 2″ elasticized strap just proximal to wrist crease; use piece of adhesive foam to further stabilize forearm in orthosis and prevent migration. Foam should not overlap orthosis edges; avoid excessive compression over radial sensory nerve.
- Proximal strap: 2″ elasticized strap placed just distal to elbow crease.
- Note there is no strap proximal to elbow crease—this permits elbow flexion.

Survey Completed Orthosis

- Smooth and slightly flare all edges.
- Check for complete clearance of wrist and desired elbow motion.

PATTERN PEARLS 3–23 TO 3–24

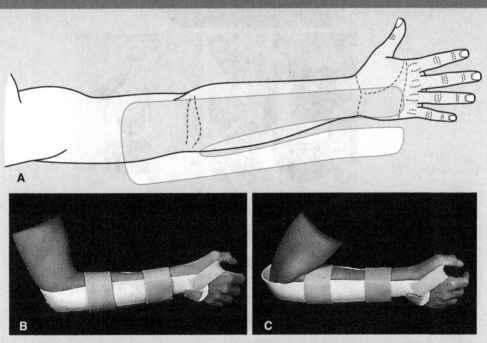

FIGURE PP3–23 **A–C,** A "sugar tong" design to restrict forearm rotation.

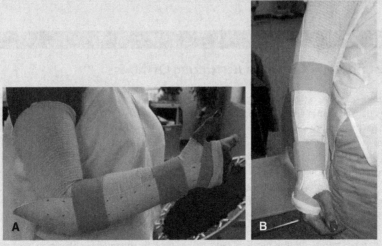

FIGURE PP3–24 **A and B,** Elbow extension restriction orthosis with wrist included to restrict forearm rotation.

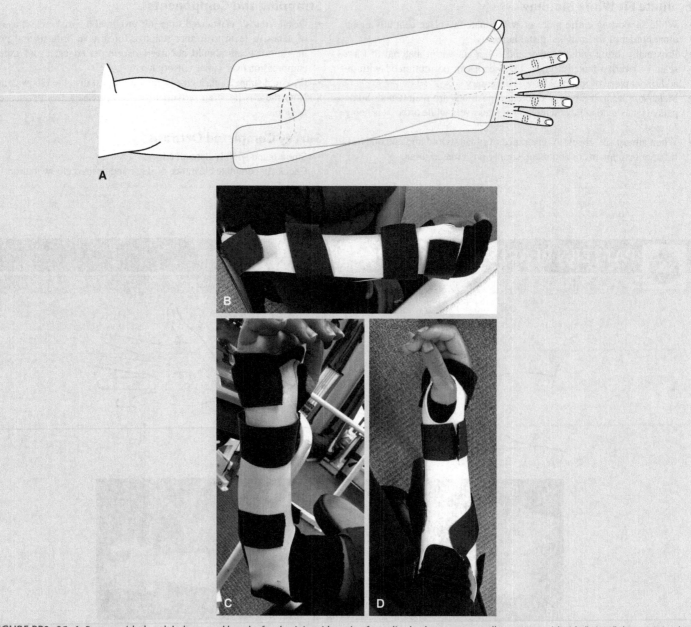

FIGURE PP3–25 A, Pattern with thumb hole; general length of orthosis in mid-section from distal palmar crease to elbow crease with side "wings" that are joined together dorsally to limit elbow extension **(B). C and D,** Gravity assist positioning is key during fabrication—have patient seated with elbow at 90° flexion and forearm neutral. Fully clear the elbow crease volarly to allow unrestricted elbow flexion.

CLINICAL PEARL 3–12

Elbow Flexion Mobilization, Extension Restriction Orthosis

The dynamic elbow flexion orthosis with restricted elbow extension shown here is an example of the combined use of a mobilization orthosis with a restrictive component (see Chapter 2); it was designed for a patient who was referred 3 weeks after a biceps tendon repair. The orthosis segments were fabricated following instructions for the circumferential humerus and forearm orthoses. A hinge connects the segments, with the axis positioned at the elbow joint. Rubber band traction passively positions the elbow in flexion, and the hinge is set to restrict a specific amount of active elbow extension (similar to dynamic orthosis for digital flexor tendon injuries). The patient periodically exercises within the orthosis limits (restricted active elbow extension with passive elbow flexion via the rubber band). Note that the hinge not only acts as an anchor for the rubber bands and a blocking mechanism to elbow extension but also prevents the proximal and distal orthosis segments from migrating toward each other when under tension from the rubber band. A static component can be added to immobilize the elbow between exercise sessions. The orthosis can be further secured to the shoulder girdle via a figure-8–type strap. Note: This protocol must be reviewed by the referring physician prior to implementation. Be mindful to monitor for any signs of ulnar nerve compression at the elbow caused by elbow flexed positioning.

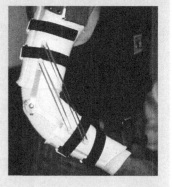

CHAPTER 03: RESTRICTION ORTHOSES DISCUSSION POINTS

1. What is the purpose of a restriction orthosis?
2. Give examples of the appropriate diagnosis and functional goals for:
   - A digit extension restriction orthosis
   - An RF and SF MCP extension restriction orthosis
   - An elbow flexion restriction orthosis
3. What diagnoses would be most appropriate for a forearm rotation restriction orthosis?
4. Describe two different thumb MP restriction orthoses and the rationale for use.

REFERENCES

Chinchalkar S., & Yong S. A. (2004). An ulnar boost splint for midcarpal instability. *The Journal of Hand Therapy*, 17, 377–379.

Garcias-Elias M. (2008).The non-dissociative clunking wrist: A personal view. *The Journal of Hand Surgery*, 33, 698–711.

Lichtman D., Gaenslen E. S., & Pollock G. R. (1997). Midcarpal and proximal carpal instabilities. In Lichtman D. M. & Alexander A. H. (Eds.), *The wrist, diagnosis and treatment* (pp. 316–328).

O'Brien M. (2013). An innovative orthotic design for midcarpal instability, non-dissociative: Mobility with stability. *The Journal of Hand Therapy*, 26, 363–364.

Skirven T. M. (2011). Rehabilitation for carpal ligament injury and instability. In Skirven T., Osterman L., Fedorczyk J., & Amadio P. (Eds.), *Rehabilitation of the hand* (6th ed., pp. 1013–1023). Philadelphia, PA: Elsevier.

Skirven T. M., & DeTullio L. M. (2006). Carpal fractures and instabilities. In Burke S. L., Higgins J. P., & McClinton M. A. (Eds.), *Hand and upper extremity rehabilitation: A practical guide* (pp. 461–474). Elsevier.

4 Nonarticular Orthoses

MaryLynn A. Jacobs, MBA, MS, OTR/L, CHT
Noelle M. Austin, MS, PT, CHT

1 Digit- and Thumb-Based Orthoses

PROXIMAL OR MIDDLE PHALANX ORTHOSIS (FO) (Fig. 4–1)

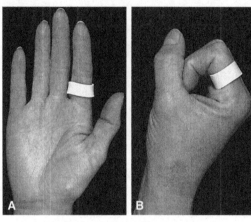

FIGURE 4–1

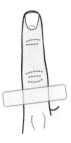

FIGURE 4–2

COMMON NAMES

- Pulley ring
- Pulley protection splint

ALTERNATIVE ORTHOSIS OPTIONS

- Circumferential taping or strapping

PRIMARY FUNCTIONS

- Protect ruptured pulley.
- Protect pulley reconstruction.

ADDITIONAL FUNCTIONS

- Enhance tendon function (prevent bowstringing at or about A2 and A4 pulley regions) secondary to sacrificed, irreparable, or stretched out pulley mechanism.

Common Diagnoses and General Optimal Positions

Flexor tendon injury with pulley reconstruction (zones I and II)

Iatrogenic injury to pulley secondary to flexor tendon repair or tenolysis

FABRICATION PROCESS

Pattern Creation (Fig. 4–2)

- Measure circumference of digit segment involved (e.g., proximal or middle phalanx).
- Measure width of segment involved; corresponding width of orthosis should be approximately one-half or one-third that of segment.
- Consider using strapping material for the dorsal component if edema or getting the ring over an enlarged joint presents as an issue.

Refine Pattern

- Accommodate for use of circumferential wrappings (Coban™, Performance Health) or wound dressings beneath orthosis.
- Orthosis should allow unimpeded flexion of metacarpophalangeal (MCP), proximal interphalangeal (PIP), and/or distal interphalangeal (DIP) joints.

Options for Material

- Use 1/16″ material, which provides adequate support.
- Consider use of 1″ thermoplastic tapes such as Orficast® (North Coast Medical) or QuickCast2 (Performance Health).
- If strapping is used across dorsum of segment, consider a thin strapping material or an elasticized material such as neoprene that can be trimmed to the appropriate width.

Cut and Heat

- While material is heating, position patient with forearm supinated and digits slightly abducted.
- Protect patient with recent flexor tendon repair in wrist/hand extension restriction orthosis (dorsal blocking orthosis) during the fabrication process.

Evaluate Fit While Molding

- Mold the warm material of choice around proximal or middle phalanx.
- For patient with no edema or with no wraps/dressings, consider circumferential design in which ring is overlapped and/or sealed circumferentially. Otherwise, leave gap over dorsum of phalanx for orthosis removal; small strap can be applied to join ends of orthosis.
- For patients with enlarged PIP or DIP joints, be sure to leave gap over dorsum for orthosis removal.
- Allow material to completely set before removing.

Strapping and Components

- If strap is necessary, it should be approximately the same width as orthosis dorsally.
- Small metal homemade rivet attachment can be used to secure one end of strap.

- Some elasticized strapping materials (e.g., neoprene) will adhere directly to thermoplastic therefore eliminating traditional closure techniques.

Survey Completed Orthosis

- Assure the patient is able to safely don and doff the orthosis.
- Smooth borders and round strap ends.
- Check for unimpeded joint motion.
- Remember that orthosis will need to be modified as edema or wound dressings worn beneath orthosis change.

PATTERN PEARLS 4–1 TO 4–3

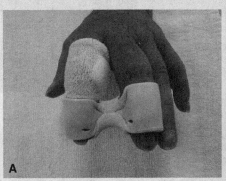
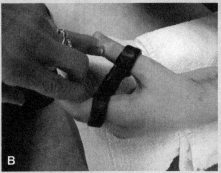

FIGURE PP4–1 A, Modification of design used to maintain digit abduction to facilitate wound healing. **B,** Similar design used to assist in maintaining thenar web space postsurgery.

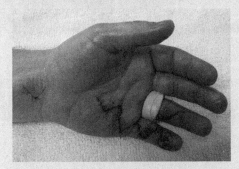

FIGURE PP4–2 Circumferential orthosis used to support pulley repair status post–flexor tendon repair.

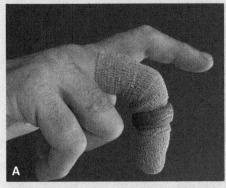
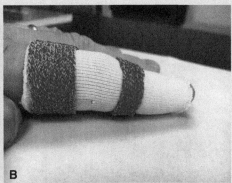

FIGURE PP4–3 A, Orficast® (North Coast Medical, Morgan Hill, CA) used over elasticized wrap after A4 pulley reconstruction. **B,** Multiple pulley ring orthoses used to support an A2 and A4 annular pulley reconstruction. These are shown worn over a single layer of digit stockinette.

CLINICAL PEARL 4–1

Alternative Options for Pulley Protection

A clinician might encounter an edematous digit and fear that the pulley ring will not be easily applied or removed. A patient may also have an enlarged joint, therefore making the ease of application challenging and the intimate fit required about the pulley impossible.

Consider the following:

A–C, Fabricate a volar orthosis (one-half to two-thirds the circumference of the digit) and add a small strap. The strap can either be elastic based or traditional loop material depending on the need. In the case shown, a small segment of foam **(C)** was added to the dorsal strap in order to provide a snug fit.

D and E, A similar volar one-half circumference orthosis fabricated using elastic therapeutic tape for closure. The tape adheres well to the skin, keeping the pulley ring in place.

F, Neoprene adhered to warm thermoplastic material and can be considered for a flexible closure option.

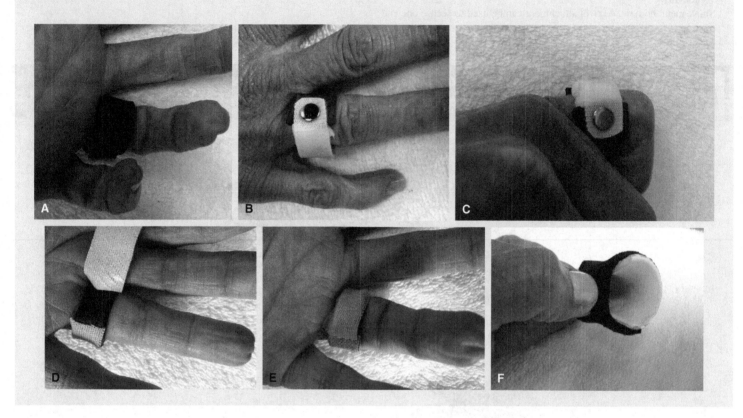

PROXIMAL AND/OR MIDDLE PHALANX STRAPS (FO) (Fig. 4–3)

COMMON NAMES

- Buddy straps
- Buddy splint
- Buddy taping

ALTERNATIVE ORTHOSIS OPTIONS

- Prefabricated
- Ring-designed orthoses
- Taping
- Thermoplastic material
- Relative motion orthoses

PRIMARY FUNCTIONS

- Adjoin affected digit to border unaffected digit, minimizing lateral stress and allowing range of motion (ROM) and some function.

ADDITIONAL FUNCTIONS

- Facilitate passive and active ROMs of affected digit via active motion of adjacent digit.
- Use in combination with hand-based orthosis to prevent rotation of digit.

Common Diagnoses and General Optimal Positions
PIP collateral ligament injury
PIP dislocation
Volar plate injury
Stiff digit
Sagittal band injury

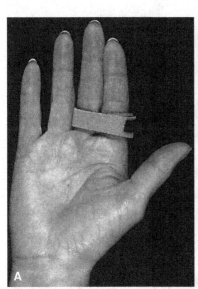
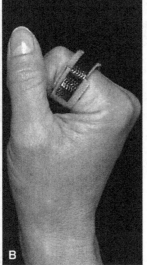

FIGURE 4–3

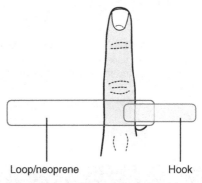

Loop/neoprene   Hook

FIGURE 4–4

FABRICATION PROCESS

Pattern Creation (Fig. 4–4)

- Measure approximately 6″ of ½″ soft strapping material.
- Measure 1″ to 1½″ nonadhesive hook.

Refine Pattern

- Measure width of segment involved; corresponding width of orthosis should be one-half to one-third that of segment.
- Consider additional strap at middle phalanx for added support, depending on size of digit.

Options for Material

- Soft strapping material (Rolyan® SoftStrap®, Performance Health) works best because they are nonelastic yet soft.
- Neoprene material is an option for circumstances that require a small amount of stretch.
- Nonadhesive hook material used to attach strap ends together.

Cut and Heat

- Trim both hook and strapping material according to digit(s) size.

Evaluate Fit While Molding

- Position digits slightly abducted so there is adequate working room and a decreased tendency for maceration between digits.

Strapping and Components

- From volar approach, place one end of soft strap between digits so that the end is flush with dorsum of proximal phalanx.
- Wrap the other end volar to dorsal and, again, volar to dorsal, attaching to hook.

Survey Completed Orthosis

- Trim excess length and width about digital web spaces if necessary.
- Consider use of gauze or polyester batting between fingers to reduce effects of perspiration.

 PATTERN PEARL 4-4

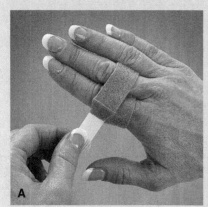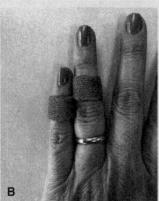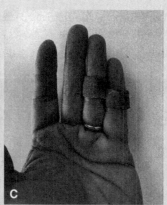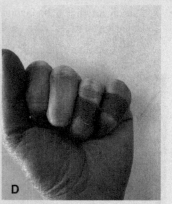

FIGURE PP4-4 A, 3pp° Buddy Loops°. **B-D,** Orficast° used to create custom buddy orthosis—fabricate separate rings first and then adhere together to allow for unrestricted digit ROM. Especially helpful when addressing the small finger. (A, Photo courtesy of 3-Point Products, Stevensville, MD.)

 CLINICAL PEARL 4-2

Additional Buddy Strapping Techniques

A and B, Sewing method. Lay soft strap on a flat surface and place the center of the hook strap in the middle of the soft strap. Stitch the strap onto the hook material at the center point. Loop each side of the soft strap material completely around the digit and back to the center, completely covering the hook material. With this design, dorsal closure leaves the soft strap on the volar surface to allow for unimpeded flexion of the digits. **C, Tape.** Use ½″ athletic tape to secure the digits together. Note the use of gauze between the fingers to prevent maceration.

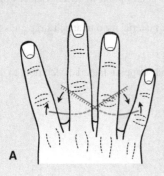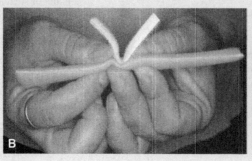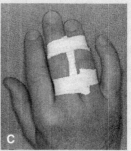

CLINICAL PEARL 4–3

Techniques for Buddy Strapping Small Finger

Buddy strapping the small finger (SF) may pose a problem because it is much shorter than the RF, and the flexion creases of the fingers do not line up. To buddy strap these fingers effectively, allowing for PIP and DIP motion, consider the following techniques.

A–C, No-sew method. Zigzag or step-cut a piece of soft strapping. Use hook to attach the loop together. The center portion of the strap should be quite narrow to decrease bulk in this area. Make sure full motion is available.

D and E, Sewing method. Fabricate two separate loops and stitch them together, off center, to the degree necessary to accommodate the digit length differential. This technique allows for a good custom fit.

F–H, Neoprene used to make a zigzag or step design about the middle phalanx. No sewing is necessary; however, careful attention should be taken cutting the pattern and the direction the material is cut (stretch vs. nonstretch direction).

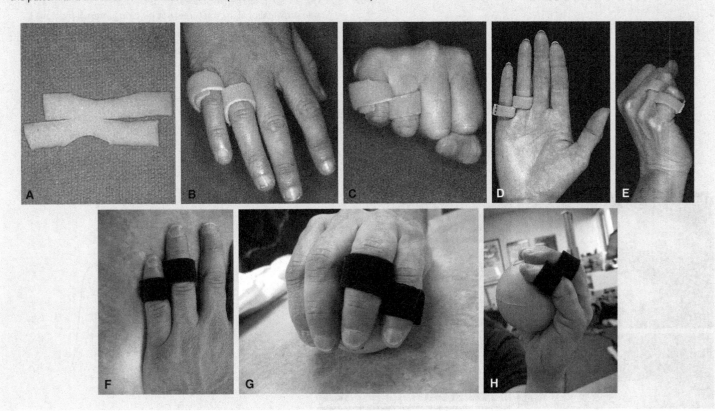

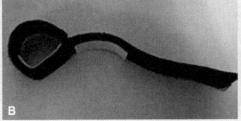

CLINICAL PEARL 4–4

Use of Neoprene and/or Microfoam™ Tape to Prevent Migration

A and B, Using a strip of Microfoam™ tape (Performance Health) can help prevent buddy straps from falling off or slipping on digits. This low-tack tape can be replaced easily as needed. Shown is strap fabricated from neoprene with seam tape for permanent closure. Beige material visualized dorsally is iron-on seam tape used to create small finger loop.

C and D, Neoprene, adhesive hook and a small rivet can suffice as another option for a buddy orthosis. **C,** Shown with rivet surrounded by adhesive hook (outlined) ready to be folded over IF to secure in place **(D)** orthosis in place

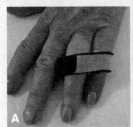
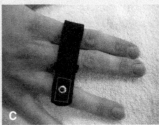
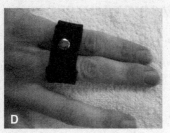

PROXIMAL OR MIDDLE PHALANX CIRCUMFERENTIAL ORTHOSIS (FO) (Fig. 4–5)[a]

COMMON NAMES

- Proximal phalanx fracture brace
- Middle phalanx fracture base
- Clamshell fracture brace

ALTERNATIVE ORTHOSIS OPTIONS

- Cast
- Digit immobilization orthosis

PRIMARY FUNCTIONS

- Support and protect proximal or middle phalanx during healing while allowing motion of proximal and distal joints.

Common Diagnoses and General Optimal Positions

Stable proximal phalanx fractures (not requiring internal fixation)

Unstable fractures requiring surgical fixation: pinning at 1–2 weeks post-surgery, depending on fracture stability; screw fixation 3–5 days postsurgery, depending on fracture stability

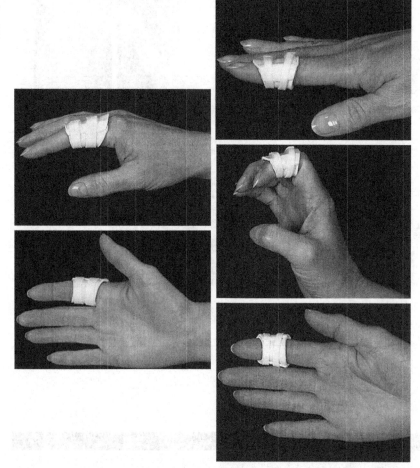

FIGURE 4–5

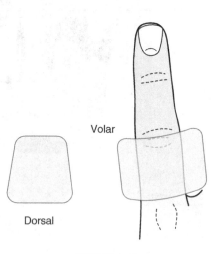

Volar

Dorsal

FIGURE 4–6

[a]Described by Kim Oxford, MOT, OTR, CHT, and David H. Hildreth, MD, University of Texas Health Science Center.

FABRICATION PROCESS

Pattern Creation (Fig. 4–6)

- Mark pattern as close to digit length and circumference as possible.
- If patient cannot fully extend the involved PIP joint or is in pain, consider measuring unaffected digit.
- For more distal fractures, extend lateral supports to distal end of PIP joint.
- For more proximal fractures, extend material volarly and dorsally on MCP joint.

Refine Pattern

- Remember to accommodate for use of circumferential edema reduction wrappings such as Coban™ or wound dressing beneath orthosis.
- Orthosis should allow unimpeded flexion of MCP, PIP, and DIP joints.

Options for Material

- Important to use a coated material
- Elastic- or plastic-based thermoplastic 1/16″ material
- Thermoplastic tapes

Cut and Heat

- Cut volar and dorsal pieces of material and heat.
- Apply Coban™ or compression garments as necessary before orthosis application.
- Position digits slightly abducted so there is adequate working room.

Evaluate Fit While Molding

- Fabricate volar portion of orthosis and allow to set before applying dorsal piece.
- For dorsal piece, lay warmed material over proximal phalanx, slightly overlapping it onto volar piece.
- Once completely set, pop orthosis apart.

Strapping and Components

- Use one or two ¼″ to ½″ straps for optimal closure. This allows application of gentle circumferential pressure.

Survey Completed Orthosis

- Smooth borders, especially between digital web spaces.
- Check for irritation of adjacent digits and possible neurovascular compromise.

CLINICAL PEARL 4–5

Circumferential Phalanx Orthosis

Middle or proximal phalanx nondisplaced shaft fractures can sometimes be managed with a circumferential orthosis design. Before application, examine the PIP for proximal phalanx injuries or the DIP for middle phalanx injuries to be sure that the joint is not enlarged, which would make this orthosis impossible to remove. Choose a 3/32″ or 1/16″ material that will readily adhere to itself once the coating has been disrupted.

Cut a strip of material the full length and approximately ¼″ more than the circumference of the segment being treated. Have the patient supinate the hand and slightly abduct the digits. Place the center of the warmed material over the volar proximal or middle phalanx and bring it around both the ulnar and the radial borders. Pinch the entire length of the ends together dorsally (this can also be done volarly). Carefully cut the excess material. Turn attention back to the volar aspect while still warm and check that the volar MCP/PIP or PIP/DIP creases are cleared to allow motion.

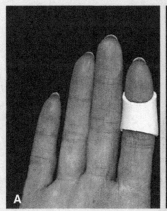
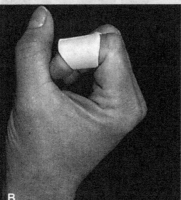
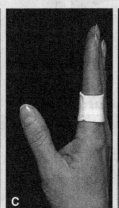
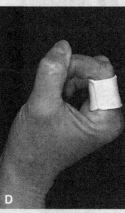

CLINICAL PEARL 4–6

Hinged Digit Orthosis

Hinged PIP orthosis can be fabricated easily by first making two nonarticular phalanx orthoses. These are then connected by means of a homemade hinge shown utilizing Orficast® which was rolled and crimped at the joint level. This orthotic design can protect PIP joint from lateral forces during flexion/extension ROM.

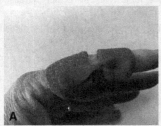
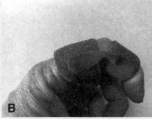
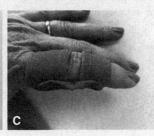
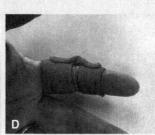

RELATIVE MOTION ORTHOSIS (FO) (Fig. 4–7A–D: RM FLEX; E–H: RM EXT)

COMMON NAMES

- Relative motion (RM) extension or flexion orthosis
- Yoke splint
- Merritt splint
- Active redirection orthosis
- Finger figure-8 orthosis

ALTERNATIVE ORTHOSIS OPTIONS

- MCP immobilization orthosis (used for increasing PIP/DIP active ROM
  - MCP extension—promote distal flexion
  - MCP flexion—promote distal extension

PRIMARY FUNCTIONS

- Protect extensor tendon injury/repair
- Address stiffness at PIP joints
- Prevent compensatory joint mechanics commonly seen with joint deficits

- Resolve active PIP extension lag (RM flexion orthosis)
- Resolve active PIP flexion deficits (RM extension orthosis)
- Maintain ROM gains from exercise session
- Limit full flexion at the MCP joint(s) to facilitate motion at IP joints

Common Diagnoses	General Optimal Positions
Acute/chronic boutonniere	MCP flexion
Acute/chronic sagittal band rupture	MCP extension
PIP joint stiffness	PIP flexion stiffness: MCP extension PIP extension stiffness: MCP flexion
Tendon injury/repair	Extensor tendon: MCP extension Flexor tendon: MCP flexion

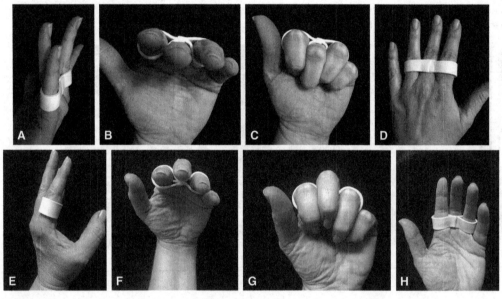

FIGURE 4–7

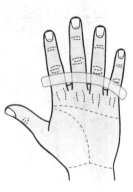

FIGURE 4–8

FABRICATION PROCESS

Pattern Creation (Fig. 4–8)

- Length of strip: measure circumference of the hand at MCP joint level (6″–8″).
- Width of strip should be approximately ½″ (slightly shorter than length of proximal phalanx so this will vary per patient) to allow for maximal pressure distribution on proximal phalanges.

Refine Pattern

- Remember to accommodate for use of circumferential edema wraps such as Coban™ if needed.
- Orthosis should allow unimpeded flexion of MCP, PIP, and DIP joints.

Options for Material

- Thickness of material should be minimized and depends on patient and strength during use.
- Elastic- or plastic-based thermoplastics, 1/16″ or 3/32″ thickness.
- 1/8″ material may be appropriate for larger hands and when more rigidity is required.
- Material may be folded in half lengthwise to further increase the thickness and final strength of orthosis.
- May choose material without protective coating to allow for adhesion of overlapped segments.
- Materials with coating will need to have this protective barrier removed to allow for segments to be adhered together.
- Avoid perforated materials since the edges of the perforations would likely be irritating between the digits.
- Thermoplastic tapes such as Orficast® provide a low profile option—double the thickness and smooth out the edges to maximize comfort.

Cut and Heat

- Cut strip of material when it is fully heated so edges will self-seal creating a smooth border.
- Remember to apply Coban™ or any compression garments as necessary before orthosis application.
- Position digits slightly abducted so there is adequate working room.

Evaluate Fit While Molding

- Preposition with affected MCP in either relative extension or flexion depending on purpose of orthosis.
- RM EXTENSION orthosis: place midsection of strip over VOLAR proximal phalanx of affected digit.
- RM FLEXION orthosis: place midsection of strip over DORSAL proximal phalanx of affected digit.
- Wrap material around adjacent digits and connect at affected digit either volarly (RM EXT) or dorsally (RM FLEX)—trim away excess material.
- Appreciate the normal descent on ulnar side of hand during molding process—distal transverse arch—to create functional position.

- To allow for easy donning/doffing make sure the "rings" are able to easily slide over the PIP joints—may need to enlarge these during the molding process or after fabrication process.
- Once completely cool/hard remove have patient flex and extend digits to be sure the desired motion is achieved.

Strapping and Components

- Ideally do not use strapping to allow for a low maintenance orthosis that can get wet.
- If edema or enlarged PIP joints are a concern, may fabricate with "open rings" to prevent excess circumferential pressure and utilize loop closure dorsally.
- With RM flexion orthosis—may use foam piece under the dorsal ring overlying the proximal phalanx to dissipate any excessive pressure.

Survey Completed Orthosis

- Smooth borders, especially between digital web spaces.
- Check for irritation of adjacent digits and possible neurovascular compromise.

CLINICAL PEARL 4–7

Relative Motion Orthosis to Facilitate Active PIP Joint Motion

Note: Chapter 7 is dedicated to Relative Motion Orthoses. Commonly, patients with stiff PIP joints compensate with excessive motion proximally at the MCP joints. The use of these "ring-type" orthoses worn between exercise sessions can enhance functional use as well as help patients maintain gains from therapy sessions by preventing compensatory motions with activities of daily living (ADLs).

With PIP flexion deficits, patients may hyperflex at the MCP joints when attempting to make a fist. **A,** The use of a relative motion orthosis (RMO) can be an effective way to facilitate PIP joint flexion and minimize this abnormal movement pattern during functional use or exercise. This technique is most effective when addressing limitations of the MF or RF (but the design can be modified for other digits; always include three digits in orthosis for best results). Cut a 6″ by ½″ strip of thermoplastic material. Thickness depends on size of hand; use thinnest possible to minimize bulk. Width should be slightly shorter than the length of the proximal phalanx. Heat, and place the central portion over the volar proximal phalanx of the involved digit. The other two ends will wrap dorsal to volar about the adjacent digits, forming two rings. The MCPs of the uninvolved digits are held in slight flexion while the involved digit is positioned in relative MCP extension while the orthosis sets. Check that the orthosis borders do not interfere with active movement of the involved digit. Note that the orthosis must allow unimpeded MCP and PIP motion. While the patient flexes, they should feel the gentle pressure of the material at the proximal phalanx encouraging PIP joint flexion. **B,** Placing a DIP immobilization orthosis can further isolate PIP flexion efforts.

C and D, Similarly, with active PIP extension deficits (extension lag), an orthosis fabricated for purpose of encouraging active PIP extension can be used. For this design, once the strip of material is heated, the middle portion of the orthosis is placed dorsally on the affected digit's proximal phalanx. The other two ends will wrap volar to dorsal about the adjacent digits, forming two rings. The MCPs of the uninvolved digits are held in slight extension while the involved digit is positioned in relative MCP flexion while the orthosis sets. This is a helpful adjunct to manual PIP extension blocking exercises because the orthosis will provide blocking pressure over the proximal phalanx with active efforts, minimizing the tendency for the MCP joint to hyperextend.

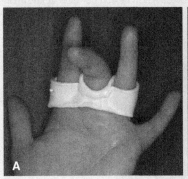
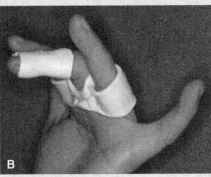
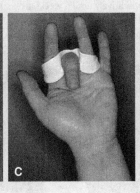
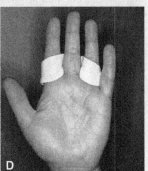

CLINICAL PEARL 4–8

Pencil for Positioning

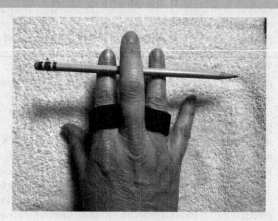

Utilizing a pencil to hold the affected digit in ideal position can prevent loss of MCP extension or flexion after the material has been wrapped appropriately.

CLINICAL PEARL 4–9

RM at Middle Phalanx

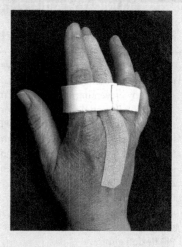

A helpful adjunct to RM orthoses with the aim of improving a PIP active extension lag is the addition of therapeutic taping. Application of tape with stretch directly over the PIP joint (no tension over DIP of MCP joint) can act as an assist for PIP extension. This can be worn directly under the RM orthosis to maximize the ability to reduce this troublesome lag.

CLINICAL PEARL 4–10

Therapeutic Taping with RM Orthosis

RM design used at middle phalanx level to assist with regaining active/passive finger extension in this patient status post trigger finger release of middle finger. She did not show up postoperatively until 4 weeks after surgery and had been positioning middle finger protectively in flexion during that entire time. Orthosis was utilized during the day to allow adjacent digits to actively assist with extension and preventing reverting back into the flexed posture. Notice use of therapeutic taping dorsally to assist in activation of extensors (A-D).

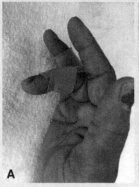
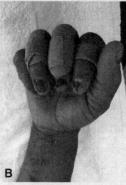
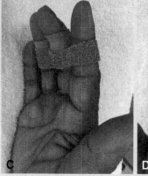
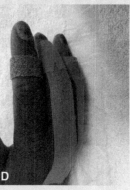

A   B   C   D

CLINICAL PEARL 4–11

Blocking Further Motion With RM Orthoses

An additional segment of thermoplastic can be added to the RM orthosis to either limit end range of MCP flexion (**A,B**) or PIP flexion (**C,D**). This might be appropriate when treating a patient with a sagittal band injury or trigger finger.

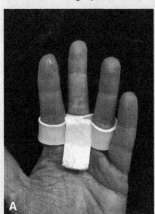
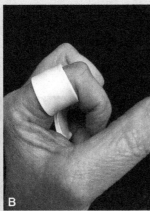
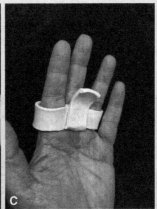
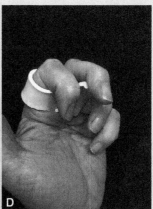

EXPERT PEARL 4–1

Relative Motion Alternative
DEBBIE FISHER, MS, OTR, CHT
Texas

Small hair curler sticks (0.8–1 cm) can be easily bent to be used as an RMO (**A-C**). This alternative material allows for easy adjustability, provides increased comfort for the patient, and is quick and simple to customize.

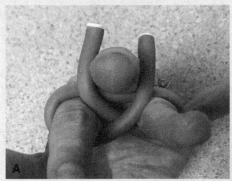
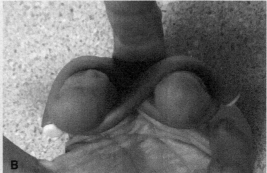
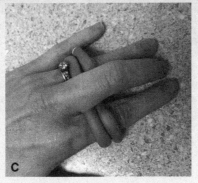

Use of a Relative Motion Orthosis for Regaining PIP Joint Flexion or Extension

HandLab: Clinical Pearls

JUDY C. COLDITZ, OT/L, CHT, FAOTA
North Carolina

Therapists have traditionally used both orthotic intervention and passive range of motion to improve joint motion before focusing on active motion. Since injury to a finger usually creates greater stiffness in one joint, the looser joint(s) moves the most and the stiffer joint(s) moves the least. This is obviously detrimental to the stiffer joint(s) regaining motion.

An alternative way to improve PIP joint motion is to restrict motion at the MP joint so it can neither hyperextend nor hyperflex. In other words, the force for extension or flexion is diverted to the PIP joint because it cannot be taken up by the hypermobile MP joint. (In the case of the little finger, the motion at the CMC joint must also be restricted.)

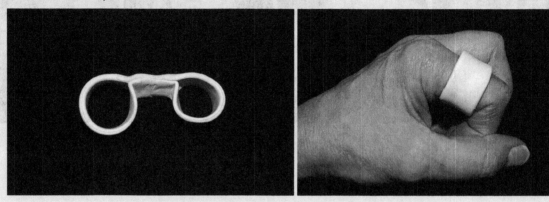

Example of an active redirection orthosis used to regain PIP joint flexion.

It is my belief that this "active redirection" can mobilize a stiff joint without additional passive modalities as long as the active redirection occurs for prolonged periods of time. The focused duration of active redirection causes a change in the resistance of the stiff joint while also retraining the motor cortex to activate finger motion in a different pattern. Retraining is the key to a patient's ability to retain the motion gained.

In recent years, the use of a small orthosis that holds one MP joint in a position relative to the adjacent MP joints has become the standard of treatment for extensor tendon injuries in zone 5 and 6. This orthosis is referred to by a variety of names: relative motion orthosis, ICAM (immediate controlled active motion), yoke orthosis, and Merritt orthosis (after one of the original authors).[1]

Active redirection to mobilize a stiff PIP joint uses the same orthotic design, but the purpose is to control the MP joint of the stiff finger. At times this includes a relative position of the adjacent MP joint(s), but not always.

Facilitating PIP Joint Extension

If you place a pencil/pen over the dorsum of your proximal phalanx and under the two adjacent fingers, you will block the MP joint of the finger in the middle in greater flexion. This blocked position of the MP joint assures that the force of the extensor digitorum communis is not allowed to act at the MP joint but is diverted to act along with the interosseous and lumbrical muscles at the PIP joint to gain extension. The orthosis is constructed to block the MP joint.

This design works well for the two middle fingers when only three fingers need to be included, but the border digits cannot be adequately stabilized unless all fingers are included (see below).

Facilitating PIP Joint Flexion

Holding the MP joint of a finger with a stiff PIP joint in extension will assure that powerful extrinsic flexor force is directed toward the PIP joint, preventing the intrinsic muscles from overpowering by hyperflexing the MP joint. This can easily be achieved by positioning one of the two middle fingers' MP joints in more extension than the adjacent joints, but it becomes more challenging on the border digits.

Orthotic Design

The purpose of the active redirection orthosis is to control the position of the MP joint. Often it is trial and error with the orthotic design to determine what is required to adequately stabilize the MP joint. Someone who is hypermobile may need a design that is different from someone who has more limited normal joint motion.

Below are some suggestions to use as a starting point; the orthosis for your patient may need to be different. The drawings are cross sections of the right hand. See what design works best for the balance of motion in your patient!

CHAPTER 4

Index finger

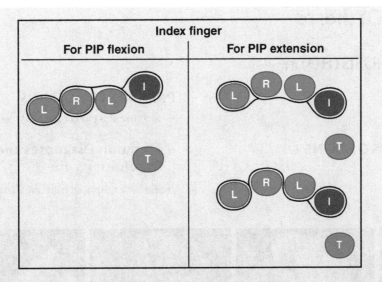

Ring finger

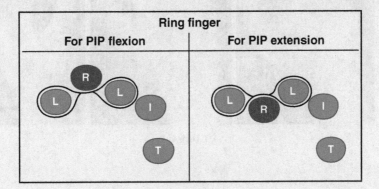

Long finger

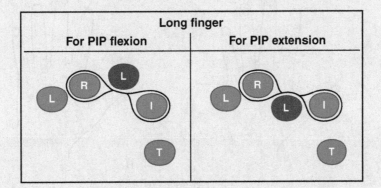

Little finger

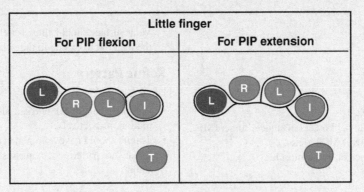

[1]Howell J. W., Merritt W. H., & Robinson S. J. (2005). Immediate controlled active motion following zone 4-7 extensor tendon repair. *Journal of Hand Therapy, 18*(2), 182–190. Clinical Pearls reprinted with permission from Clinician's Classroom at BraceLab.com written by Judy Colditz OT/L CHT FAOTA, copyright HandLab/BraceLab, Raleigh NC. No. 26, August 2013.

2 | Hand-Based Orthoses

METACARPAL ORTHOSIS (HO) (Fig. 4–9)

COMMON NAMES

- Metacarpal fracture brace

ALTERNATIVE ORTHOSIS OPTIONS

- Cast
- Galveston fracture brace
- Prefabricated orthosis

PRIMARY FUNCTIONS

- Stabilize and protect involved metacarpal during fracture healing.

Common Diagnoses and General Optimal Positions

Stable/nondisplaced metacarpal fracture

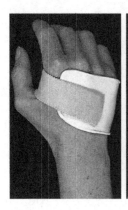
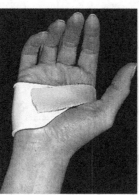
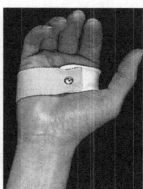
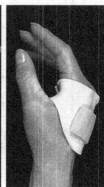
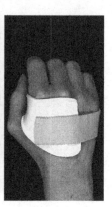

FIGURE 4–9

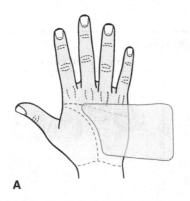
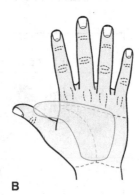

A   B

FIGURE 4–10

FABRICATION PROCESS

Pattern Creation

Ulnar Design (Fig. 4–10A)

- Mark proximal border at wrist crease.
- Mark just proximal to volar and dorsal borders of middle finger (MF), ring finger (RF), and small finger (SF) MCP joints.
- Volar surface should allow clearance of thenar muscles.

Radial Design (Fig. 4–10B)

- Mark proximal border at wrist crease
- Mark just proximal to volar and dorsal borders of second and third metacarpals.

- Volar surface should allow for clearance of thenar muscles yet allow for the material to extend to the volar aspect of the third metacarpal.

Refine Pattern

Ulnar Design

- Proximal and distal borders should allow full wrist and MCP joint motion, respectively.
- Thumb should have unimpeded motion.
- Make sure pattern encompasses third metacarpal for increased orthosis stability.

Radial Design

- Proximal and distal borders should allow full wrist and MCP joint motion, respectively.
- Thumb should have unimpeded motion.

Options for Materials

- Use lightly perforated material that retains some degree of flexibility when set. Orthosis must bend slightly to be removed for hygiene; perforations help prevent skin maceration.
- Material should provide intimate fit about metacarpals, provide stability and protection, and prevent orthosis migration.
- Materials that can be reheated and remolded several times are a good option if ongoing orthosis modifications become necessary to accommodate for fluctuations in edema.
- Thermoplastic tapes in larger formats such as 3 inches and greater.

Cut and Heat

- For ulnar design, position extremity with shoulder forward flexed and internally rotated, elbow flexed, and forearm pronated to achieve gravity-assisted position (ulnar side of hand facing up).
- For radial design, position forearm in neutral rotation to achieve gravity-assisted position.

Evaluate Fit While Molding

Ulnar Design

- Place material centrally on ulnar aspect of hand just distal to wrist.
- On volar surface, material should rest just proximal to distal palmar crease and on dorsal surface just proximal to MCP joints.

- Allow gravity to assist while gently contouring and encompassing third to fifth metacarpals.

Radial Design

- Place material centrally on radial aspect of hand just distal to wrist.
- On volar surface, material should rest just proximal to distal palmar crease and on dorsal surface just proximal to MCP joints.
- Allow gravity to assist while gently contouring and encompassing second to third metacarpals.

Strapping and Components

- Both ulnar and radial designs may need a wrist strap to prevent migration; soft or elasticized strapping works well.
- For ulnar design, use custom (trimmed) soft foam strap through first web space to maximize comfort and prevent skin irritation caused by friction (as sometimes seen with traditional loop material).
- For radial design, use elasticized strap on ulnar border to accommodate variations in muscle bulk during active hand use.

Survey Completed Orthosis

- Smooth proximal and distal borders.
- Make sure there is no irritation from strap material in first web space with thumb motion.

 PATTERN PEARLS 4–5 TO 4–10

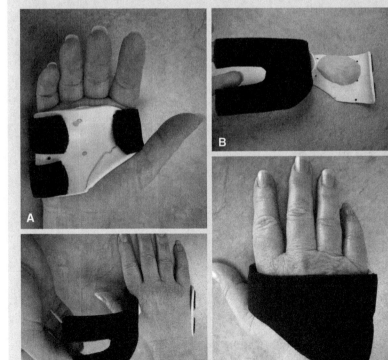

FIGURE PP4–5 A–D, Circumferential design using thermoplastic volarly and neoprene dorsally to cushion bony anatomy. **A and B,** Note the elastomer used beneath the orthosis to address scar mobility. The elastomer was applied after the orthosis was formed and the perforations in the thermoplastic were used for the elastomer to seep through in order to anchor in place as it cured and hardened the 3-inch-wide neoprene dorsal strap was modified on the ulnar border to "cut out" two tabs for a more secure closure.

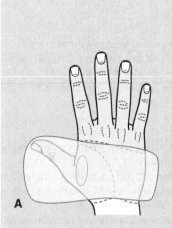
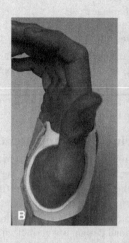
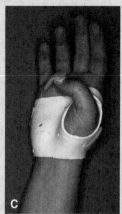

FIGURE PP4-6 A and B, Thumbhole incorporated into the radial design, increasing stability of the orthosis on the hand. **C,** A nonarticular radial approach is used for composite flexion mobilization (dynamic via rubber band) utilizing adhesive hook with a loop and monofilament line.

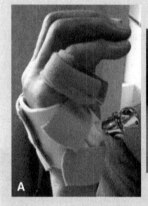
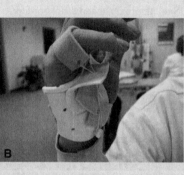
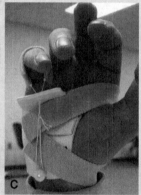

FIGURE PP4-7A-C A, Ulnar-based design used for SF MCP flexion mobilization orthosis using a static progressive approach. **B and C,** Also an ulnar base with a dynamic approach using rubber band traction and a "homemade" thermoplastic outrigger.

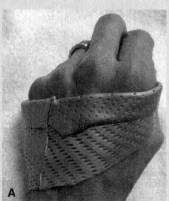
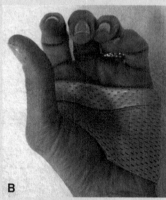

FIGURE PP4-8 A and B, Orfit® material pinched together, then cut, forming a seam used to create circumferential design.

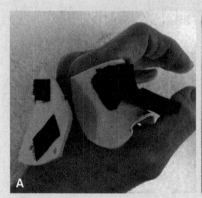
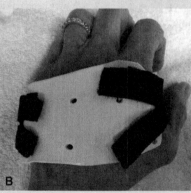
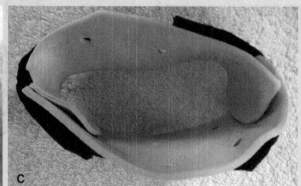

FIGURE PP4-9 A-C, Clamshell design. Note in **C** the intimate fit and contour of the thermoplastic material about the arches of the hand. This careful attention to molding will result in proper fit and minimal orthosis movement.

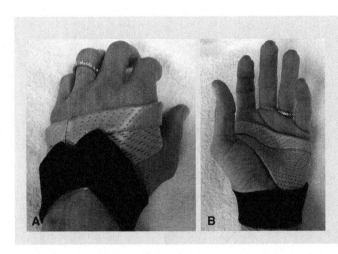

FIGURE PP4–10 A and B, Elasticized strap (neoprene) about wrist for stabilization.

3 | Forearm-Based Orthoses

FOREARM ORTHOSIS (WHO or EO) (Fig. 4–11)

COMMON NAMES

- Forearm fracture brace
- Clamshell forearm splint

ALTERNATIVE ORTHOSIS OPTIONS

- Cast/functional casting
- Prefabricated orthosis

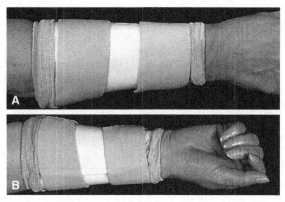

FIGURE 4–11

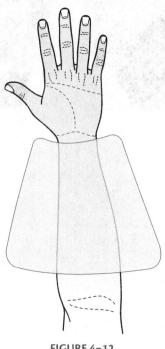

FIGURE 4–12

PRIMARY FUNCTIONS

- Stabilize and protect radius and/or ulna during fracture healing by applying gentle, circumferential compression to surrounding soft tissues.

ADDITIONAL FUNCTIONS

- Can be used as transitional protective device for forearm fractures after healing has occurred, when patient must return to work and/or sports.

Common Diagnoses and General Optimal Positions

Radius and/or ulna shaft fractures

FABRICATION PROCESS

Pattern Creation (Fig. 4–12)

- Measure circumference of proximal border just distal to elbow flexion crease and add 1″.
- Measure circumference of distal border just proximal to ulnar styloid and add 1″.
- Connect proximal to distal borders to account for length of orthosis.

Refine Pattern

- Be sure to allow enough material for approximately 1″ overlap.
- In general, patients may find it easier to pull straps toward them rather than away; thus, overlap material on ulnar forearm from volar to dorsal.

Options for Materials

- Use coated material to avoid permanent bonding of overlapped section and to allow orthosis to pop apart.
- For adults, 3/32″ material is adequate to stabilize forearm.
- For young children, 1/16″ material can be used.
- Lightly perforated material with some degree of memory may help provide intimate fit about forearm yet allow some flexibility for ease of removal and to increase air exchange.

Cut and Heat

- Position forearm in neutral rotation to achieve gravity-assisted position if diagnosis allows.

Evaluate Fit While Molding

- Place warm material on towel; position so that wide section is applied proximally, and narrow section is applied distally.
- Gently apply to forearm, keeping in mind desired overlap area.
- Begin evenly and lightly stretching material around forearm and overlapping it onto itself.
- Do not overstretch material, which may disrupt material's protective coating, causing inadvertent adherence.
- Once overlapped, apply constant moving pressure along length of orthosis until material is set.
- Remove orthosis when completely set, pop apart overlapped section, and remove from patient.

Strapping and Components

- Consider use of 1″ or 2″ self-adhesive D-ring straps, because they allow firm and easy closure.

- Attach D-rings so patient can tighten orthosis by directing pull of straps toward body.
- Alternatively, 2″ elasticized straps allow patient to control compression placed on arm.
- Line entire length of inside seam with Moleskin (Performance Health) or other thin liner. Overlap liner onto itself by approximately 1″ to minimize potential of pinching forearm skin between orthosis pieces.
- Consider lining proximal and distal borders with soft liner, such as Moleskin or Microfoam™ tape (Performance Health) to reduce migration.

Survey Completed Orthosis

- Stockinette or TubiGrip™ (Performance Health) under orthosis can provide comfort, aid with edema, and minimize orthosis irritation.
- Check for possible bony irritation and/or neurovascular compromise.
- Instruct patient to remove orthosis for hygiene only and to follow physician's protocol.

CHAPTER 4

PATTERN PEARLS 4–11 TO 4–15

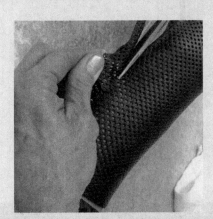

FIGURE PP4–11 Circumferential design (elastic-coated material, Orfit® Colors™, North Coast Medical) using a pinch/cut technique to form seam.

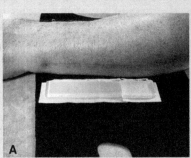
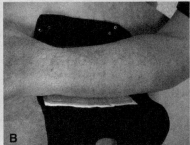
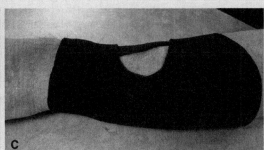

FIGURE PP4–12 A–C, Neoprene used to protect ulna osteotomy with silicone inserted over incision site.

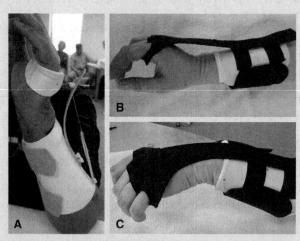

FIGURE PP4–13A–C Forearm orthosis used as base for various mobilization orthoses. **A,** Shown with a dynamic rubber band traction, utilizing neoprene for dynamic wrist and digit extension **(B)** and wrist functional flexion **(C)**. Note the Microfoam™ tape on the distal border of the orthosis.

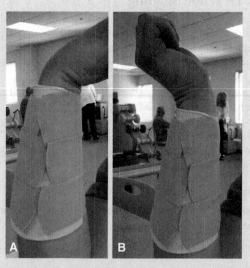

FIGURE PP4–14A,B Make certain to allow for full clearance of wrist motion. **A,** Wrist flexion. **B,** Wrist extension.

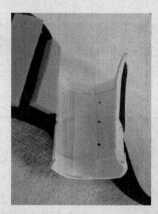

FIGURE PP4–15 Microfoam™ tape (Performance Health) along the borders and several strips along the length is combined with open cell foam on the strapping to further help prevent orthosis migration.

 CLINICAL PEARL 4–12

Use of Elasticized Sleeve to Help Molding Process

A light elasticized cotton sleeve can be used to secure circumferential orthosis such as a forearm guard or a proximal forearm orthosis. This technique allows for even pressure distribution while the material is setting. Do not use a size that is too tight, which may cause the orthosis' borders to dig in, possibly causing skin irritation. As noted in **(C)** the stockinette should end just before the proximal (in this case) border so that there is no risk of the orthosis edges to be directed in toward the skin. The patient can gently open and close the fist while the material is hardening, allowing the design to incorporate proximal forearm musculature.

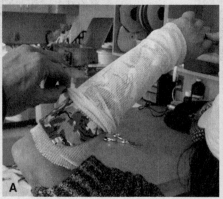
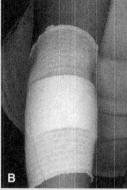
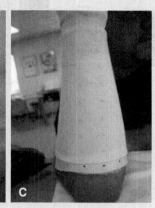

CLINICAL PEARL 4–13

Protective Playing Orthosis

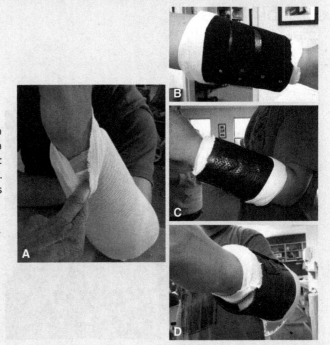

A, High dense foam padding can be added prior to fabrication and held in place with compressive stockinette. Thermoplastic material can then be applied. **B–D,** Shown here is a football player returning to sport with this protective orthosis status post fracture of the midshaft of the ulna. Neoprene straps were used to provide a snug fit. Note the foam and the use of small rivets to anchor one end of the neoprene straps for secure closure.

CLINICAL PEARL 4–14

Circumferential Designs and Material Adherence

With circumferential designs, there are several techniques for preventing the thermoplastic material from adhering to itself. The best material of choice is one that has a coating; however, these materials will often "stick" together if they have been overstretched or overheated.

When there is no choice but to use uncoated material, try one of these techniques. (1) Do not overstretch the orthosis material. (2) Do not be too aggressive when pressing the pieces together. (3) Apply a wet Ace™ wrap or similar to the bottom piece (with an extra inch overlap directly onto the skin) and then wrap around gently over the entire orthosis **(A)**. (4) Place a wet paper towel between the pieces just before overlapping **(B and C)**. (5) Apply a thin layer of hand lotion on the warmed material's surface just before overlapping.

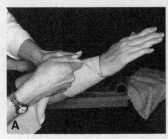
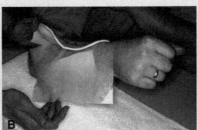
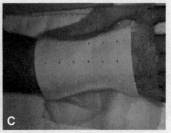

EXPERT PEARL 4–3

Strapping Option
SABRINA CASSELLA, MEd, OTR/L, CHT
Massachusetts

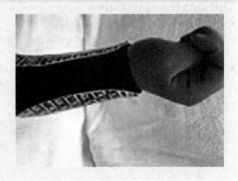

Simply adhere neoprene directly to thermoplastic. Remove protective coating and dry heat area to prepare for adherence. Stretch in strap provides comfortable option.

PROXIMAL FOREARM ORTHOSIS (EO) (Fig. 4–13)

COMMON NAMES

- Tennis elbow strap
- Tennis elbow cuff
- Golfer's elbow strap

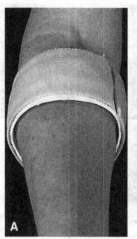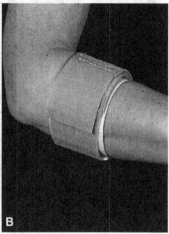

FIGURE 4–13

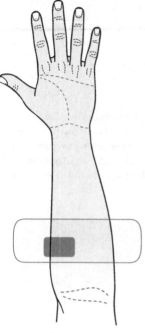

FIGURE 4–14

- Lateral epicondylitis strap
- Medial epicondylitis strap
- Counterforce brace

ALTERNATIVE ORTHOSIS OPTIONS

- Prefabricated orthosis
- Taping
- Neoprene orthosis

PRIMARY FUNCTIONS

- Decrease stress at proximal attachment of wrist extensors or flexors during functional use by providing counterforce and dispersing pressure about muscle bellies.

Common Diagnoses and General Optimal Positions

Lateral epicondylitis (tennis elbow)

Medial epicondylitis (golfer's elbow)

FABRICATION PROCESS

Pattern Creation (Fig. 4–14)

- Measure circumference of proximal forearm 1″ to 1½″ below epicondyles; subtract 1″ to obtain circumference of orthosis.
- Width of orthosis should be approximately 2½″.

Refine Pattern

- Check length and width.

Options for Materials

- Use 1/16″ or 3/32″ material.
- Gel- or foam-lined thermoplastic materials eliminate added step of lining material over muscle bellies.
- When using traditional material, adhesive-backed foam or gel can be applied to molded thermoplastic in area over muscle bellies to disperse pressure.

Cut and Heat

- Position patient with elbow gently flexed, forearm neutral to slight pronation for lateral epicondylitis, or neutral with slight supination for medial epicondylitis.
- Heat thermoplastic material.
- Note that some gel- and foam-lined materials can be heated in sealed plastic bag to prevent water from saturating lining (refer to manufacturer's instructions for details).

Evaluate Fit While Molding

- Make sure there is adequate width and length. Should the orthosis be applied too tightly, there is a risk of radial nerve irritation (radial tunnel or radial sensory nerve irritation).

Lateral Epicondylitis

- Rest warm material over proximal extensor muscle bellies approximately two fingerbreadths distal to lateral epicondyle.
- Wrap material from ulnar aspect of arm to radial volar aspect, leaving slight opening along ulnar border. Stockinette can be used to allow material to set with even pressure distribution.
- Once material is secured on proximal forearm, have patient lightly open and close fist to get contouring about muscle bellies.

Medial Epicondylitis

- Rest warm material over proximal flexor muscle bellies approximately two fingerbreadths distal to medial epicondyle.
- Once material is secured on proximal forearm, have patient lightly open and close fist to get contouring about muscle bellies.

Strapping and Components

- After material has set, apply adhesive foam or gel on portion of orthosis that will be resting over flexor and/or extensor muscle bellies.
- Adhesive hook is applied to nearly full circumference of orthosis to provide even pressure distribution throughout orthosis.

- Consider that use of 2″ elasticized strap to allow orthosis to accommodate for forearm musculature is contracting and relaxing.
- Apply strap with even tension across entire circumference of orthosis.
- D-ring strap also works well for this type of orthosis.
- Direction of strap application should provide for easy donning and doffing.

Survey Completed Orthosis

- Smooth borders of orthosis's edges.
- Instruct patient in appropriate strap tightness and caution regarding signs of neurovascular compromise.
- Mark proximal and distal ends of orthosis and review proper orthosis placement.

 PATTERN PEARLS 4–16 TO 4–19

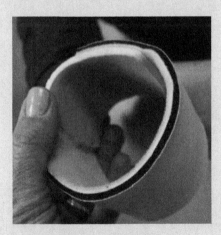

FIGURE PP4–16 A foam-lined thermoplastic (approximately 2.5″ by 2.5″) over extensor or flexor muscle bellies with imbedded 2.5″ neoprene strap to secure.

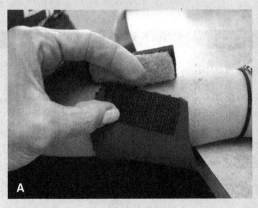 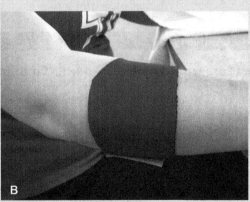

A   B

FIGURE PP4–17 A and B, Custom neoprene strap uses adhesive hook/loop for closure. Sew corners of hook and loop for longevity.

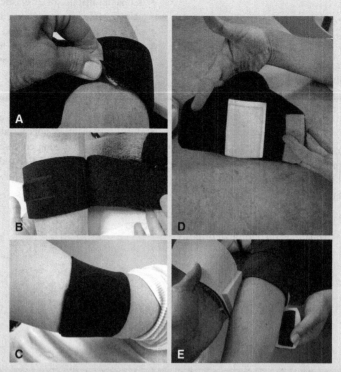

FIGURE PP4–18 A–C, Custom neoprene strap combined with adhesive silicone gel lining. The silicone gel acts as an antiskid element for the neoprene to help keep it in place and as a shock absorber during forearm muscular activity. **D,** Another type of adhesive backed silicone applied to a proximal forearm orthosis. **E,** High dense foam can also be considered for gentle compression over the proximal flexor or extensor muscle groups.

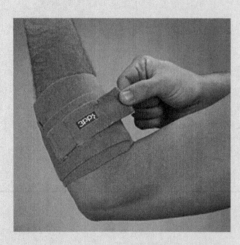

FIGURE PP4–19 3pp® Tennis elbow strap. (Photo courtesy of 3-Point Products.)

CLINICAL PEARL 4–15

Proximal Forearm Orthosis to Address Combined Medial and Lateral Epicondylitis

Two pieces of silicone gel or 3/8″ foam (2″ by 2″) can be added to a circumferential design to place pressure simultaneously over the proximal extensor and flexor muscle bellies. Occasionally, some patients present with lateral and medial epicondylitis simultaneously, likely because of overcompensating with the opposing muscle-tendon group.

4 | Arm-Based Orthoses

HUMERUS ORTHOSIS (SO or EO) (Fig. 4–15)

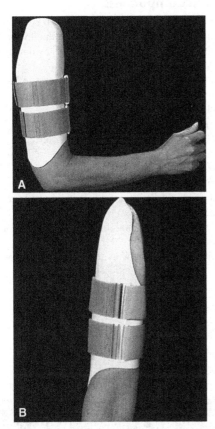

FIGURE 4–15

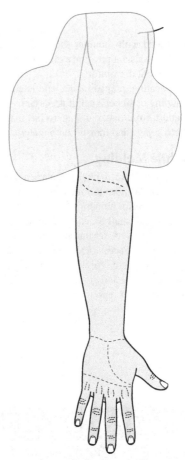

FIGURE 4–16

COMMON NAMES

- Humeral fracture brace
- Sarmiento humerus brace

ALTERNATIVE ORTHOSIS OPTIONS

- Zipper-designed orthosis
- Cast/functional casting
- Prefabricated orthosis
- Sling

PRIMARY FUNCTIONS

- Stabilize and protect humerus during fracture healing by applying gentle, circumferential compression to surrounding soft tissues.

Common Diagnoses and General Optimal Positions

Humeral shaft fracture

FABRICATION PROCESS

Pattern Creation (Fig. 4–16)

- Location of fracture along shaft dictates length of orthosis.
- For proximal shaft fractures, orthosis pattern should extend to proximal edge of acromion process, and distal edge can terminate just above elbow crease.
- For distal shaft fractures, orthosis pattern should extend just distal to acromion process, and distal edge can terminate over epicondyles medially and laterally.
- Both designs should support medial arm to axilla.

Refine Pattern

- Proximal border should allow nearly full shoulder motion.
- Distal border should allow unimpeded elbow motion.
- Check that there is enough material to encompass humerus circumferentially and add 1″ to 1½″ extra for overlap.
- Avoid irritation to epicondyles, olecranon, axilla, and ulnar nerve at cubital tunnel.

Options for Materials

- Use coated material so overlapped section can be popped open.
- For larger arms, ⅛″ or 3/32″ materials provide needed support.

- For smaller arms, 3/32″ or 1/16″ materials provide adequate support.
- Remember that elastic materials tend to shrink around the immobilized part; do not remove until orthosis is completely set.
- Use lightly perforated material that retains some degree of flexibility when set. Orthosis must bend slightly to be removed for hygiene; perforations help prevent skin maceration.

Cut and Heat

- Position patient seated with shoulder supported in slight abduction, it may help to have the assistant position extremity during fabrication process to minimize patient discomfort.
- While material is heating, prepad medial and lateral epicondyles using self-adhesive padding or silicone gel, if necessary.
- Carefully cut pattern from material. Pattern has many curves; try to be accurate in pattern design and transfer onto material.

Evaluate Fit While Molding

- Supporting entire piece of warm material, place along anterior humerus, aligning cut out for axilla and anterior elbow appropriately; open section is positioned along posterior humerus.
- If bracing for proximal shaft fracture, simultaneously extend warm material over humeral head to acromion process.
- If bracing for distal shaft fracture, extend material distally over epicondyles, making sure not to interfere with elbow mobility.
- Using both hands, carefully and gently stretch material anterior to posterior, under axilla, and over onto itself.

- Do not overstretch material, which may disrupt material's protective coating, causing inadvertent adherence.
- Gently flare material around proximal segment with careful attention to axilla (do not overlap material, which tends to irritate this sensitive region) and along distal borders.

Strapping and Components

- Use 2″ self-adhesive D-ring straps, because they allow firm and easy closure; patient can make adjustments according to comfort.
- Attach D-rings so patient can tighten orthosis by directing pull of straps toward body.
- Line inside of orthosis with Moleskin or other thin liner. Overlap liner onto itself by approximately 1″ to minimize potential of pinching forearm skin between orthosis pieces.
- Line proximal and distal borders with Microfoam™ tape or self-adhesive gel liners to decrease distal migration.

Survey Completed Orthosis

- Some patients may benefit from wearing stockinette or TubiGrip™ beneath orthosis to minimize orthosis irritation and aid with controlling perspiration.
- Check for migration and possible bony irritation or neurovascular compromise.
- Instruct patient to remove for hygiene only and to follow physician's protocol.

PATTERN PEARLS 4–20 TO 4–24

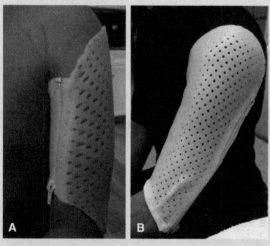

FIGURE PP4–20 **A and B,** Rolyan® AquaForm™ Humerus Fracture Brace (Performance Health). Note the seam in **B** made during fabrication to accommodate for the narrowing of the distal segment of the upper arm.

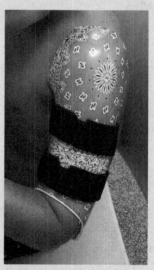

FIGURE PP4–21 Elasticized circumferential strapping is an excellent choice for orthosis closure and additional fracture stabilization.

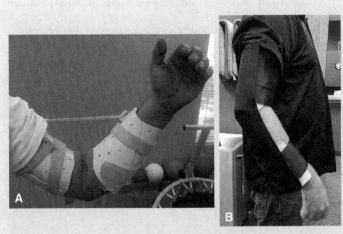

FIGURE PP4–22A,B Forearm and humeral nonarticular orthoses can be joined together to form a mobilization orthosis. **A,** Use of rubber band traction for elbow flexion. **B,** Use of neoprene for terminal elbow extension.

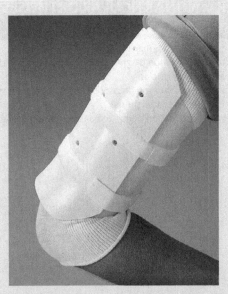

FIGURE PP4–24 Rolyan® preformed humerus brace. (Photo courtesy of Performance Health.)

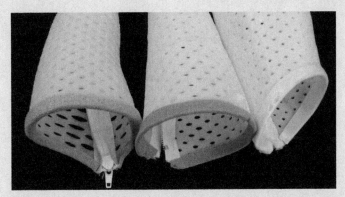

FIGURE PP4–23 Lining proximal and distal ends of a nonarticular orthosis may assist in reducing migration and minimizing tissue irritation.

CLINICAL PEARL 4–16

Preventing Skin Irritation From Overlapped Segments

Lining the inside overlapped edge of circumferentially designed orthosis with Moleskin (Performance Health) or a similar material may reduce the potential for irritation at the orthosis/skin interface. The key is to overlap the lining onto itself to form an extra 1″ to 2″ soft flap on the inside of the orthosis. This technique can be used for most circumferential designs. **A,** Shown using an adhesive back thin foam. **B,** Shown with overlapped elastic therapeutic tape.

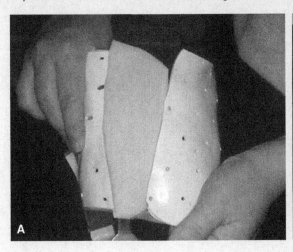

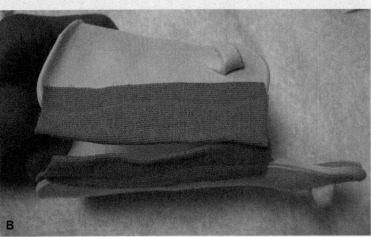

CHAPTER 4

CHAPTER 4: NONARTICULAR ORTHOSES DISCUSSION POINTS

1. What is the purpose of a nonarticular orthosis?
2. Describe the most common diagnosis, and the purpose of a circumferential proximal phalanx orthosis.
3. Give an example of a common diagnosis for a hand fracture that would be treated with a nonarticular orthosis?
   - Name two key fabrication points to consider during the fabrication process.

- Describe the important fabrication modifications for a radial design and an ulnar design.
4. Give an example of a common diagnosis for an upper arm injury that would be managed with a nonarticular orthosis.
5. Describe two or more fabrication considerations when constructing a circumferential humerus orthosis.

Index

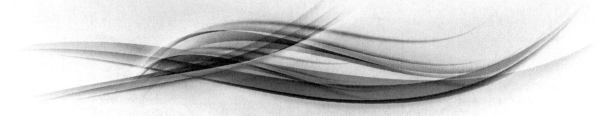

Note: Page numbers followed by "f" indicate figures and "t" indicate figures.

SLIP
SHEET

SLIP
SHEET